an atlas of the human brain and spinal cord

an atlas of the human brain and spinal cord

E. G. MIKE BERTRAM, M.Sc., Ph.D.

Professor and Associate Chairman, Department of Anatomy, and Head, Division of Basic Neurology, University of Toronto, Faculty of Medicine, Toronto, Ontario, Canada

KEITH L. MOORE, Ph.D., F.R.S.M.

Professor and Chairman, Department of Anatomy, University of Toronto, Faculty of Medicine, Toronto, Ontario, Canada
Formerly Professor and Head of Anatomy, University of Manitoba, Faculty of Medicine, Winnipeg, Manitoba, Canada

SANS TACHE

WILLIAMS & WILKINS
Baltimore/London

Made in the United States of America

Reprinted 1983

Library of Congress Cataloging in Publication Data

Bertram, Ewart G.
An atlas of the human brain and spinal cord.

Includes index.
1. Central nervous system--Atlases. I. Moore, Keith L. II. Title. [DNLM: 1. Brain--Anatomy and histology--Atlases. 2. Spinal cord--Anatomy and histology--Atlases. WL 17 B548c]
QM455.B53 611'.8'0222 82-2587
ISBN 0-683-00610-X AACR2

Composed and printed at the
Waverly Press, Inc.
Mt. Royal and Guilford Aves.
Baltimore, Md. 21202, U.S.A.

To our gracious wives,
Lee
and
Marion
and to students in neuroanatomy

Preface

The prime purpose for writing a scientific book is to give valuable, organized information about a particular subject, and to indicate what is most important for students to know. Although there are several atlases of the human central nervous system available that illustrate neuroanatomical structures, we believe they do not completely fulfill the purpose of helping the beginning student or the graduate student to develop a **three-dimensional image of the complex neuroanatomical relationships of structures** in the brain and the spinal cord. It is for this reason that we have produced this *Atlas of the Human Brain and Spinal Cord* for students in the neurosciences with the hope that it will provide an improved understanding of the anatomy of the central nervous system. It will also be helpful to other health science students and to other persons who are interested in the structure and function of the brain.

For many years we have had dissected demonstration specimens of the brain in our laboratory, which are sealed in clear plastic containers containing 10% formalin. Each specimen has an accompanying photograph that has all the **important structures labeled and clearly illustrated.** In addition to this, several brains were serially sectioned in the horizontal, coronal, and sagittal planes and then stained, photographed, and sealed in clear plastic containers. In each of these series, all the important structures were also labeled on accompanying photographs.

Many of our students, neurological and neurosurgical colleagues, urged us to prepare a photographic atlas of comparable dissections of the brain so that neuroscientists and medical students elsewhere could benefit from this three-dimensional approach.

All specimens illustrated in this atlas were carefully dissected to show the **natural anatomical relationships of the structures** in the brain. The dissections were photographed and the salient features in each dissection numbered. **The photographs have not been retouched or changed in any way.** They are true representations of each dissection; hence, any skillful dissector should be able to reproduce them. The structures on the plates were numbered instead of labeled so that students may use them for review purposes.

The legend on the facing page to each photograph gives the identity of the numbered structures in boldface print. Each structure has a short explanatory note describing the **important information** about it. These notes also describe the meaning of Latin and Greek words, the morphology or composition of the structure, and its origin, termination, course, and relations. **It is not intended to be a substitute for a textbook**; it is a concise photographic guide to learning the essential information about the central nervous system.

Many times the legends of different figures describe the same structures and some information is repeated. This was done deliberately because we believe that **repetition is a beneficial aid to learning.** The order of presentation of the dissections is from general surface features to internal structures of the cerebrum. As the dissections progress from superficial to deep areas, each underlying structure is revealed so that a clear, three-dimensional understanding of its relationship is obtained. These dissections are correlated with views of the same structures in the serial sections included at the back of the atlas.

The terminology in this atlas adheres to the internationally accepted *Nomina Anatomica*, 4th ed., approved by the Tenth International Congress of Anatomists at Tokyo in August, 1975. In accordance with international agreement, the terminology in this atlas departs from strict Latin in some cases by anglicizing terms or by using direct English translations. Although eponyms have been omitted in the *Nomina Anatomica*, those commonly used by neuroscientists and others have been included in parentheses in this Atlas, *e.g.*, **lateral sulcus** (fissure of Sylvius). Similarly, commonly used old terms are included in parentheses, *e.g.*, **superior cerebellar peduncle** (brachium conjunctivum) to facilitate the efforts of clinicians who wish to adopt the new terminology and to enable students to understand the terms they are likely to hear some neuroscientists use. In this way, it is hoped that the transition from the old terminology to the new will occur smoothly in a reasonable time.

Sincere thanks are due to the following medical students: Mary Nowaks, Tom Zwimpfer, Ab. Guha, and Paul Waldon. A gratifying result of preparing many of these dissections is that several of these students have been motivated to pursue careers in neurosurgery and neurology. **Mr. Stephen Toussaint,** Chief Technician in the Division of Gross Anatomy in our department also prepared some of the dissections. We owe him special thanks for the excellent photographs he took for this atlas.

Mrs. Laine Eljas, our neurological technician, stained the serial sections, numbered, and inserted the pointers and numbers on all the photographs with great skill. She made a very valuable contribution.

Our colleague, **Dr. D. L. McRae,** Professor Emeritis of Radiology, a specialist in neuroradiology, and Dr. Perry Cooper, of Sunnybrook Hospital, Toronto, Canada, provided the computerized tomography sections (CT scans), which were photographed by Mr. John Kozie, B.Sc., Director of Photographic Services, University of Toronto. In addition, Dr. McRae's comments, suggestions, and constructive criticisms were invaluable during the preparation of the atlas. We were also grateful to Mrs. A. Agur for proofreading some of the manuscript.

We wish to thank most sincerely Dr. M. B. Carpenter, Professor and Head of Anatomy in the Uniformed Services University of the Health Sciences, and Williams & Wilkins who kindly consented to let us use some illustrations from Carpenter's *Human Neuroanatomy*, 7th ed.

Finally, our secretaries, **Mrs. Jill Weinheimer** and **Mrs. Marion Moore** deserve our most sincere thanks and appreciation. They worked very faithfully and with great patience, often under pressure, when trying to read our handwritten notes and edited manuscripts. Marion also spent many hours proofreading the final copy.

We wish to express our gratitude to **Sara Finnegan**, President of the Medical Book Division and to **Toni Tracy**, Editor-in-Chief of Williams & Wilkins who were most helpful during the planning and preparation of this atlas.

E. G. Bertram
K. L. Moore

Toronto, Canada

Contents

Introduction

The anatomy of the central nervous system (CNS) is well illustrated in this atlas. The CNS, consisting of the brain and spinal cord, develops from the neural tube. Early in embryonic life three swellings, the **primary brain vesicles**, appear at the cranial end of the neural tube. These vesicles, called the prosencephalon, the mesencephalon and the rhombencephalon, form the brain, and the remainder of the neural tube forms the spinal cord. At about the end of the fifth week of embryonic development, two of these brain vesicles (the prosencephalon and the rhombencephalon) develop **secondary brain vesicles** as follows: the telencephalon and the diencephalon are derived from the prosencephalon, and the metencephalon and the myelencephalon originate from the rhombencephalon. The mesencephalic vesicle does not divide. It is from these brain vesicles that the major divisions of the adult brain are formed as follows:

Telencephalon—the massive cerebral hemispheres
Diencephalon—the thalamus, hypothalamus, subthalamus, and epithalamus
Mesencephalon—midbrain
Metencephalon—pons and cerebellum
Myelencephalon—medulla oblongata

The anatomy of each major division of the adult brain is presented and illustrated first, and then horizontal, coronal, and sagittal serial sections are displayed, thereby completing a three-dimensional demonstration.

The **cerebral hemispheres** consist of the cortex, the medullary center, and the basal ganglia (nuclei) and contain cavities called **lateral ventricles.** The cortex has many convolutions of gyri and sulci and several important areas of functional localization. The **medullary center** consists of a solid mass composed of association fibers (fasciculi), commissural fibers (*e.g.*, the corpus callosum, and the anterior commissure), and projection fibers (corticospinal, corticobulbar, and corticopontine, etc.). The **basal ganglia** (nuclei) are the caudate, the lentiform, the amygdaloid, and the claustrum. The caudate and lentiform nuclei, which comprise the **corpus striatum**, have important relations with the projection fibers and the thalamus. The horns of the lateral ventricles project into the frontal, occipital, and temporal lobes of the cerebral hemispheres.

The **diencephalon** is buried in the basal and medial areas of each hemisphere and encloses the narrow third ventricle. Each division of the diencephalon (thalamus, hypothalamus, subthalamus, and epithalamus) is subdivided into nuclear areas.

The **brain stem** consists of three major divisions: the **midbrain**, the **pons**, the **medulla oblongata.** Contained throughout the brain stem are: (1) the motor and/or sensory nuclei of the cranial nerves; (2) nuclear areas associated with the motor system (red, substantia nigra, olivary, and reticular); (3) ascending (sensory) pathways; and (4) descending (motor) pathways.

The **cerebellum** or "little brain" consists of the cerebellar cortex, the medullary center, various nuclei (dentate, emboliform, globose, and fastigial), and contains part of the fourth ventricle. The important **cerebellar peduncles** (superior, middle, and inferior), consisting of afferent and efferent fibers, join the cerebellum to the brain stem.

The **spinal cord** consists of (1) a central core (medullary center) of H-shaped gray matter that is subdivided into various nuclear areas which have a sensory or a motor function; and (2) an outer cortical area (cortex) made up of ascending (sensory) pathways, (*e.g.*, lateral and ventral spinothalamic, spinotectal, spinocerebellar tracts, and descending (motor) pathways (*e.g.*, corticospinal, vestibulospinal, reticulospinal) tracts.

The **blood vessels of the brain** consist of four main arteries, left and right (the vertebrals and the internal carotids), and their branches.

The stained, horizontal, coronal, and sagittal serial sections show the neuroanatomical structures and their relationship to each other throughout the brain.

Terminology is important to the understanding of the descriptions throughout this atlas and it helps in the comprehension of neuroanatomical relations:

Rostral (L., beak)—refers to structures directed toward the front or the nose.

Caudal (L., tail)—refers to structures directed toward the inferior (lower) end.

Superior—refers to structures at the uppermost part of the cerebral hemispheres.

Inferior—refers to the lowermost part of the cerebral hemispheres.

Dorsal—refers to structures close to the posterior surface of the body, or the back.

Ventral—refers to structures close to the anterior surface, or the front.

Ipsilateral (L. *ipsi*, same)—tracts or structures that project to other structures on the same side.

Contralateral (L. *contra*, against)—tracts or structures that project to other structures on the opposite side.

Medial—indicates a structure that is located toward the median plane of the brain or the spinal cord.

Lateral—indicates structures located away from the median plane of the brain or spinal cord.

Coronal (frontal) is a vertical plane or section that is parallel to the coronal suture of the skull.

Median is a vertical plane or section passing through the sagittal suture of the skull and dividing the brain along its midline into two symmetrical halves.

Sagittal is any vertical section that parallels the median plane.

Parasagittal (Gr. *para*, alongside or near) is a plane, section, or structure that is near the median (midsagittal) plane.

Horizontal is a section intersecting both the coronal and median planes at right angles.

Transverse—denotes planes of section at right angles to the long axis of a structure. Transverse sections are cut through the brain stem and the spinal cord to study their internal structure.

In our medical school, as well as in many others in North America, the dural coverings and reflections, the venous sinuses, and the structure of the cranium are studied in the Gross Anatomy course. Consequently, they are not illustrated in this atlas.

The photographs of the dissections reveal all the major structures, pathways, and nuclear areas that a skilled dissector is able to isolate; therefore, the atlas will serve as a useful guide for students in preparing good dissections or will be helpful to students in courses where dissections are not done.

The concise notes in the legends on each numbered structure in the photographs can serve as a means of **self study** because they give the student cryptic information essential for every medical student to know.

1

General Features of the Brain

Primary Brain Vesicles

P, **prosencephalon** (G. *pros*, before + *enkephalos*, brain)—forebrain
M, **mesencephalon** (G. *mesos*, middle + *enkephalos*, brain)—midbrain
R, **rhombencephalon** (G. *rhombos*, a lozenge-shaped figure + *enkephalos*, brain)—hindbrain

In the developing embryo, growth and differentiation are the greatest at the rostral end of the neural tube from which the large complex brain develops. Toward the end of the 4th week, three swellings (rostral, middle, and caudal), the primary brain vesicles, which are called the **prosencephalon** (forebrain), **mesencephalon** (midbrain), and **rhombencephalon** (hindbrain), develop at the rostral end of the neural tube.

Secondary Brain Vesicles

During the 5th week of development, the caudal and rostral primary vesicles each divide into two swellings so there are five secondary brain vesicles as follows:

From **rhombencephalon:**

1. **Myelencephalon** (G. *myelos*, marrow + *enkephalos*, brain)—the "marrow brain."
2. **Metencephalon** (G. *meta*, after + *enkephalos*, brain)—the "after brain."

From mesencephalon (no division):

3. **Mesencephalon** (G. *mesos*, middle + *enkephalos*, brain)—the "midbrain."

From **prosencephalon:**

4. **Diencephalon** (G. *dia*, through, between + *enkephalos*, brain)—the "interbrain."
5. **Telencephalon** (G. *telos*, end + *enkephalos*, brain)—the "endbrain."

Derivatives of Secondary Brain Vesicles

Telencephalon becomes the

6. **Cerebral hemispheres** (right shown)—consisting of the olfactory system, the corpus callosum, the cerebral cortex, and the medullary centers.

Diencephalon becomes the

7. **Thalamus, Epithalamus, Hypothalamus, and Subthalamus** (not seen in photograph).

Mesencephalon is the

8. **Midbrain**

Metencephalon becomes the

9. **Pons**
10. **Cerebellum**

Myelencephalon becomes the

11. **Medulla Oblongata**

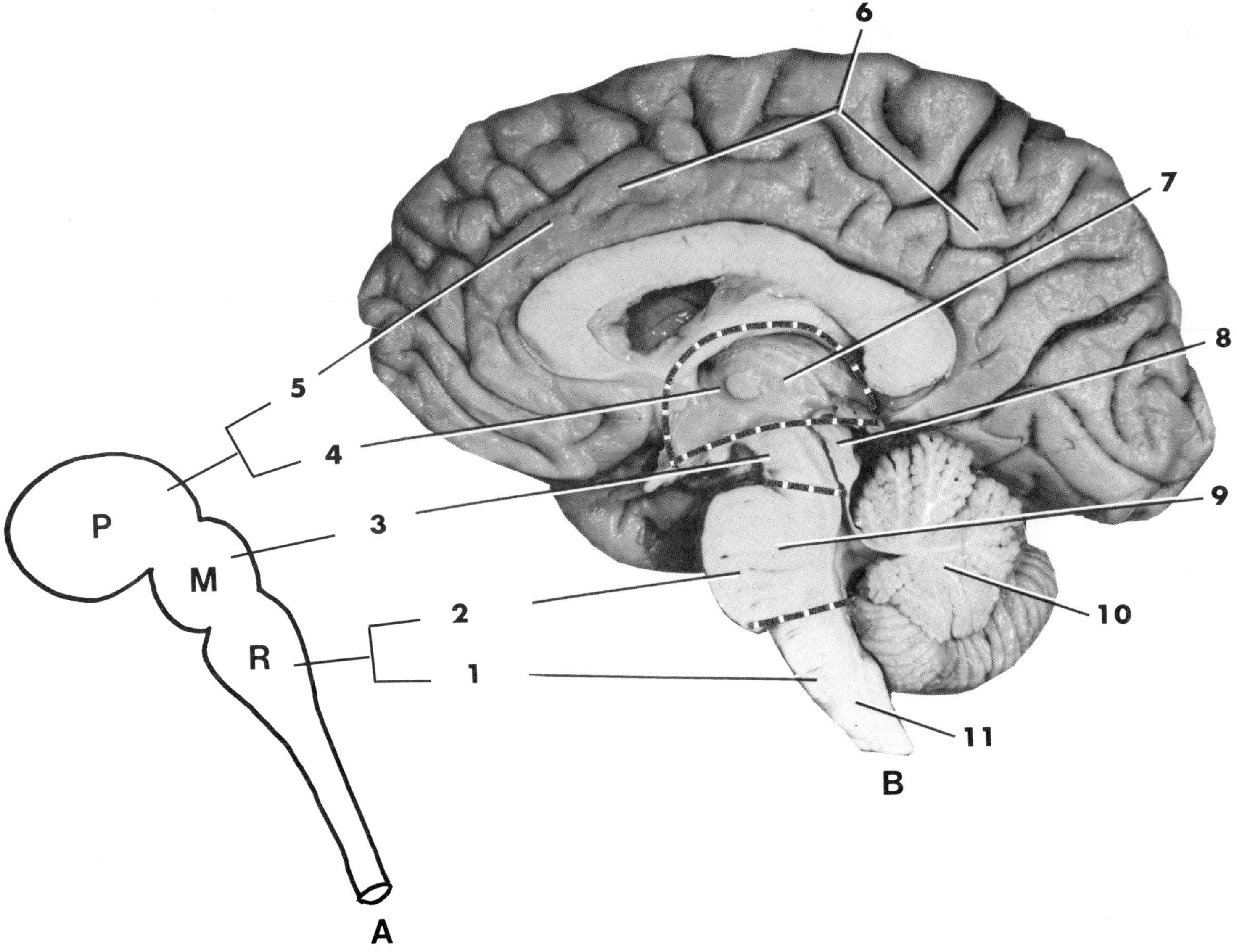

Figure 1 Shows the various regions of the brain which developed from the primary and secondary brain vesicles. *A*. Schematic representation of the primary brain vesicles. *B*. Regions of the mature brain as seen in midsagittal section.

1. **Medulla Oblongata** (L. *medulla,* marrow, from *medius,* middle)—caudal part of the brain stem that developed from the secondary brain vesicle called the myelencephalon. The medulla is about 3 cm long and widens gradually in a rostral direction. It is concealed superiorly by the cerebellum (**10**).
2. **Pons** (L. bridge)—the part of the brain stem that developed from the secondary brain vesicle known as the metencephalon. It appears to constitute a bridge between the right and left halves of the cerebellum. For a better view of the pons, see no. **2**, Fig. 3*A*.
3. **Temporal Pole**—the convex anterior end of the temporal lobe of the cerebral hemisphere. It is located in the anterior part of the middle cranial fossa and is protected by the wings of the sphenoid bone.
4. **Superficial Middle Cerebral Vein**—runs inferiorly and anteriorly along the lateral sulcus in the subarachnoid space and drains into the cavernous sinus.
5. **Frontal Pole**—the convex anterior end of the frontal lobe of the cerebral hemisphere. It is protected by dura mater and the frontal bone of the skull. It is located in the anterior part of the anterior cranial fossa.
6. **Left Cerebral Hemisphere**—(only a small part of it is indicated) the cerebral hemispheres constitute the largest part of the brain. They develop from the secondary brain vesicle called the telencephalon. Each hemisphere consists of a highly convoluted gray cortex overlying the white matter (medullary center) and neuronal masses known as basal ganglia (nuclei). The hemispheres occupy most of the interior of the skull.
7. **Superior Cerebral Veins**—eight to 12 in number, these veins course superiorly in the subarachnoid space, over the lateral surface of the cerebral hemisphere to drain into the superior sagittal sinus.
8. **Preoccipital Notch**—an ill-defined indentation on the inferior border of the cerebral hemisphere that is produced by upward pressure of the ridge of the petrous portion of the temporal bone on the soft cerebral hemisphere. It is used as a landmark for establishing the boundaries of the occipital lobe.
9. **Occipital Pole**—convex posterior end of the occipital lobe lying superior to the tentorium cerebelli and the cerebellum. The occipital bone of the skull and the dura mater overlie it.
10. **Cerebellum**—this "little brain" develops from the secondary brain vesicle called the metencephalon. It lies on the dorsal aspect of the pons (**2**) and medulla (**1**). It is separated from the posterior part of the cerebral hemispheres by a dural fold and the tentorium cerebelli.
11. **Spinal Cord (Rostral End)**—as the cervical portion of the spinal cord passes through the foramen magnum of the skull, it immediately enlarges to form the medulla (**1**) which is the caudal portion of the brain stem.

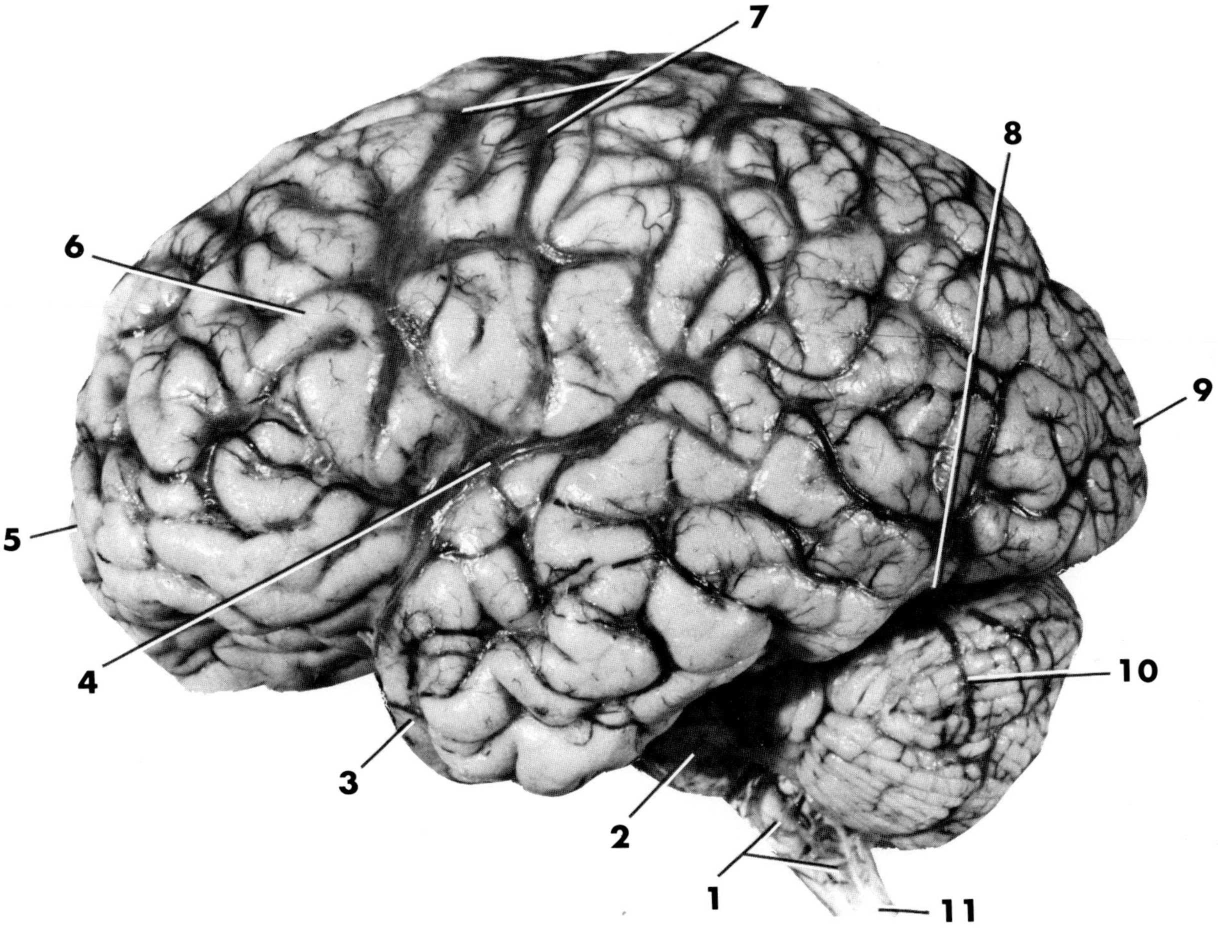

Figure 2 Lateral view of the left side of the brain showing some of its general features. The transparent arachnoid membrane covering the cerebral hemispheres is intact, and the superficial cerebral blood vessels in the subarachnoid space can be seen clearly through the arachnoid. The white patches on the surface of the cerebral hemisphere represent areas of reflected light from the moist, shiny surface of the arachnoid.

1. **Medulla Oblongata**—caudal part of the brain stem that developed from the secondary brain vesicle, called the myelencephalon. It is located in the posterior cranial fossa.

2. **Pons**—the middle portion of the brain stem (midbrain, pons, and medulla) that developed from the secondary brain vesicle, called the metencephalon. It also is located in the posterior cranial fossa.

3. **Mammillary Body** (right)—on the posterior ventral portion of the exposed hypothalamus. These two distinct swellings are located in the interpeduncular fossa, posterior to the tuber cinereum and the optic chiasma (**6**) (see also no. **9**, Fig. 16*B*).

4. **Temporal Lobe of Right Cerebral Hemisphere**—the part of the cerebral hemisphere that occupies the middle cranial fossa. It developed from the primary prosencephalon and the secondary telencephalic brain vesicle. It is separated from the frontal and parietal lobes by the lateral sulcus.

5. **Right Optic Nerve (C.N. II)**—located between the eyeball and the optic chiasma. Ganglionic fibers from the retina conduct visual impulses to the brain via this nerve.

6. **Optic Chiasma**—located anterior to the tuber cinereum (**12**) and the infundibulum (pituitary stalk) of the hypothalamus. It consists of a lateral area of uncrossed fibers coursing from one optic nerve to the ipsilateral optic tract, and a medial area of crossed fibers coursing from each optic nerve to the contralateral optic tract.

7. **Frontal Lobe of Right Cerebral Hemisphere**—this forepart of the cerebral hemisphere develops from the primary prosencephalic and the secondary telencephalic brain vesicles. It is located in the anterior cranial fossa posterior to the frontal bone of the skull. The lateral sulcus separates it from the temporal lobe, and the central sulcus separates it from the parietal lobe.

8. **Longitudinal Cerebral Fissure**—separates the anterior, posterior, and superior parts of the cerebral hemispheres. The falx cerebri (fold of dura mater) is located in this fissure.

9. **Olfactory Bulb**—an ovoid structure on the inferior surface of the frontal lobe in the anterior cranial fossa. It lies on the cribriform plate of the ethmoid bone and the adjacent part of the frontal bone. Olfactory nerve fibers from the olfactory mucosa in the se end in this structure.

10. **Olfactory Tract**—consists of nerve fibers that course from the olfactory bulb on the inferior surface of the frontal lobe to the olfactory cortex in the frontal and temporal lobes.

11. **Lateral Sulcus (Fissure of Sylvius)**—a deep furrow that begins on the ventral and inferior surfaces of the cerebral hemisphere and curves onto the lateral surface of the cerebral hemisphere. It separates the temporal lobe from the frontal and parietal lobes. The insula is located in its depths (no. **9**, Fig. [illegible]).

12. **Tuber Cinereum and Infundibular Stem (Cut)**—the part of the ventral portion of the hypothalamus that is bounded by the optic chiasma, the optic tracts, and the mammillary bodies. The infundibular stem (cut) arises from this eminence and forms the pituitary stalk, thereby attaching the pituitary gland (hypophysis cerebri) to the brain (see also no. **6**, Fig. 16*B*).

13. **Interpeduncular Fossa**—the deep space between the left and right cerebral peduncles (not shown as they are masked by the temporal lobes) of the midbrain. Because many blood vessels penetrate the floor of this fossa, it is sometimes called the posterior perforated substance (see also no. **9**, Fig. 38).

14. **Flocculus**—small irregular cerebellar mass on the ventral surface of the cerebellum that is located lateral to the junction of the pons and the medulla. It functions in balance and equilibrium and is *part of the flocculonodular lobe*.

15. **Cerebellum**—this "little brain" is located on the dorsal aspect of the pons and the medulla in the posterior cranial fossa. Like the pons, it develops from the secondary metencephalic and primary rhombencephalic brain vesicles.

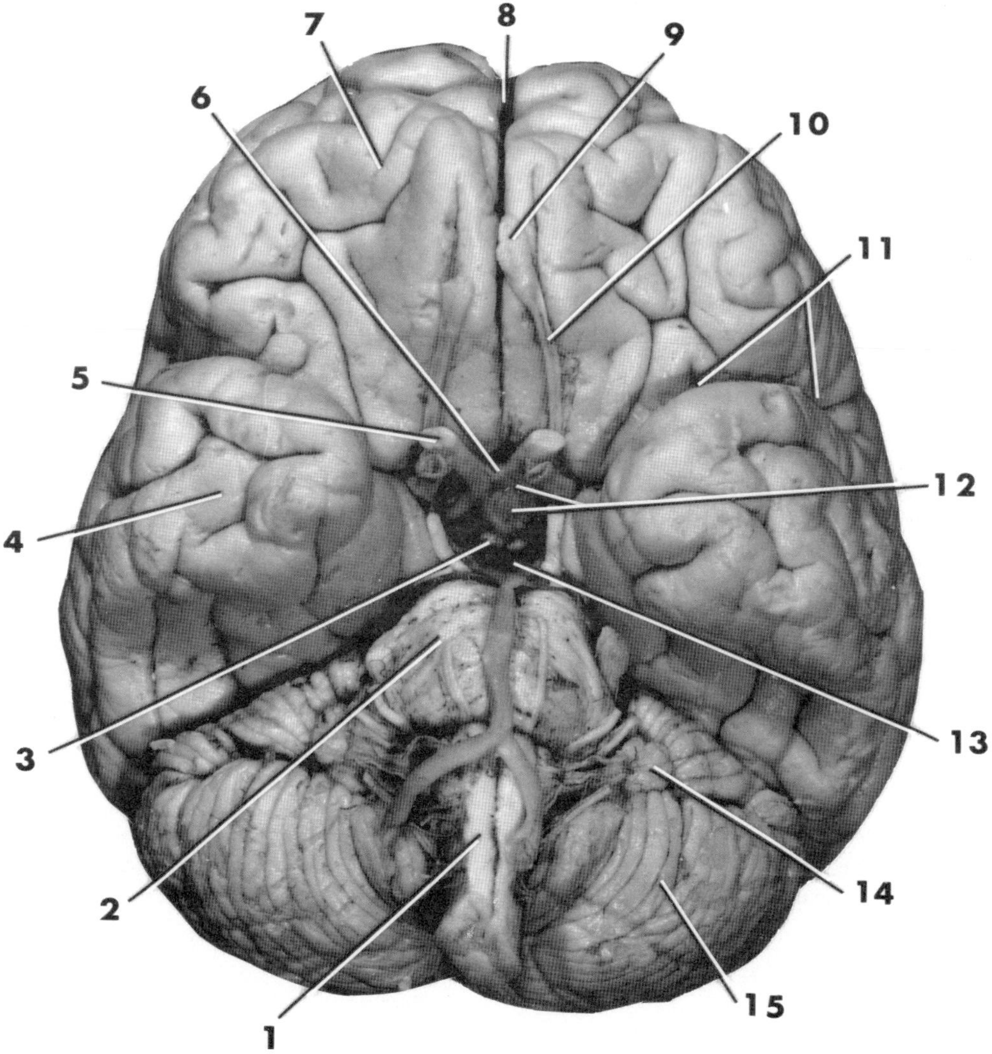

Figure 3*A* Ventral (basal) view of the brain showing some of the general features of the cerebrum and the brain stem.

1. **Pyramid**—this elongated pyramid-shaped column of fibers is located on each side of the ventral median fissure on the ventral surface of the medulla. It consists of descending motor tract fibers.
2. **Vertebral Artery** (right)—enters the skull through the foramen magnum and runs anterosuperiorly on the medulla to join the left vertebral artery and form the basilar artery (**5** and no. **4**, Fig. 65) at the caudal border of the pons.
3. **Vagus Nerve (C.N. X)**—a mixed nerve with sensory and motor components. Its fibers enter and leave the brain stem with the C.N. IX and C.N. XI fibers in the dorsolateral sulcus. These three nerves leave the skull through the jugular foramen.
4. **Facial Nerve (C.N. VII)**—a mixed nerve with sensory and motor components. Its fibers enter and leave the caudal border of the pons laterally with the C.N. VIII. These two nerves enter the interior of the skull through the internal acoustic (auditory) meatus.
5. **Basilar Artery**—formed by the union of the two vertebral arteries. It ends at the rostral border of the pons by dividing into the two posterior cerebral arteries (**9** and no. **5**, Fig. 65).
6. **Trochlear Nerve (C.N. IV)**—this motor nerve is the only cranial nerve to emerge from the dorsal surface of the brain stem. It curves around the lateral surface of the midbrain and courses with C.N. III between the posterior cerebral and the superior cerebellar arteries.
7. **Internal Carotid Artery**—a terminal branch of the common carotid artery. It enters the skull through the carotid canal, courses through and above the cavernous sinus, and terminates by forming the anterior and middle cerebral arteries.
8. **Oculomotor Nerve (C.N. III)**—this cranial nerve supplies all of the extraocular muscles with the exception of two that are supplied by C.N. IV and C. N. VI. It emerges at the rostral border of the pons in the interpeduncular fossa.
9. **Posterior Cerebral Artery**—one of the two terminal branches of the basilar artery. It supplies the medial and inferior surfaces of the temporal and occipital lobes, as well as a peripheral strip on the lateral surface.
10. **Trigeminal Nerve (C.N. V)**—a mixed nerve with a large sensory and a small motor component. Its fibers enter and leave the pons laterally, at the junction of the basal pons and the middle cerebellar peduncle.
11. **Abducens Nerve (C.N. VI)**—a motor nerve to one eye muscle (*lateral rectus*). Its fibers emerge from the caudal border of the pons.
12. **Auditory (Vestibulocochlear) Nerve (C.N. VIII)**—a special sensory nerve. Fibers from the internal ear enter the interior of the skull via the internal acoustic meatus and enter the brain stem with fibers of C.N. VII laterally, at the caudal border of the pons.
13. **Glossopharyngeal Nerve (C.N. IX)**—a mixed nerve with sensory and motor components. It emerges from the medulla with C.N. X and C.N. XI in the dorsolateral sulcus.
14. **Spinal Accessory Nerve (C.N. XI)**—a motor nerve, the fibers of which emerge from the dorsolateral sulcus of the medulla with C.N. IX, and C.N. X. These three nerves exit from the skull through the jugular foramen.
15. **Decussation of Pyramids**—approximately 85% of the pyramidal fibers cross in the ventral medial fissure (no. **17**, Fig. 38) to the contralateral side of the caudal medulla or to the upper cervical spinal cord.

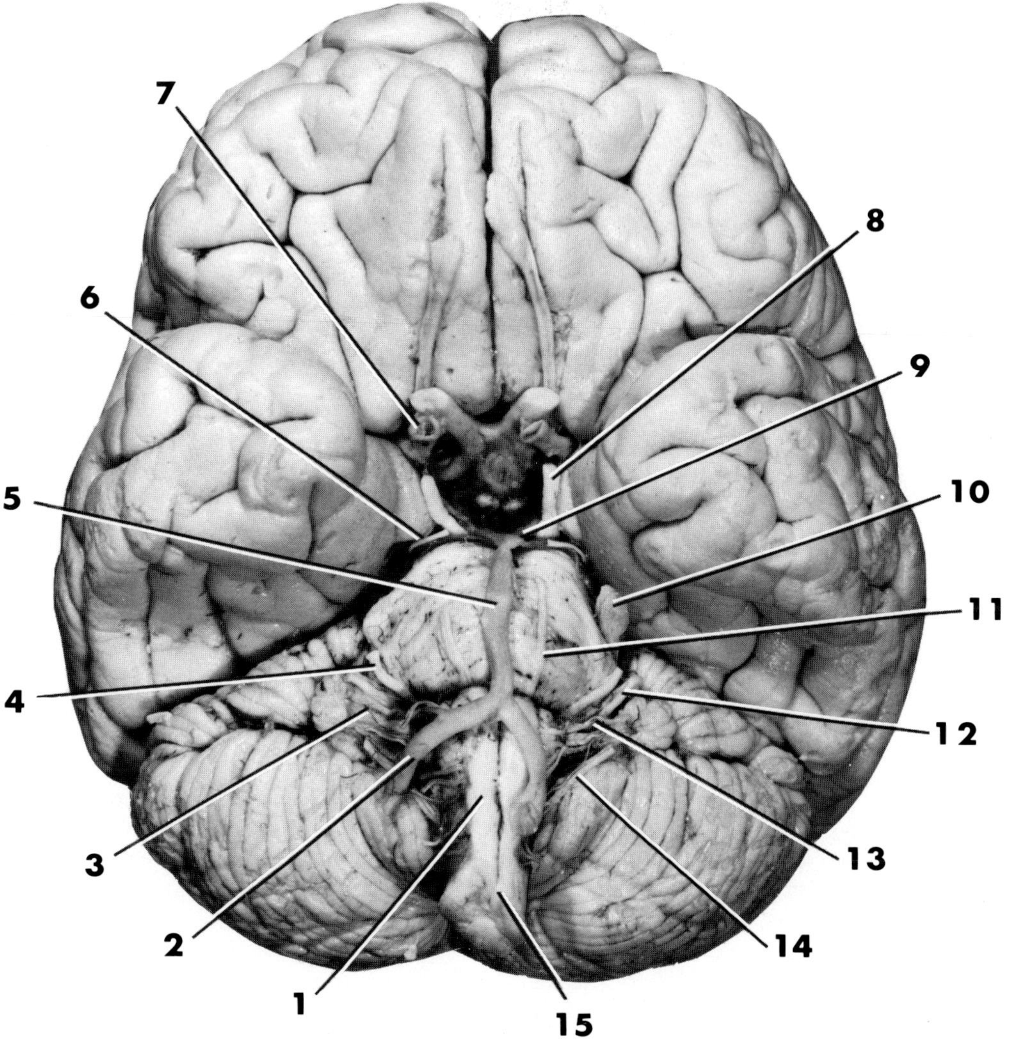

Figure 3*B* Ventral (basal) view of the same brain showing more detailed features of the cerebrum and the brain stem.

1. **Brain Stem**—consists of **(a)** the **medulla oblongata,** the expanded wedge-shaped structure which is a continuation of the cephalic end of the spinal cord after it has passed through the foramen magnum; **(b)** the **pons,** the middle portion of the brain stem, which consists of a basal portion, the fibers of which extend into the cerebellum and a tegmental area **(c);** and the **midbrain,** the rostral portion of the brain stem which is located immediately caudal to the diencephalon. A portion of the midbrain extends obliquely beneath the diencephalon (thalamus and subthalamus).
2. **Fornix (Column of)**—this bundle of fibers is part of the limbic system that connects the hippocampus with nuclear areas of the hypothalamus. Its fibers curve from the dorsal surface of the thalamus inferiorly and anterior to the interventricular foramen (see no. **6,** Fig. 4*B*).
3. **Septum Pellucidum**—this membrane, sometimes double, is located between the anterior part of the corpus callosum and the fornix. It separates parts of the anterior horns and variable other parts of the lateral ventricles.
4. **Frontal Pole (of Cerebral Hemisphere)**—the forepart of the frontal lobe, the largest part of the cerebral hemisphere. It is located in the anterior cranial fossa, where it is protected by the meninges and the frontal bone. The frontal lobe is not well demarcated from the parietal lobe on the medial surface of the hemisphere. A line drawn from the central sulcus inferiorly to the corpus callosum separates these lobes.
5. **Diencephalon (Thalmus, Epithalamus, Subthalamus, and Hypothalamus**—located between the cerebral hemispheres and the midbrain. Much of it is buried in the ventral and median portions of each cerebral hemisphere. It forms the lateral walls of the third ventricle. The **hypothalamus (a)** is the part of the diencephalon that lies inferior to the **thalamus (b)** and the hypothalamic sulcus. It is the only part of the diencephalon that is exposed on the basal surface of the brain. Although it occupies only a small portion of the brain, it has many important functions. The thalamus is a large ovoid mass of gray matter forming the major part of the diencephalon. It is situated on each side of the third ventricle and inferior to the body of the lateral ventricle and the body of the fornix. It has important sensory and motor functions.
6. **Central Sulcus (Fissure or Sulcus of Rolando)**—an important landmark on the lateral surface of the cerebral hemisphere. It extends over the superior border for a short distance on the medial surface. The general sensory area lies immediately posterior to the sulcus, and the motor area lies immediately anterior to it. If an imaginery line were extended inferiorly from this sulcus to the corpus callosum, it would separate the frontal lobe from the parietal lobe.
7. **Area of Parietal Lobe (of Cerebral Hemisphere)**—on the medial surface this lobe can be separated from the frontal lobe as outlined above **(6),** and it can easily be separated from the occipital lobe **(9)** by the parietooccipital sulcus **(8)**. The parietal lobe is protected by the meningeal coverings and the overlying parietal bone.
8. **Parietooccipital Sulcus**—this prominent sulcus on the medial surface of the cerebral hemisphere extends inferiorly to the calcarine sulcus (no. **3,** Fig. 9*A*) and superiorly onto the lateral surface for a short distance.
9. **Occipital Lobe**—is the caudal area of the cerebral hemisphere. The parietooccipital sulcus separates it on the medial surface from the parietal lobe. The occipital bone and meninges cover and protect this lobe.
10. **Cerebral Aqueduct (of Sylvius)**—this canal passes through the midbrain between the tectum and cerebral peduncles and connects the third and fourth ventricles (see also no. **6,** Fig. 43).
11. **Cerebellum ("Little Brain")**—situated on the dorsum of the pons and medulla. It consists of a midline structure, the **vermis (a),** and two lateral structures, the **cerebellar hemispheres (b,** right shown). It has an important controlling function in fine movement and equilibrium.

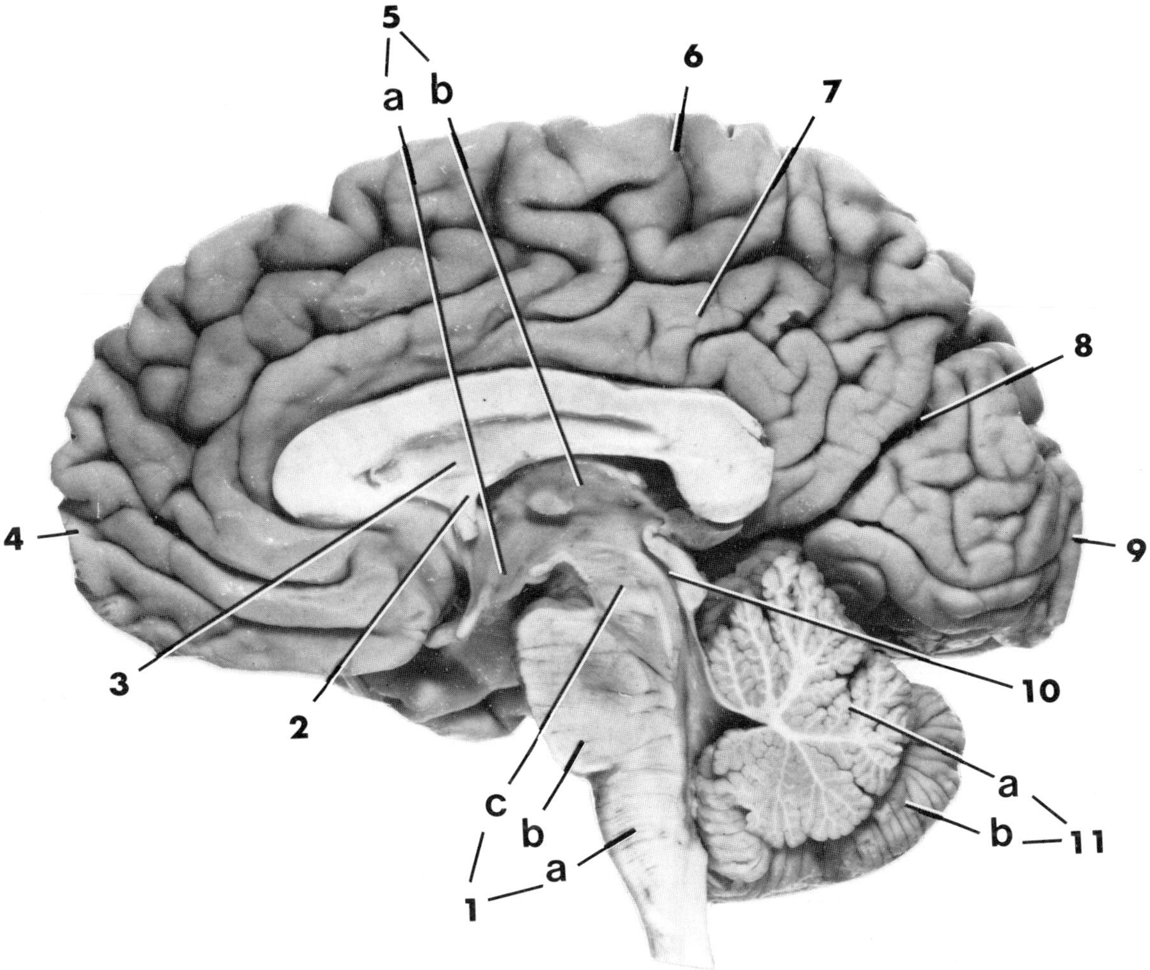

Figure 4*A* Medial view of the right half of the brain sectioned in the median (midsagittal) plane to show some of the general features of the cerebrum and the brain stem.

1. **Massa Intermedia**—a bridge of gray matter connecting the left and right thalami across the third ventricle. It is present in approximately 70% of brains.
2. **Mammillary Body**—one of a pair of distinct swellings located in the interpeduncular fossa posterolateral to the midline tuber cinereum and the optic chiasma. The mammillary bodies and the tuber cinereum are the only parts of the hypothalamus that are exposed on the ventral surface of the brain.
3. **Optic Chiasma**—located anterior to the tuber cinereum (no. **12,** Fig. 3*A*). Parts of the hypothalamus and the third ventricle are anterior, superior, and posterior to it. Fibers from the medial half of each retina cross from the optic nerve to the opposite optic tract.
4. **Lamina Terminalis**—represents the rostral end of the embryonic neural tube and limits the third ventricle anteriorly. It extends from the optic chiasma to the anterior commissure (**5**).
5. **Anterior Commissure**—commissural fibers cross the midline and pass through the cerebral basal ganglia on their way to the temporal lobe.
6. **Interventricular Foramen (of Monro)**—located between the lateral and third ventricles. It is bounded anteriorly by a column of the fornix (see Fig. 4A, No. 2) and posteriorly by the anterior tubercle of the thalamus.
7. **Corpus Callosum** (L. body + *callosus,* hard)—this large body of compact reciprocal commissural fibers connects similar areas of each cerebral hemisphere. It is divisible into different regions, the anterior region—the **genu (a),** which thins out to form the **rostrum (b);** the large central region, the **body (c);** and the enlarged posterior area, the **splenium (d).**
8. **Stria Medullaris Thalamicus**—part of the epithalamus which consists of fibers that stream along the dorsomedial border of the thalamus to the habenular trigone, located at the base of the pineal body **(9).**
9. **Pineal Body (Gland)**—shaped like a pine cone, it is part of the epithalamus and is attached to the diencephalon by the pineal stalk into which the third ventricle extends as the pineal recess.
10. **Tectum (Roof)**—the dorsal surface of the midbrain has four rounded elevations, the *paired superior and inferior colliculi* (corpora quadrigemina). The colliculi make up the roof (L. *tectum*) and indicate the extent of the midbrain on the dorsal surface.
11. **Superior Medullary Velum**—this sheet of pia mater and ependymal cells stretches from one superior cerebellar peduncle to the other, forming the forepart of the roof of the fourth ventricle (see also no. **15,** Fig. 56).
12. **Fourth Ventricle**—the large ventricle between the cerebellum and the pons and the medulla. Its floor is formed by the dorsal surface of the tegmental area of the pons and the open medulla. Its roof is formed by the vermis, the superior cerebellar peduncles, and the thin sheet of the superior medullary velum and the inferior medullary velum.
13. **Lateral Recess**—the lateral recess of the fourth ventricle extends laterally ventral to the cerebellar peduncles to communicate with the subarachnoid space as the lateral aperture of the fourth ventricle. Usually this aperture contains part of the choroid plexus of the fourth ventricle.

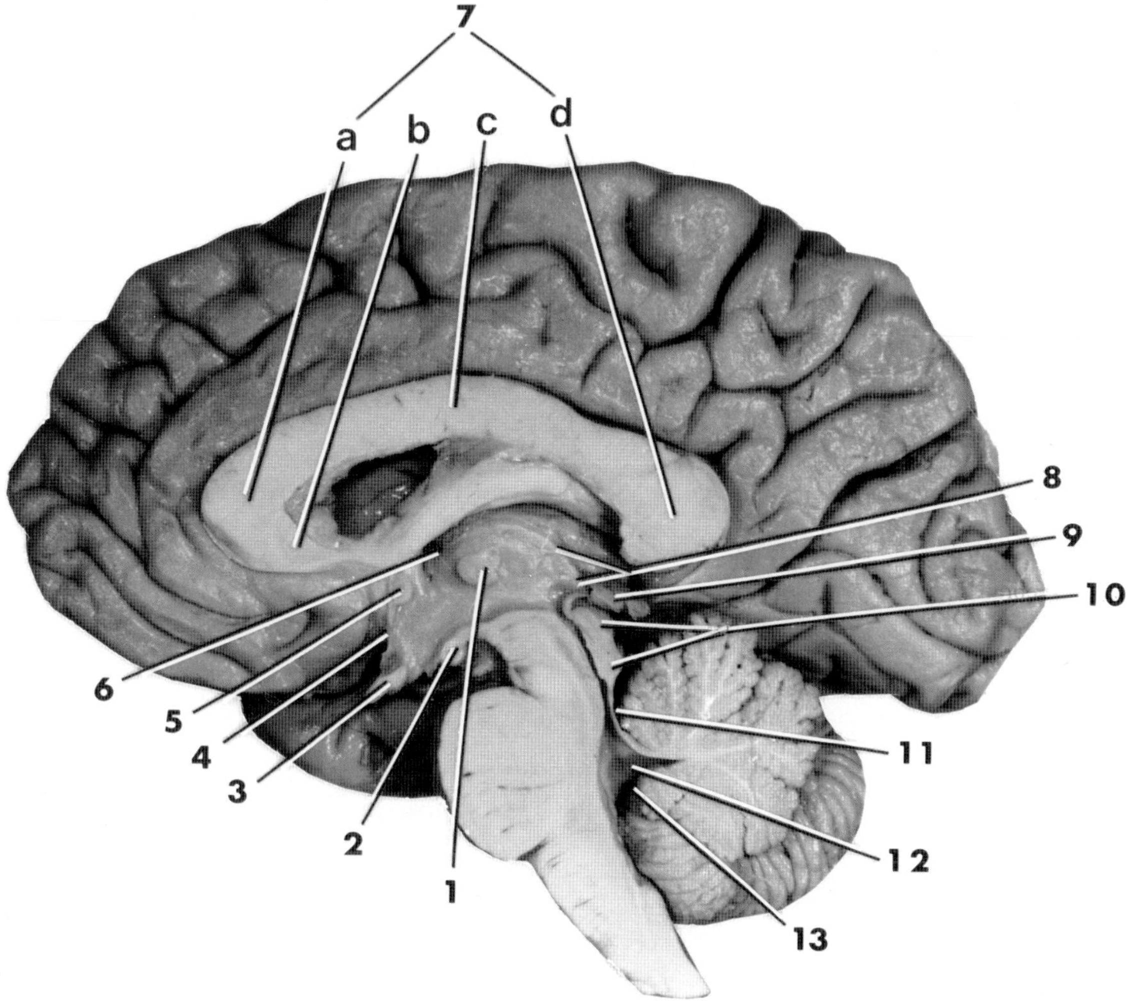

Figure 4*B* Medial view of the right half of the same brain sectioned in the median (midsagittal) plane showing more detailed features of the cerebrum and the brain stem.

2

Lobes, External Configurations, and Functional Localization of the Major Areas of the Cerebrum

Surface Markings

These are used for determining the boundaries of the lobes of the cerebral hemispheres.

1. **Preoccipital Notch**—An ill-defined indentation on the inferior border of the cerebral hemisphere that is produced by upward pressure of the ridge of the petrous portion of the temporal bone on the soft cerebral hemisphere.

2. **Parietooccipital Sulcus (Fissure)**—a prominent sulcus on the medial surface of the cerebral hemisphere that intersects the superior border, approximately 4 cm from the occipital pole, and continues a short distance on the dorsolateral surface.

3. **Central Sulcus (Fissure, Sulcus of Rolando)**—a prominent groove sloping downward and forward from about the midpoint of the superior border of the hemisphere. It stops short of the lateral sulcus. This important landmark separates the frontal lobe from the parietal lobe.

4. **Lateral Sulcus (Fissure of Sylvius)**—a deep furrow directed superiorly and posteriorly on the lateral surface of the hemisphere. It is an important landmark which separates the frontal lobe from the temporal lobe.

Lobes

A. **Occipital Lobe**—on the lateral surface of the cerebral hemisphere. It is limited anteriorly and separated from the parietal (**B**) and temporal (**D**) lobes by an imaginary line which joins the parietooccipital sulcus (**2**) with the preoccipital notch (**1**).

B. **Parietal Lobe**—on the lateral surface of the hemisphere. It is limited anteriorly by the central sulcus (**3**) and its imaginary projection to the lateral sulcus (**4**); inferiorly by the lateral sulcus and its posterior imaginary projection; posteriorly by the upper half of the imaginary line extending from the parietooccipital sulcus (**2**) to the preoccipital notch.

C. **Frontal Lobe**—on the lateral surface of the cerebral hemisphere. It is limited posteriorly by the central sulcus (**3**) and its imaginary projection (*dotted lines*) to the lateral sulcus (**4**) and inferiorly by the lateral sulcus.

D. **Temporal Lobe**—on the lateral surface of the cerebral hemisphere. It is limited superiorly by the lateral sulcus (**4**) and its imaginary posterior projection (*dotted lines*) and posteriorly by the lower half of the imaginary line (*dotted line*) joining the parietooccipital sulcus (**2**) with the preoccipital notch (**1**). The temporal lobe occupies the middle cranial fossa of the skull.

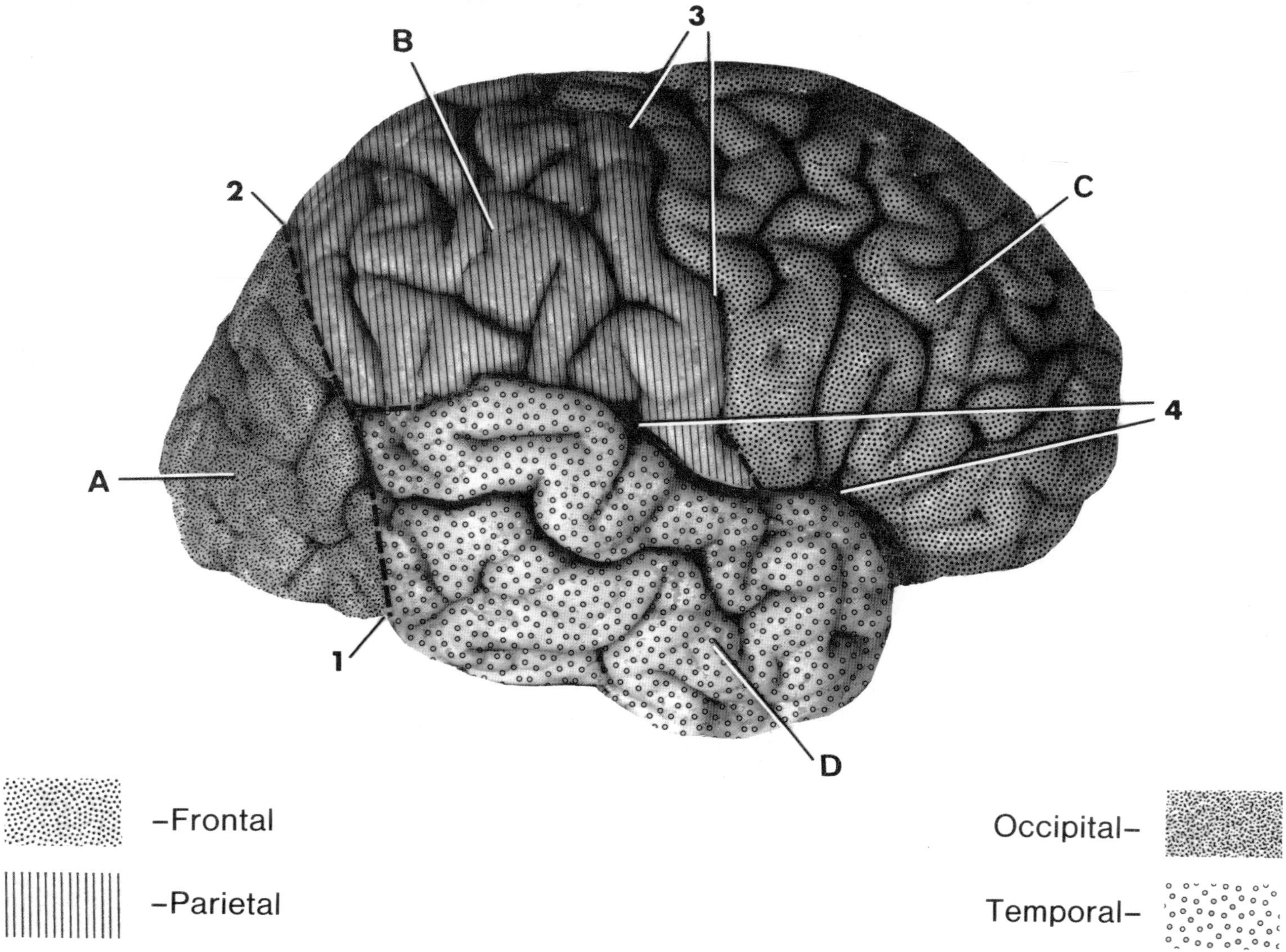

Figure 5 Lateral view of the right cerebral hemisphere demonstrating the boundaries and surface areas of the four lobes.

Surface Markings

These are used for determining the boundaries of the lobes of the cerebral hemispheres.

1. **Preoccipital Notch**—an ill-defined indentation on the inferior border lying on the cerebral hemisphere that is produced from the weight of the very soft cerebral hemisphere lying on the ridge of the petrous portion of the temporal bone.
2. **Calcarine Sulcus**—begins inferior to the posterior end of the corpus callosum and follows an arched course to the occipital pole. This sulcus is an important landmark for the visual cortex, most of which lies in the walls of the sulcus.
3. **Parietooccipital Sulcus (Fissure)**—a prominent fissure on the medial surface of the cerebral hemisphere. It begins at the calcarine sulcus, passes upward and backward to intersect the superior border, about 4 cm in front of the occipital pole, and extends for about 1.5 cm on the superolateral surface.
4. **Central Sulcus (Fissure of Rolando)**—commences on the medial surface of the hemisphere about 2 cm inferior to the superior border. It courses upward and indents the superior border just posterior to its midpoint and then courses downward and forward over the lateral surface, stopping just short of the lateral sulcus (no. **9**, Fig. 7*B*).
5. **Corpus Callosum** (L. *corpus*, body + *callosus*, hard)—a midline structure which is the main commissure of the cerebral hemispheres. It has the following main structures: a large body, a splenium, a genu, and a rostrum. Parts of the corpus callosum form the boundaries of some of the lobes on the medial surface of the hemisphere.
6. **Lateral Sulcus (Fissure of Sylvius)**—begins as a very deep furrow (space) on the inferior surface of the cerebral hemisphere and extends laterally, separating the frontal and temporal lobes to reach the lateral surface of the hemisphere. On the lateral surface it is directed posteriorly and superiorly into the parietal lobe. Much of the lateral sulcus is the boundary line of some cerebral lobes.
7. **Hippocampal Sulcus**—a deep sulcus resting against the lateral side of the midbrain and separating the parahippocampal gyrus from the dentate gyrus. It forms one of the boundaries of the temporal lobe.

Lobes

A. **Occipital Lobe**—on the medial surface of the cerebral hemisphere. It is limited anteriorly and superiorly by the parietooccipital sulcus (**3**) and the anterior (precalcarine) half of the calcarine sulcus (**2**). These sulci separate the occipital lobe from the parietal lobe (**B**). Inferiorly, the occipital lobe is demarcated from the temporal lobe (**D**) by an imaginary line (*dotted*) extending from the anterior end of the calcarine sulcus (**2**) to the preoccipital notch (**1**).

B. **Parietal Lobe**—on the medial surface of the cerebral hemisphere. It is separated from the occipital lobe by the parietooccipital sulcus (**3**) and the anterior half of the calcarine sulcus (**2**). It is bounded in front by an imaginary line (*dotted*) extending from the central sulcus (**4**) inferiorly to the corpus callosum (**5**). The corpus callosum forms its inferior boundary.

C. **Frontal Lobe**—on the medial surface of the cerebral hemisphere. It is bounded posteriorly by an imaginary line extending from the central sulcus (**4**) to the corpus callosum (**5**) and arbitrarily separating it from the parietal lobe (**B**). The large medial surface of the frontal lobe envelops the anterior half of the corpus callosum.

D. **Temporal Lobe**—on the medial and inferior surfaces of the cerebral hemisphere. It is bounded posteriorly by an imaginary line (*dotted*) extending from the anterior end of the calcarine sulcus (**2**) to the preoccipital notch (**1**) demarcating it from the occipital lobe. It is bounded superiorly by the hippocampal sulcus (**7**).

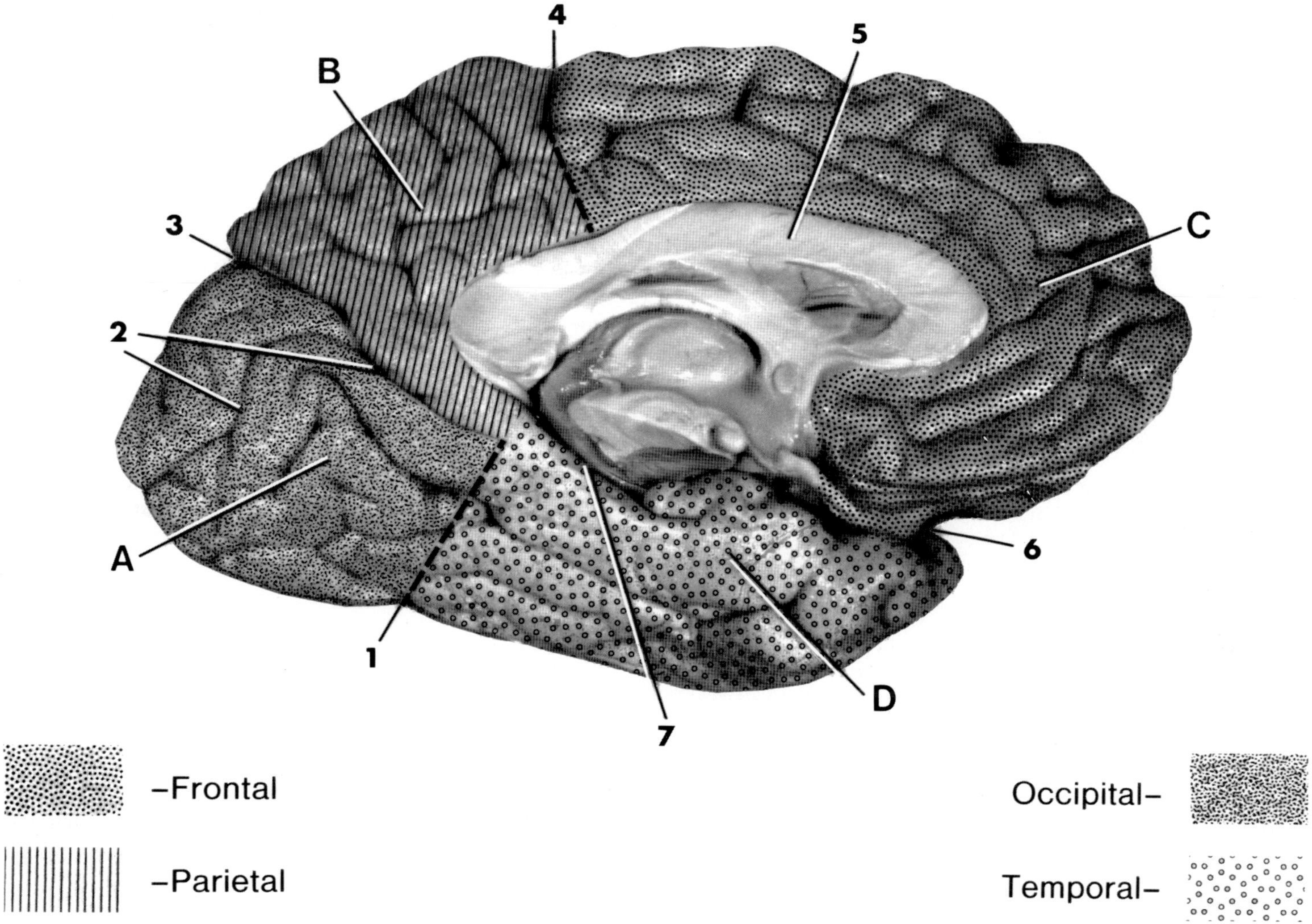

Figure 6 Medial and inferior view of the left cerebral hemisphere demonstrating the boundaries and surface areas of the four lobes.

1. **Middle Temporal Gyrus**—located between the superior (**10**) and inferior (**2**) temporal gyri. It is separated from these gyri by the superior and middle temporal sulci.
2. **Inferior Temporal Gyrus**—located between the middle (**1**) and fusiform (no. **3**, Fig. 9*B*) gyri. It forms much of the inferior border of the temporal lobe and extends onto the medial surface.
3. **Inferior Parietal Lobule**—located posterior to the postcentral gyrus (**5**) and inferior to the superior parietal lobule (**4**), which is separated from it by the intraparietal sulcus.
4. **Superior Parietal Lobule**—located posterior to the postcentral gyrus and superior to the intraparietal sulcus.
5. **Postcentral Gyrus**—located in the parietal lobe between the central sulcus (no. **5**, Fig. 7*B*) and the postcentral sulcus. It parallels the precentral gyrus (**6**). Its cortex is concerned with general somesthetic sensation.
6. **Precentral Gyrus**—located in the caudal portion of the frontal lobe. It is separated from and parallels the central sulcus (no. **5**, Fig. 7*B*). Much of the somatomotor area is located in this gyrus.
7. **Superior Frontal Gyrus**—located anterior to the precentral gyrus. It forms the superior border of the frontal lobe and curves from its lateral surface onto its medial surface.
8. **Middle Frontal Gyrus**—the part of the frontal lobe lying between the superior (**7**) and inferior (**9**) frontal gyri and anterior to the precentral gyrus (**6**).
9. **Inferior Frontal Gyrus**—located inferior to the middle frontal gyrus. The anterior ascending and anterior horizontal rami of the lateral sulcus (no. **9**, Fig. 7*B*) divide the posterior portion of this gyrus into:
   a. **Pars Orbitalis**—the part of the inferior frontal gyrus which is separated from the pars triangularis by the anterior horizontal ramus of the lateral sulcus (no. **9c** Fig. 7*B*).
   b. **Pars Triangularis**—the part of the inferior frontal gyrus which is located between the pars opercularis (**c**) and the pars orbitalis (**a**). **Broca's motor speech area** is located in the cortex of the pars triangularis and pars opercularis (**b** and **c**).
   c. **Pars Opercularis**—the part of the inferior frontal gyrus located immediately anterior to the precentral gyrus and separated from the pars triangularis (**b**) by the anterior ascending ramus of the lateral fissure (no. **9b**, Fig. 7*B*).
10. **Superior Temporal Gyrus**—forms the inferior wall of the lateral sulcus. It is separated from the middle temporal gyrus by the superior temporal sulcus.

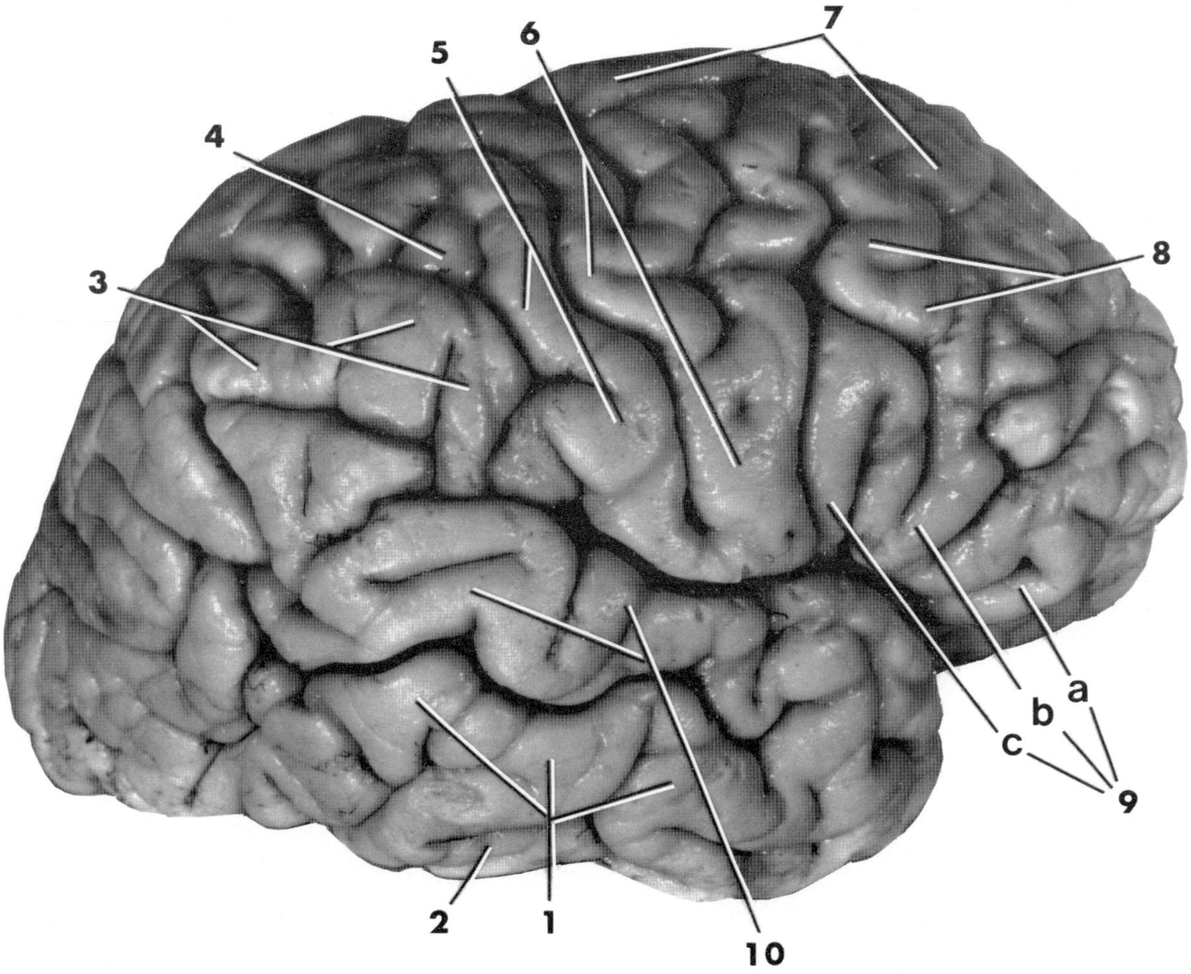

Figure 7A Lateral surface of the right cerebral hemisphere showing the main gyri of the lobes.

1. **Middle Temporal Sulcus**—separates the middle temporal gyrus from the inferior temporal gyrus (see nos. **1** and **2**, Fig. 7*A*). It runs parallel to the superior temporal sulcus (**2**).

2. **Superior Temporal Sulcus**—separates the superior temporal gyrus from the middle temporal gyrus (see nos. **10** and **1**, Fig. 7*A*). It runs parallel to the lateral sulcus and extends into the inferior parietal lobule. The cortex surrounding this terminal portion of the sulcus forms the angular gyrus.

3. **Parietooccipital Sulcus (Fissure)**—a prominent fissure on the medial surface of the cerebral hemisphere (see no. **4**, Fig. 9*A*). It extends a short distance onto the dorsolateral surface, intersecting the superior border approximately 4 cm from the occipital pole.

4. **Postcentral Sulcus**—parallels the central sulcus (**5**). These sulci bound the postcentral gyrus (see no. **5**, Fig. 7*A*).

5. **Central Sulcus (Fissure, Sulcus of Rolando)**—an important landmark for the sensorimotor cortex. The general sensory area lies posterior to it in the postcentral gyrus (no. **5**, Fig. 7*A*), and the motor area is located anterior to it in the precentral gyrus (no. **6**, Fig. 7*A*). The central sulcus slopes downward and forward stopping short of the lateral sulcus. It indents the superior border of the cerebral hemisphere and extends a short distance into the paracentral lobule (no. **7**, Fig. 9*B*) on the medial surface.

6. **Precentral Sulcus**—parallels the central sulcus. It is often broken into two or more parts. The central and precentral sulci outline the precentral gyrus (see no. **6**, Fig. 7*A*).

7. **Superior Frontal Sulcus**—courses somewhat parallel to the superior border of the cerebral hemisphere. This sulcus separates the superior frontal gyrus from the middle frontal gyrus (see nos. **7** and **8**, Fig. 7*A*).

8. **Inferior Frontal Sulcus**—located above and runs parallel to the lateral sulcus. It is often broken into two or more parts and separates the middle frontal gyrus from the inferior frontal gyrus (see nos. **8** and **9**, Fig. 7*A*).

9. **Lateral Sulcus (Fissure of Sylvius)**—begins as a very deep furrow on the inferior surface of the hemisphere and extends laterally between the frontal and temporal lobes. On reaching the lateral surface, it divides into three rami (**a**, **b**, and **c**). The posterior ramus (**a**) is the main part of the fissure and is directed posteriorly and superiorly into the parietal lobe. The ascending ramus (**b**) and the anterior ramus (**c**) project only a short distance into the inferior frontal gyrus, dividing it into three portions: pars orbitalis, pars triangularis, and pars opercularis (see nos. **9a**, **b**, and **c**, Fig. 7*A*).

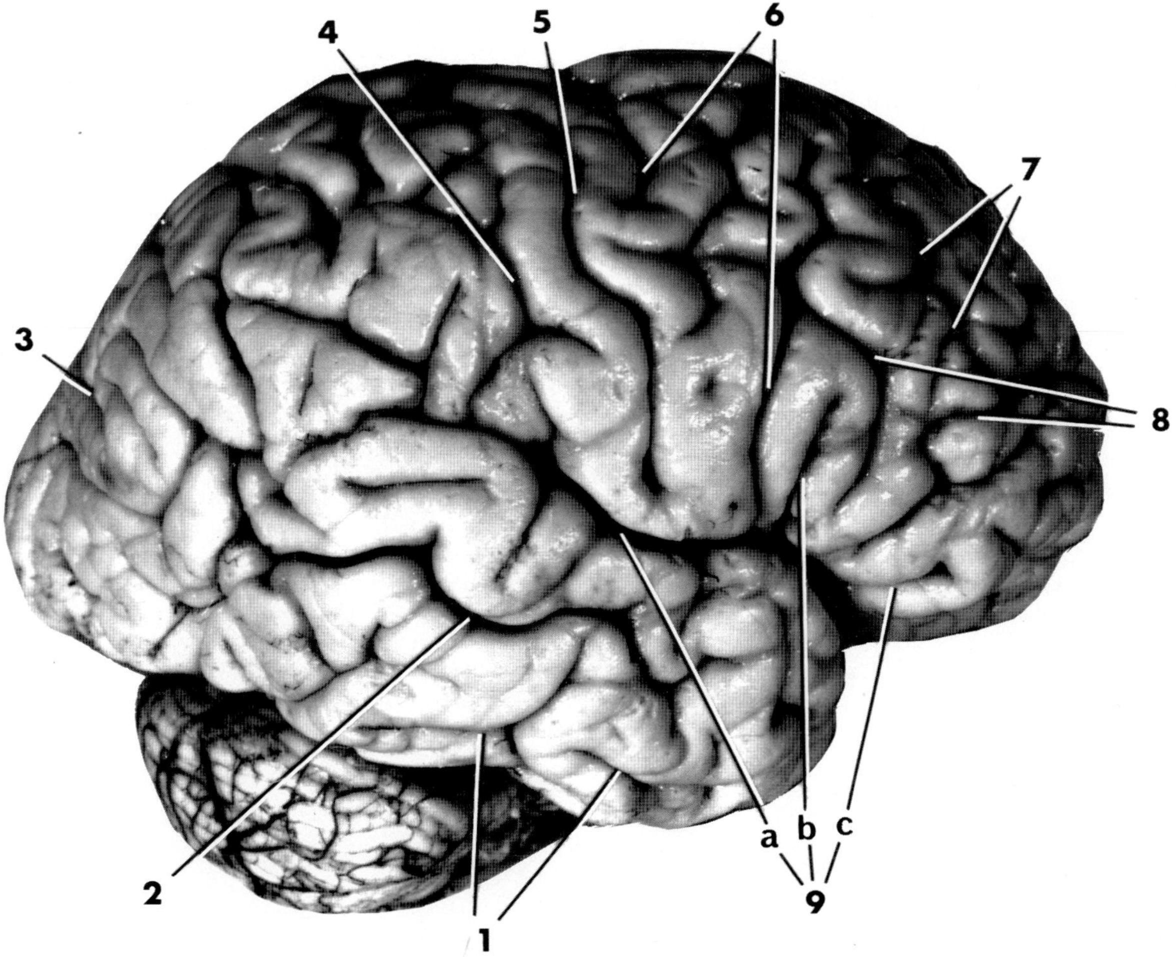

Figure 7*B* Lateral surface of the right cerebral hemisphere of the same brain showing the sulci of these lobes. The cerebellum is also shown inferior to the occipital and temporal lobes.

1. **Superior Temporal Gyrus**—forms the inferior wall of the lateral sulcus. It is separated from the middle temporal gyrus (**2**) by the superior temporal sulcus. Some of the primary and association auditory cortex is located in this gyrus.
2. **Middle Temporal Gyrus**—located between the superior and inferior temporal gyri. It is separated from these gyri by the superior and middle temporal sulci.
3. **Occipital Pole**—convex posterior end of the occipital lobe, lying superior to the cerebellum and separated from it by the tentorium cerebelli.
4. **Postcentral Gyrus**—located in the parietal lobe between the central sulcus and the postcentral sulcus, it parallels the precentral gyrus (**5**). Its cortex functions for general somesthetic sensation (see no. **5**, Fig. 7*A*).
5. **Precentral Gyrus**—located in the caudal portion of the frontal lobe. It parallels the postcentral gyrus and is separated from it by the central sulcus. Much of the somatomotor area is located in this gyrus and in the central sulcus (see no. **6**, Fig. 7*A*).
6. **Medullary Center (of Frontal and Parietal Lobes)**—consists of myelinated nerve fibers of association, commissural, and projection neurons. Note that much of the cortex and the medullary center of the parietal and the frontal lobe opercula have been removed to show the insula (**9**).
7. **Superior Frontal Gyrus**—located anterior to the superior portion of the precentral gyrus. It forms the superior border of the frontal lobe and curves from its lateral surface onto its medial surface.
8. **Lateral Sulcus (Fissure of Sylvius)**—a deep fissure extending superiorly and posteriorly which separates the frontal and temporal lobes. The anterior portion of this sulcus has ascending and horizontal rami that extend into the frontal lobe. Its posterior portion extends into the parietal lobe.
9. **Insula (Island of Reil)**—located in the depths of the lateral sulcus. It is concealed by the frontal (removed), parietal (removed), and temporal opercula. The insula (*shaded area*) is outlined by a circular sulcus and is divided into two regions by a central sulcus. Several short gyri lie anterior to the central sulcus and one or two long gyri posterior to it. The specific function of the insula is unknown. It does have some general sensory and motor functions.
10. **Transverse Temporal Gyri (Heschl's Convolutions)**—formed from the superior temporal gyrus as several oblique convolutions that course posterior to the insula within the lateral sulcus. These gyri constitute the **primary auditory cortex**. There is a spatial representation in the auditory area with respect to the pitch of sounds. Impulses of low frequencies impinge on the anterolateral part of the area and impulses of high frequencies on the posteromedial part.

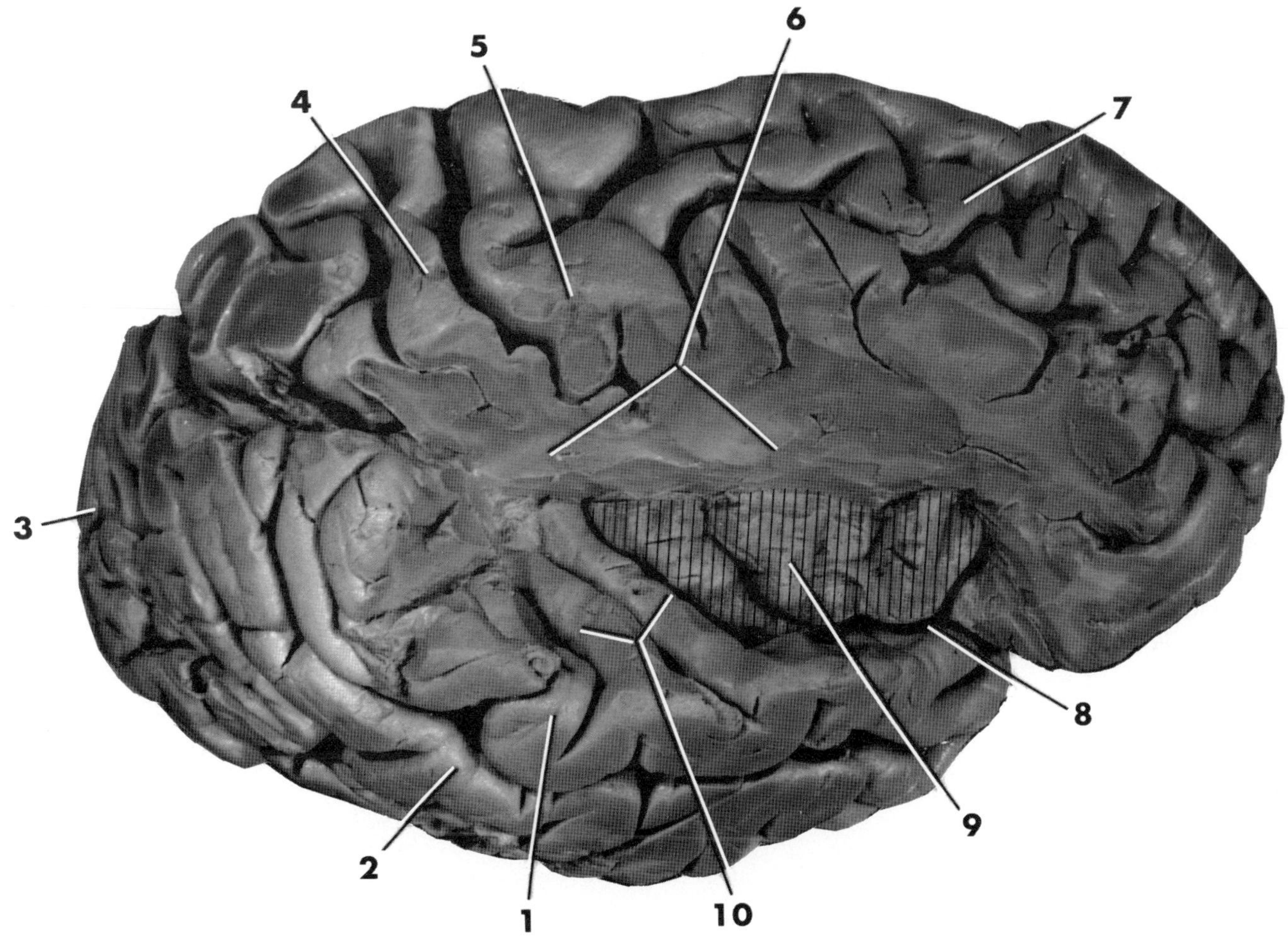

Figure 8 Superior and lateral view of the right cerebral hemisphere to show the transverse temporal gyrus (auditory cortex) and the **insula**. The parietal and frontal opercula overhanging the lateral sulcus have been removed. The superior portion of the insula is still covered by white matter.

1. **Inferior Temporal Sulcus**—intervenes between the fusiform gyrus (see no. **3**, Fig. 9*B*) and the extension of the inferior temporal gyrus (see no. **2**, Fig. 7*A*) on the inferior surface of the temporal lobe. It is often broken in two or more parts.
2. **Hippocampal Sulcus**—a deep sulcus on the medial side of the temporal lobe which rests against the lateral side of the midbrain. It separates the parahippocampal gyrus (see no. **2**, Fig. 9*B*) from the dentate gyrus.
3. **Calcarine Sulcus** (L. *calcar*, spur)—extends from the occipital pole to the splenium of the corpus callosum. It is an important landmark for the visual cortex which lies in the walls of this sulcus.
4. **Parietooccipital Sulcus (Fissure)**—extends from the calcarine sulcus (**3**) to the superior border of the cerebral hemisphere. It intersects the border approximately 4 cm from the occipital lobe and continues a short distance on the dorsolateral surface.
5. **Subparietal Sulcus**—formed by the bifurcation of the cingulate sulcus (**8**) along with the marginal sulcus (**6**). The subparietal sulcus continues into the parietal lobe. It is located superior and rostral to the calcarine sulcus and the parietooccipital sulcus.
6. **Marginal Sulcus (Ramus of Cingulate Sulcus)**—branches from the cingulate sulcus and extends superiorly to separate the paracentral lobule (no. **7**, Fig. 9*B*) from the precuneate gyrus (no. **9**, Fig. 9*B*).
7. **Central Sulcus**—an important landmark on the lateral surface of the hemisphere. This fissure intersects the superior border and continues a short distance in the paracentral lobule (no. **7**, Fig. 9*B*) on the medial surface. The cortex of the paracentral lobule, anterior to the central sulcus, has a motor function and that posterior to it, a general sensory function.
8. **Cingulate Sulcus**—intervenes between the cingulate gyrus (no. **8**, Fig. 9*B*), the extension of the superior frontal gyrus on the medial surface, and the paracentral lobule (no. **7**, Fig. 9*B*). The cingulate sulcus ends by branching into the marginal (**6**) and subparietal (**5**) sulci.
9. **Paracentral Sulcus**—a division of the cingulate sulcus (**8**) which partially separates the paracentral lobule (no. **7**, Fig. 9*B*) posterior to it from the superior frontal gyrus (no. **9**, Fig. 9*B*) anterior to it.
10. **Callosal Sulcus (Sulcus of Corpus Callosum)**—separates the corpus callosum from the cingulate gyrus. It curves around the splenium and continues as the hippocampal sulcus (**2**).
11. **Collateral Sulcus**—separates the parahippocampal and lingual gyri from the fusiform gyrus (see also nos. **2** and **4**, Fig. 9*B*).

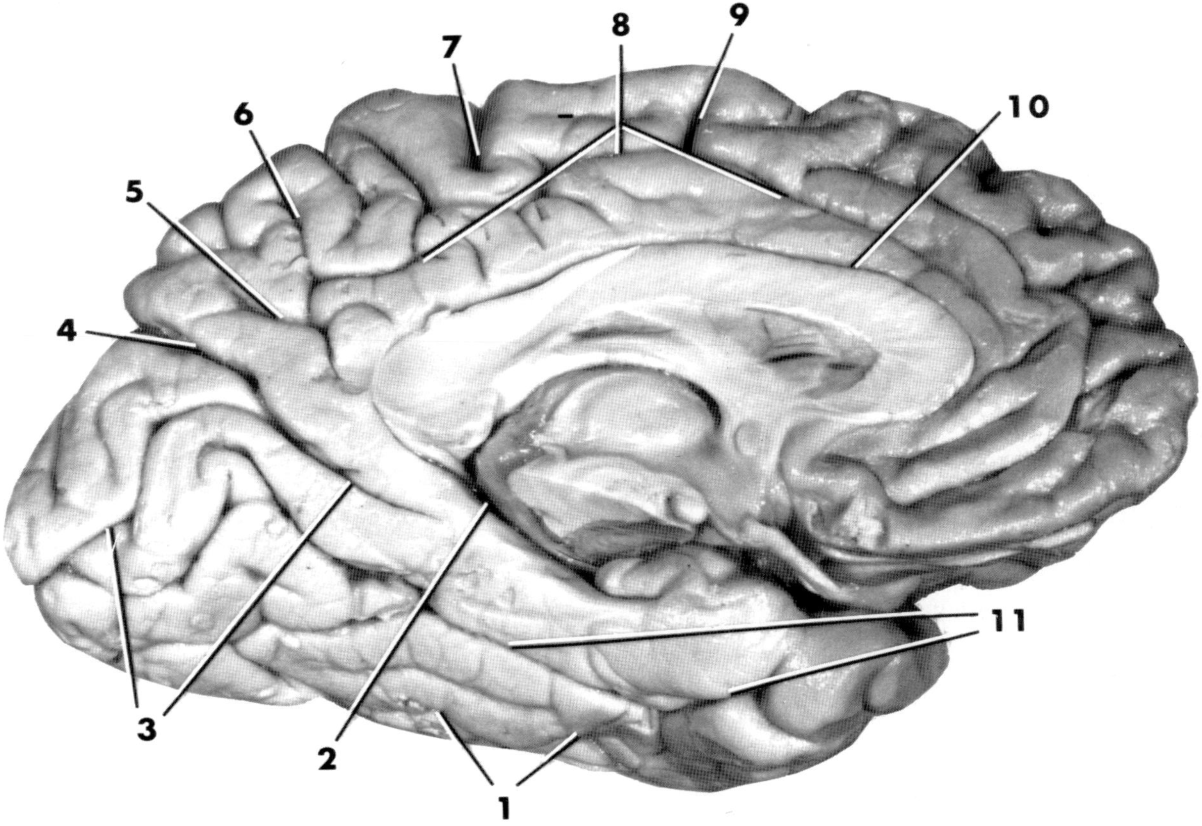

Figure 9A Sulci on the medial and inferior surfaces of the left cerebral hemisphere.

1. **Inferior Temporal Gyrus**—lies lateral to the fusiform gyrus (**3**). It is located on the inferior part of the lateral surface of the cerebral hemisphere and curves onto its inferior and medial surfaces. As it does this, it forms much of the inferior border of the temporal lobe (see no. **2**, Fig. 7*A*).

2. **Parahippocampal Gyrus**—located between the hippocampal sulcus (no. **2**, Fig. 9*A*) and the collateral sulcus (no. **11**, Fig. 9*A*). This long convolution extends from the occipital pole as the lingual gyrus (**4**), almost as far anteriorly as the temporal pole, where it hooks sharply backward as the uncus (**12**), the Latin word for hook.

3. **Fusiform Gyrus**—lies on the inferior and medial surfaces of the temporal lobe beween the parahippocampal gyrus (**2**) and the inferior temporal gyrus (**1**).

4. **Lingual Gyrus** (L. *lingua*, tongue)—the posterior area of the parahippocampal gyrus (**2**). This convolution of cortex is located inferior to the calcarine sulcus (no. **3**, Fig. 9*A*) and forms part of the visual cortex.

5. **Cuneate Gyrus (Cuneus)** (L. *cuneus*, wedge)—a triangle-shaped gyrus located between the calcarine sulcus (no. **3**, Fig. 9*A*) and the parietooccipital sulcus (no. **4**, Fig. 9*A*).

6. **Precuneate Gyrus (Precuneus)**—located posterior to the paracentral lobule (**7**) and superior to the subparietal sulcus (no. **5**, Fig. 9*A*). The parietooccipital sulcus (no. **4**, Fig. 9*A*) separates it from the cuneate gyrus (**5**).

7. **Paracentral Lobule**—the cortical region bordered by the paracentral and marginal sulci (nos. **9** and **6**, Fig. 9*A*). The central sulcus indents the superior border of the hemisphere and extends into this lobule. The cortex in the anterior half of the paracentral lobule has a motor function, and the posterior half has a general sensory function for the lower limb.

8. **Cingulate Gyrus**—begins inferior to the genu of the corpus callosum and parallels the corpus callosum as far as the splenium. It is limited by the cingulate sulcus (no. **8**, Fig. 9*A*) superiorly, and the callosal sulcus (no. **10**, Fig. 9*A*) inferiorly.

9. **Superior Frontal Gyrus**—located mainly on the dorsolateral surface of the frontal lobe (see no. **7**, Fig. 7*A*). It extends onto the medial surface of the cerebral hemisphere and forms the anterior part of its dorsal border.

10. **Subcallosal Gyrus (Area Subcallosa)**—continuous anteriorly with the superior frontal gyrus (**9**) and superiorly with the cingulate gyrus (**8**).

11. **Paraterminal Gyrus**—a small gyrus closely applied to the rostral part of the lamina terminalis. This gyrus and the subcallosal gyrus (**10**) are in close relation to the rostrum of the corpus callosum and these two (**10** and **11**) cortical fields belong to the rhinecephalon (G. nose brain).

12. **Uncus** (L. hook)—the anterior portion of the parahippocampal gyrus (**2**) hooks sharply backward on itself to form the uncus. This structure is located immediately lateral to the cerebral peduncle.

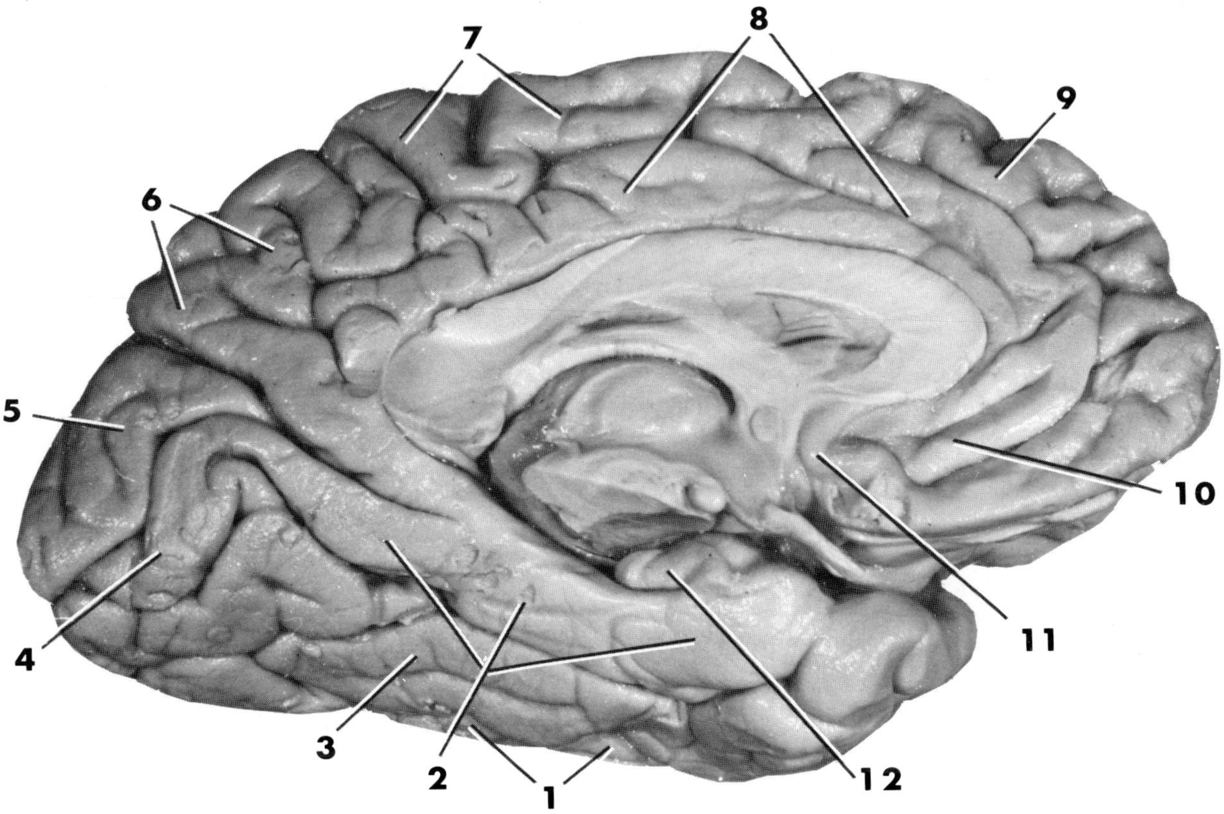

Figure 9*B* The main gyri on the medial and inferior surface of the left cerebral hemisphere.

1. **Auditory Area**—the greater part of the auditory area is located in the **transverse temporal gyrus** (Heschl's convolution) which is concealed in the floor of the lateral sulcus (no. **10**, Fig. 8). A small amount of auditory cortex is located on the free surface of the superior temporal gyrus.
2. **Visual Area**—a very small area of visual cortex (which is almost entirely on the medial surface of the cerebral hemisphere (no. **1**, Fig. 11). It is located on the lateral surface of the occipital lobe in the region of the occipital pole and is bound anteriorly by the lunate sulcus.
3. **Sensory Area (General Somesthetic Area)**—occupies the postcentral gyrus and the posterior wall of the central sulcus on the lateral surface, and the posterior part of the paracentral lobule on the medial surface (no. **2**, Fig. 11). This area of cortex is concerned with the interpretation of general sensory data from the contralateral side of the body. Like the motor cortex, the body is represented as being inverted.
4. **Motor Area**—located mainly in the precentral gyrus and the anterior wall of the central sulcus on the lateral surface of the cerebral hemisphere, and in the anterior part of the paracentral lobule on the medial surface (no. **3**, Fig. 11). The motor cortex of one cerebral hemisphere controls voluntary muscle movement in the muscles of the upper and lower limbs and lower muscles of facial expression on the opposite side of the body. The remainder of the musculature on each side of the body is influenced and controlled by the motor cortex from each hemisphere. Like the general sensory cortex, the body is represented in the motor area as being inverted.
5. **Premotor Area**—situated anterior to the motor area on the dorsolateral and medial surfaces of the cerebral hemisphere. It occupies some of the cortex of the superior, middle, and inferior frontal gyri. In general it functions in conjunction with the motor area in the contraction of the muscles of a functional group for mass or gross muscle movements in the limbs and trunk. Strong stimulation of this area can produce discrete muscle movements in the limbs.
6. **Motor Speech Area (Broca's Area)**—a cortical area occupying the pars opercularis and pars triangularis of the inferior frontal gyrus. It is developed functionally in the left hemisphere of a right-handed individual; the converse is true in a left-handed individual. Damage to this area causes motor aphasia. Most right-handed people have their speech area in the opposite hemisphere.
7. **Taste Area (Gustatory Area)**—this area is not conclusively established but is mainly found in the most ventral portion of the postcentral gyrus (upper wall of lateral sulcus), adjacent to the cortex, receiving general sensory data from the tongue and pharynx.

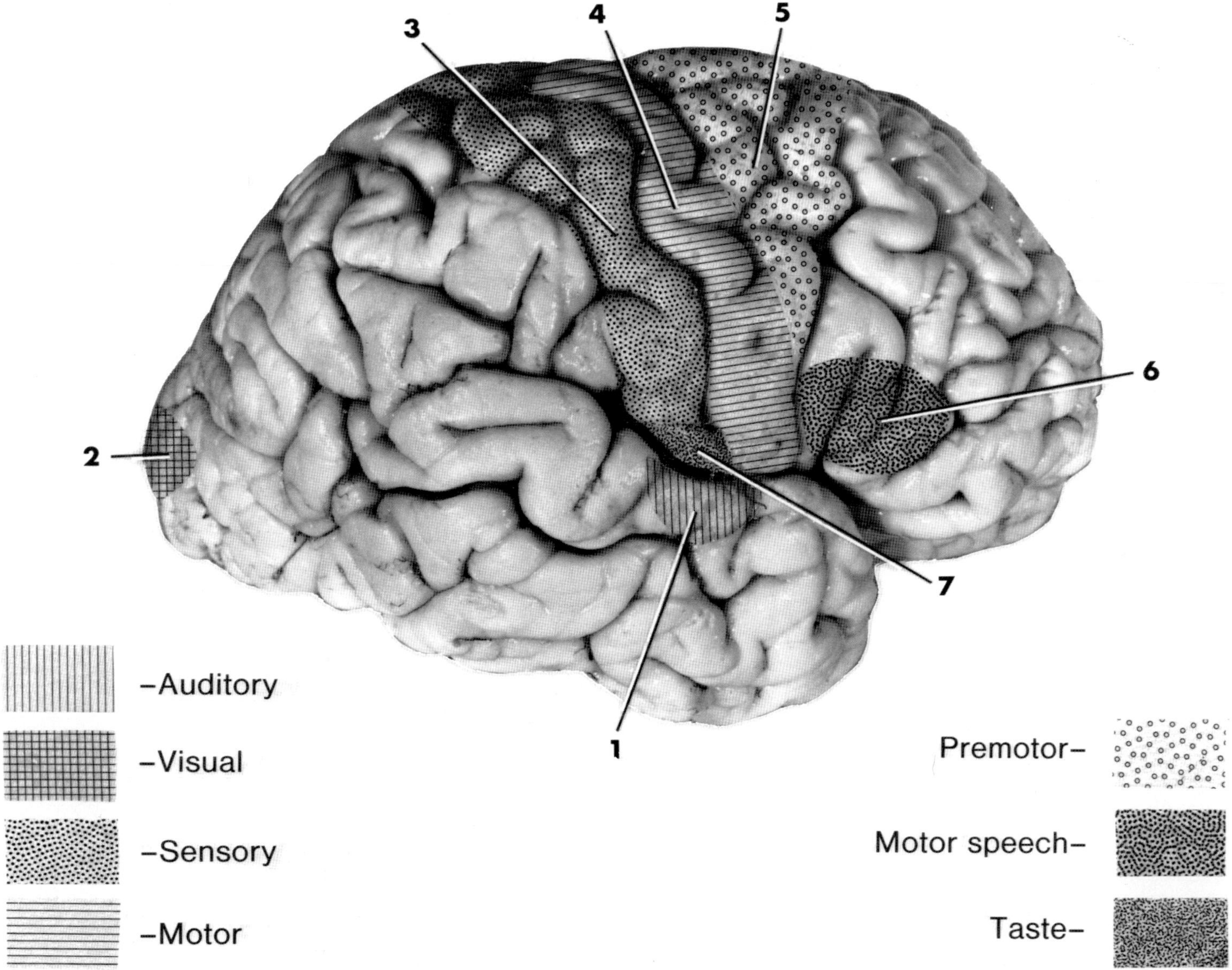

Figure 10 Some **areas of functional localization** on the dorsolateral surface of the right cerebral hemisphere.

1. **Visual Area**—located in the lips (lingual gyrus and cuneus) of the calcarine sulcus. Much of the visual cortex is buried, forming the walls of these deep sulci. A small amount of the visual area may extend onto the lateral srface at the occipital pole (see no. **2**, Fig. 10). The right visual field is appreciated by the visual cortex of the left hemisphere, and the converse is true for the left field of vision. Conscious appreciation of visual stimuli from the peripheral field of vision is located in the anterior (rostral) visual area and in the posterior (caudal) visual area for the central (acute) field of vision.
2. **Sensory Area (General, Somesthetic)**—located in the postcentral gyrus on the lateral surface (no. **3**, Fig. 10) and in the paracentral lobule posterior to the central sulcus on the medial surface of the cerebral hemispheres. The sensory cortex for the contralateral leg and foot is located in this area of the paracentral lobule. The representation of the body for general sensory data is inverted on the postcentral gyrus and posterior area of the paracentral lobule.
3. **Motor Area**—located in the precentral gyrus on the lateral surface and in the paracentral lobule in front of the central sulcus on the medial surface of the cerebral hemispheres. The motor cortex for the contralateral leg and foot is located in this area of the paracentral lobule. Like the somesthetic area, the representation of the body for motor control is inverted on the precentral gyrus and anterior area of the paracentral lobule. Damage to the cortex in the anterior area of the paracentral lobule could cause voluntary motor paralysis in the leg and foot muscles on the opposite side of the body.
4. **Premotor Area**—located in the cortex of the superior frontal gyrus that is located directly anterior to the paracentral lobule on the medial surface of the cerebral hemisphere. On the lateral surface it occupies some of the cortex directy anterior to the precentral gyrus of the superior, middle, and inferior frontal gyri. The premotor cortex functions with the motor cortex for mass muscle movement of groups of functional muscles in the limbs or trunk.
5. **Olfactory Area**—consists of two cortical areas (medial and lateral) on the medial and inferomedial surfaces of the cerebral hemisphere. The medial olfactory area (**a**) is located in the cortex of the frontal lobe, inferior to the rostrum and the genu of the corpus callosum and anterior to the lamina terminalis (cortex of subcallosal and paraterminal gyri (nos. **10** and **11**, Fig. 9*B*). The lateral olfactory area (**b**) is located in the cortex of the uncus (no. **12**, Fig. 9*B*) and adjoining region of the parahippocampal gyrus (no. **12**, Fig. 9*B*). The lateral olfactory area is the principal site for conscious appreciation of olfactory stimuli.

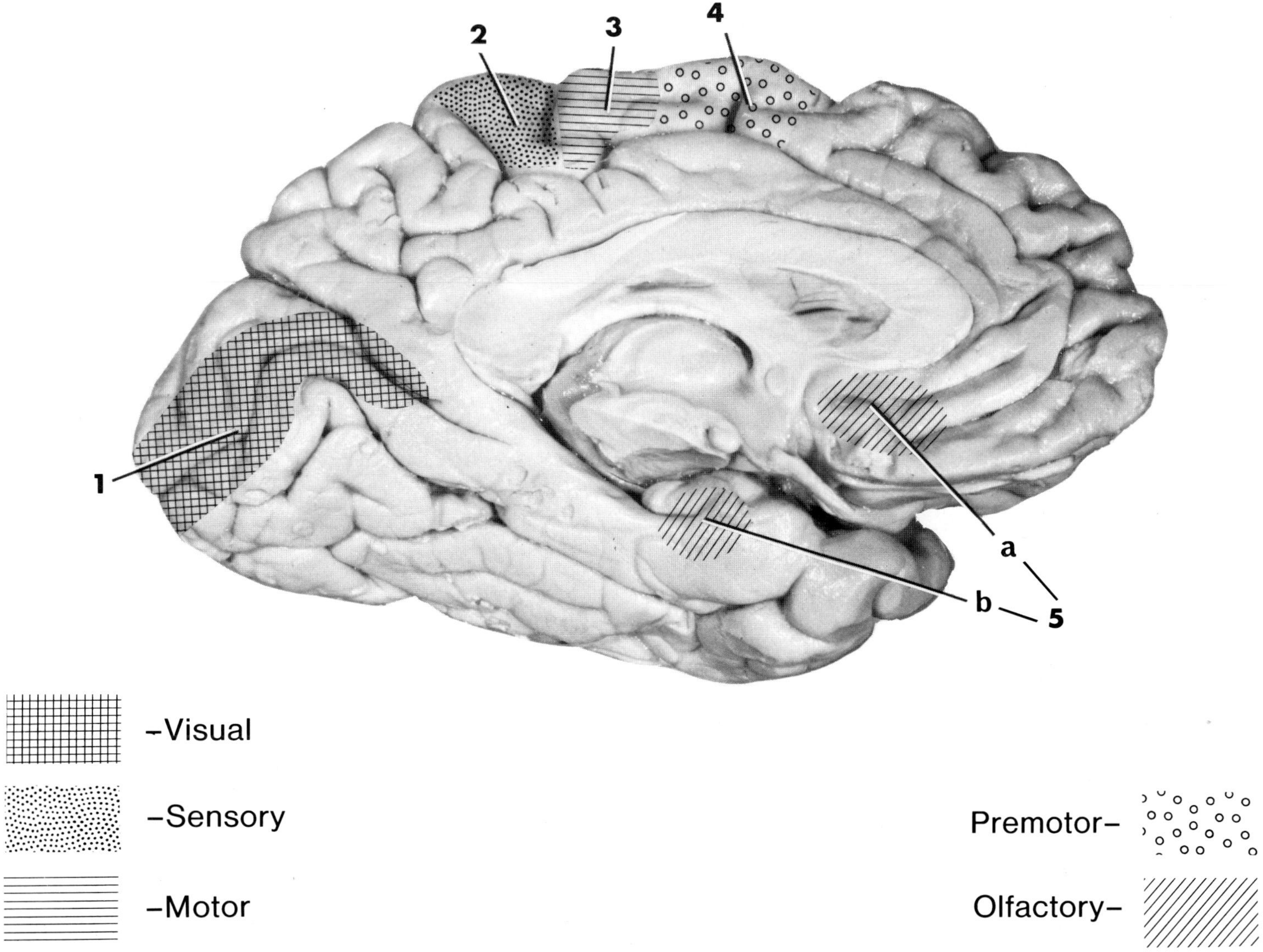

Figure 11 Some **areas of functonal localization** on the inferior and medial surfaces of the left cerebral hemisphere.

3

The Medullary Center and Basal Ganglia

1. **Insula** (L. island)—an area of cerebral cortex buried in the depths of the lateral sulcus and concealed from surface view. The cortex which normally conceals the insula has been removed.
2. **Temporal Pole**—convex anterior end of the temporal lobe. The cortex is partly removed to show its fibers.
3. **Frontal Pole**—convex anterior end of the frontal lobe which occupies the anterior cranial fossa.
4. **Superior Longitudinal Fasciculus (Arcuate Fasciculus)**—composed of long association fibers connecting the cortex of the frontal, parietal, occipital, and temporal lobes.
5. **Corona Radiata**—composed of projection fibers that converge between the lentiform and caudate nuclei and the thalamus to form the internal capsule (no. **5**, Fig. 14 and no. **2**, Fig. 16).
6. **Arcuate Fibers**—short association fibers coursing from gyrus to gyrus. The fibers are shaped like a bow, hence the term arcuate (L. *arcuatus,* bowed). See also no. **4**, Fig. 14.
7. **External Capsule (Posterior Part)**—thin layer of white matter located immediately lateral to the lentiform nucleus (see no. **7**, Fig. 13).
8. **Inferior Occipitofrontal Fasciculus**—composed of long association fibers connecting the cortex of the occipital and frontal lobes. As fibers also run in the opposite direction, this bundle is often called the frontooccipital fasciculus (see no. **8**, Fig. 14).
9. **Occipital Pole**—convex posterior end of the occipital lobe, lying superior to the cerebellum (no. **2**, Fig. 13).

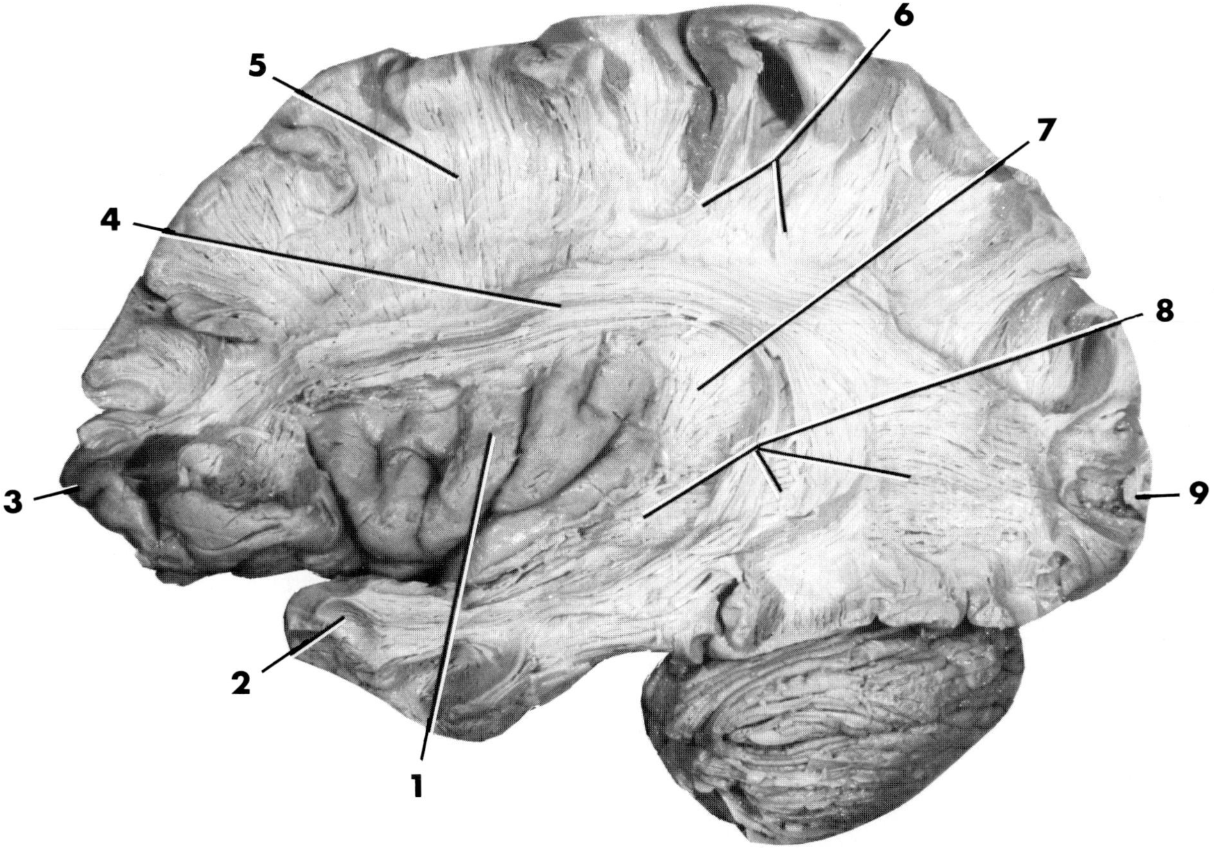

Figure 12 Medullary center of the left cerebral hemisphere showing some of its association fibers.

1. **Medulla**—caudal part of the brain stem. Also known as the medulla oblongata. (For a better view of the medulla, see no. **1**, Fig. 21).
2. **Cerebellum**—right hemisphere.
3. **Optic Radiation (Geniculocalcarine Tract)**—projection fibers coursing from the lateral geniculate body to the visual cortex and surrounding the calcarine fissure.
4. **Arcuate Fibers**—short association fibers connecting the cortex of nearby gyri.
5. **Superior Longitudinal Fasciculus (Arcuate Fasciculus)**—long association fibers interconnecting the cortex on the lateral surfaces of the frontal, parietal, occipital, and temporal lobes (see also no. **4**, Fig. 12 and no. **4**, Fig. 14).
6. **Corona Radiata**—projecting fibers coursing inferiorly from the cerebral cortex to form the internal capsule.
7. **External Capsule**—thin layer of white matter composed of projecting, commissural, and association fibers. It is located lateral to the lentiform nucleus.
8. **Inferior Occipitofrontal Fasciculus**—composed of long association fibers connecting the cortex of the lateral surface of the occipital lobe with the cortex of the inferior and lateral surfaces of the frontal lobe (see no. **7**, Fig. 16 and no. **10**, Fig. 18).
9. **Uncinate Fasciculus** (L. *uncus,* a hook)—hook-like bundle composed of long association fibers connecting the cortex of the frontal lobe with the temporal lobe (see no. **7**, Fig. 15).
10. **Basal Pons**—basal portion of the pons, part of the brain stem. The pons (L. bridge) was named because its basal or ventral surface looks like a bridge connecting the right and left cerebellar hemispheres (no. **1**, Fig. 2).

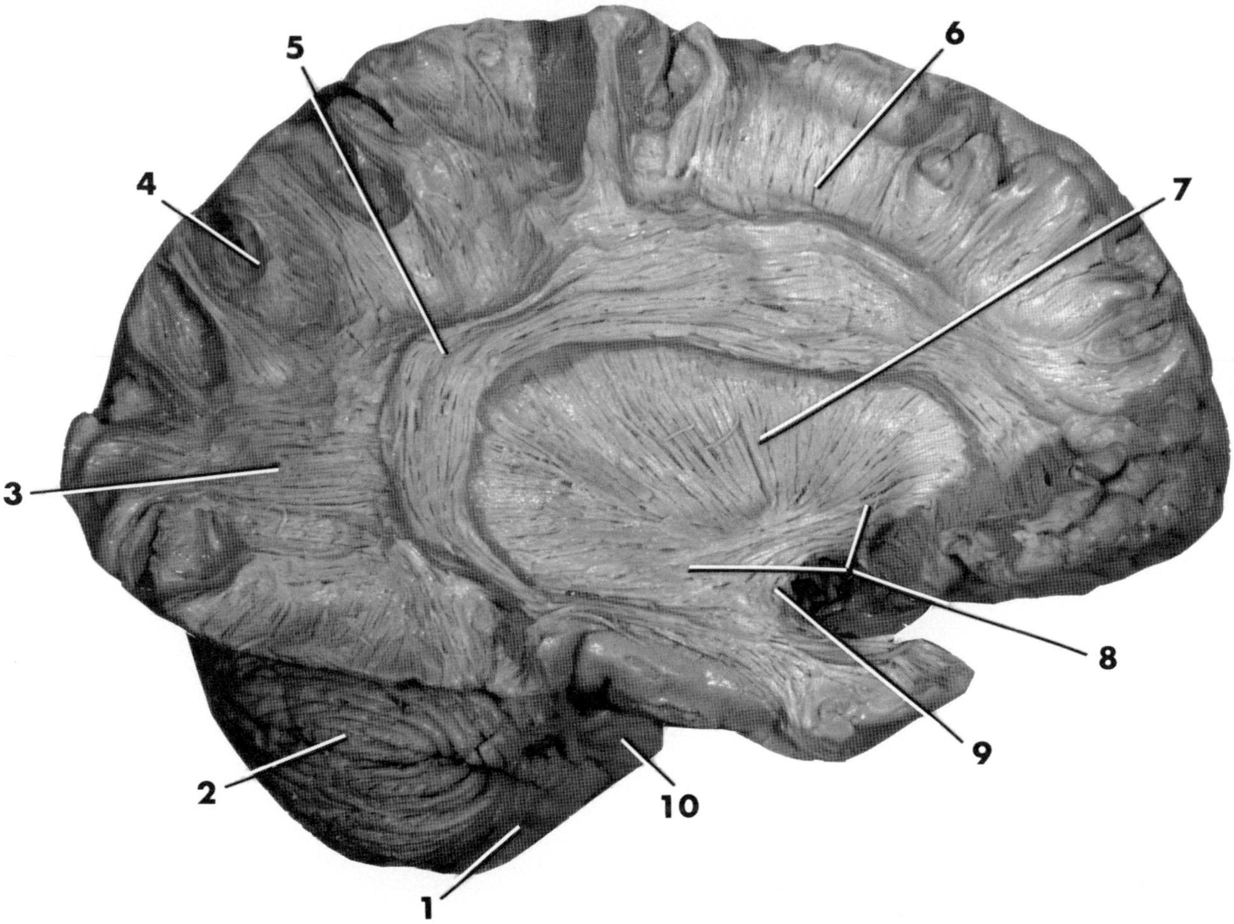

Figure 13 Medullary center of the right cerebral hemisphere after removal of the insula. Observe the long association fibers, the external capsule, and the optic radiations.

1. **Uncinate Fasciculus**—long association fibers connecting the cortex of the inferolateral frontal lobe with the temporal lobe cortex.
2. **Lentiform Nucleus (left)** (also called lenticular nucleus)—a cerebral basal ganglion located between the external and internal capsules. It consists of the putamen (outer portion) and the globus pallidus. Note the posterior portion of this nucleus has been removed to show the internal capsule (**6**).
3. **Arcuate Fibers**—short association fibers connecting the cortex of nearby gyri (see no. **3**, Fig. 16).
4. **Superior Longitudinal Fasciculus (Arcuate Fasciculus)**—long reciprocal association fibers connecting the cortex on the lateral surfaces of the frontal, parietal, occipital, and temporal lobes.
5. **Corona Radiata**—composed of projection fibers above the basal ganglia (caudate and lentiform nuclei) and the thalamus. These converging fibers become the internal capsule (see no. **2**, Fig. 16).
6. **Internal Capsule (Posterior Limb)**—exposed projection fibers from the corona radiata (**5**) which course medial to the lentiform nucleus (**2**), the posterior part of which has been removed to show the internal capsule. The posterior limb of the internal capsule is located between the lentiform nucleus and the thalamus (see also no. **6,** Fig. 19 and no. **8,** Fig. 20).
7. **Posterior Horn of Lateral Ventricle**—exposed in the occipital lobe to show the two prominent elevations in its medial wall and floor: (**a**) **bulb of posterior horn** which consists of fibers of the forceps major, and (**b**) **calcar avis** formed by the calcarine fissure.
8. **Inferior Occipitofrontal Fasciculus**—composed of long reciprocal association fibers connecting the cortex of the inferior area of the frontal lobe with the temporal and occipital lobes.

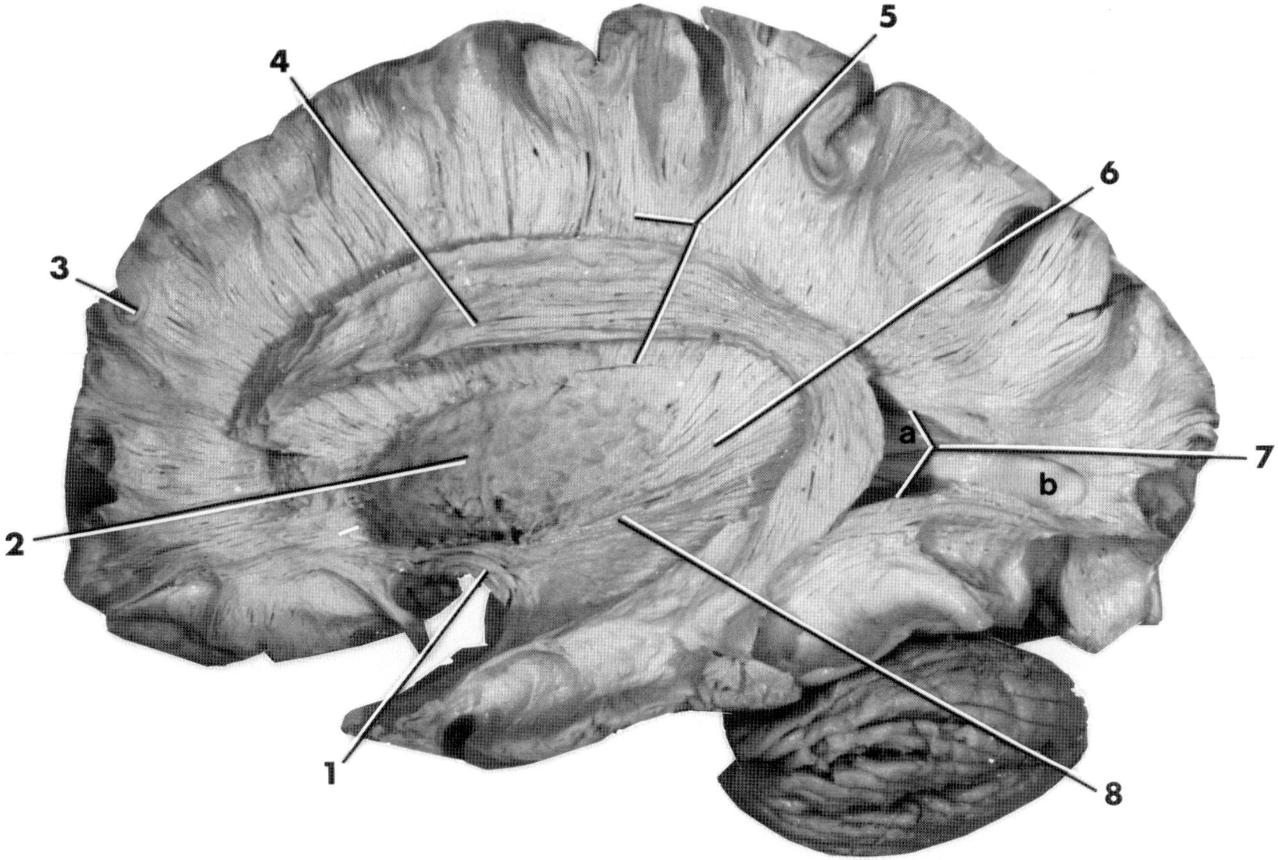

Figure 14 Medullary center of the left cerebral hemisphere. Most of the external capsule has been removed to show the lentiform nucleus. Some of the medullary center has also been removed to show the posterior horn of the lateral ventricle.

1. **External Capsule (Posterior Part)**—thin layer of white matter consisting of projection, commissural, and association fibers that cover the lateral surface of the lentiform nucleus.
2. **Optic Radiation (Geniculocalcarine Tract)**—consists of projection fibers that extend from the lateral geniculate nucleus to the visual cortex of the occipital lobe (see also no. **1**, Fig. 16 and no. **4**, Fig. 20).
3. **Lateral Part of Superior Longitudinal Fasciculus (Arcuate Fasciculus)**—consists of long reciprocal association fibers coursing in the medullary center above the insula, and connecting the cortex of the frontal, parietal, occipital, and temporal lobes (see also no. **4**, Fig. 12 and no. **5**, Fig. 13).
4. **Internal Capsule**—(exposed by removal of some of the lentiform nucleus (**6**)), consists of bundles of projection fibers (cortical afferents and efferents) which separate the caudate nucleus and the thalamus from the lentiform nucleus (**6**, see also no. **3**, Fig. 17, no. **5**, Fig. 18, and no. **8**, Fig. 20).
5. **Corona Radiata**—consists of projection fibers (cortical afferents and efferents) from the cerebral cortex coursing inferiorly in the medullary center to become the internal capsule (**4**).
6. **Lentiform Nucleus (Lateral Surface)**—a cerebral basal ganglion consisting of the putamen (outer part) and the globus pallidus (inner part). It is located beteen the external and internal capsules.
7. **Uncinate Fasciculus**—composed of association fibers connecting the association cortex of the frontal and temporal lobes (see also no. **1**, Fig. 14 and no. **9**, Fig. 18).

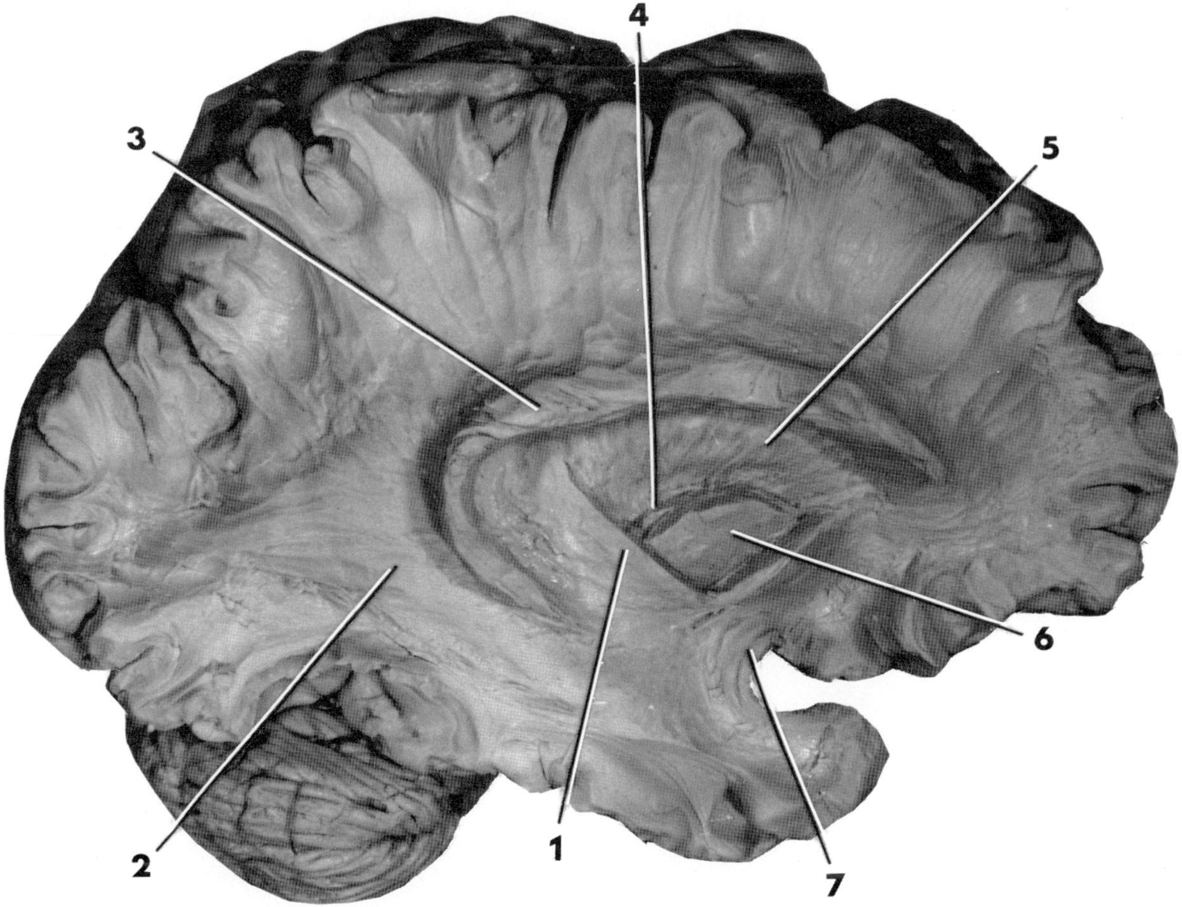

Figure 15 Medullary center of the right cerebral hemisphere showing some long association and projection fibers. Note that the caudal area of the lentiform nucleus has been removed to show the internal capsule, which consists of cortical afferent and efferent projection fibers.

1. **Optic Radiation (Geniculocalcarine Tract)**—consists of projection fibers that form part of the visual pathway connecting the lateral geniculate body with the visual cortex located in the lips of the calcarine sulcus (see also no. **6**, Fig. 17 and no. **4**, Fig. 20).
2. **Corona Radiata**—composed of projecting fibers (cortical afferents and efferents) that converge from the cerebral cortex and pass medial to the lenticular nucleus as the internal capsule (see also no. **5**, Fig. 17).
3. **Arcuate Fibers**—short association fibers that connect the cerebral cortex in nearby gyri and sulci.
4. **Cingulate Gyrus**—of opposite cerebral hemisphere. It begins inferior to the genu of the corpus callosum and extends superior to the corpus callosum as far as the splenium.
5. **Genu of Corpus Callosum** (L. *genu*, knee)—the corpus callosum, composed of commissural fibers, was removed on the left side at the level of the genu to expose the anterior horn of the lateral ventricle and the head of the caudate nucleus.
6. **Corpus Striatum**—a mass of gray matter containing important basal ganglia (nuclei). It is located in the medullary center near the base of each cerebral hemisphere. It is composed of the following: (**a**) **Head of the caudate nucleus** (L. *cauda*, a tail)—so named because it has a long tail. The head of the caudate nucleus bulges into the floor and lateral wall of the anterior horn of the lateral ventricle—many of the fibers of the anterior limb of the internal capsule (**b**) have been removed to show the connection of the head of the caudate nucleus with the lenticular nucleus; (**c**) **Putamen** (part of lenticular nucleus)—lies immediately lateral to the internal capsule. Inferior to the anterior limb of the internal capsule, the gray matter of the caudate nucleus is continuous with the gray matter of the lentiform nucleus to form the corpus striatum (L. *corpus*, body + *striatus*, furrowed or striped) (see no. **7**, Fig. 16*A*).
7. **Inferior Occipitofrontal Fasciculus**—composed of long association fibers connecting the cortex of the inferior area of the frontal lobe with the occipital lobe.

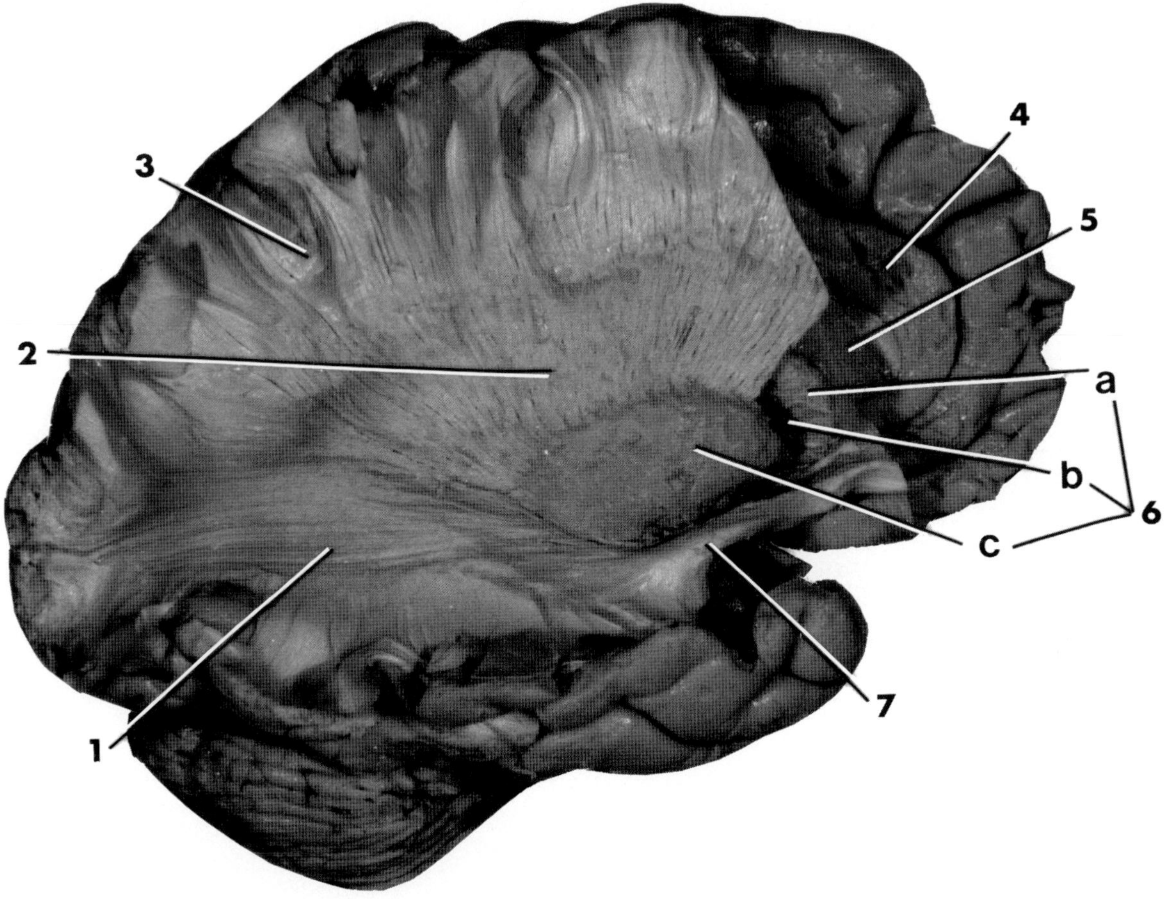

Figure 16*A* The **corpus striatum** (lentiform nucleus plus the head of the caudate nucleus), the optic radiation, and the long projection fibers coursing behind the lentiform nucleus of the right cerebral hemisphere are demonstrated. The corpus striatum was exposed by removing much of the cortex and medullary center of the frontal lobe, as well as the anterior limb of the internal capsule (projection fibers) that partially separates the lentiform nucleus and the head of the caudate nucleus.

1. **Decussation of Pyramids** (L. *decussare*, to cross in the form of an X)—site of crossing of the bundles of the corticospinal (pyramidal) tracts in the lower region of the medulla.
2. **Olive**—oval swelling of the lateral area of the medulla produced by the inferior olivary nucleus.
3. **Basal Pons**—lies between the medulla and the midbrain. Looks like a bridge (L. *pons*) extending between the right and left halves of the cerebellum.
4. **Oculomotor Nerve (C.N. III)**—oculomotor nerve, emerges from the midbrain as a series of roots between the cerebral peduncles.
5. **Amygdaloid Nucleus**—exposed by removing much of the temporal lobe. Its name means "like an almond" (L. from G. *amygdalē*).
6. **Tuber Cinereum**—a midline prominence of the base of the hypothalamus bounded by the mammillary bodies, the optic chiasma, and the beginning of the optic tracts. The name of the structure is derived from Latin and means "ashen or gray protuberance."
7. **Corpus Striatum**—an important mass of gray matter composed of basal ganglia (nuclei) of the extrapyramidal motor system. It is located on each side near the base of the cerebral hemisphere and the thalamus. It consists of (**b**) **the head of the caudate nucleus** and (**c**) **the lentiform nucleus**. The gray matter of the two nuclei is continuous inferior to the **anterior limb of the internal capsule** (**a**) which separates the dorsal portion of the head of the caudate nucleus and the putamen of the lentiform nucleus. In lower mammalian forms the gray matter intervenes between bundles of internal capsule fibers, giving the corpus striatum a striped or striated appearance—hence the name corpus striatum (see also no. **6**, Fig. 16**A**.)
8. **Basis Pedunculi (Basal Portion of Cerebral Peduncle)**—composed of projection fibers from the internal capsule.
9. **Mammillary Body**—one of a pair of small white breast-like swellings on the ventral surface of the hypothalamus.
10. **Middle Cerebellar Peduncle (Brachium Pontis)**—its fibers originate from right pontine neurons and terminate in the cortex of the right cerebellar hemisphere.
11. **Pyramid**—composed of corticospinal tract fibers, approximately 85% of which cross at the decussation of pyramids (**1**). About 15% of these fibers continue into the spinal cord on the same side.

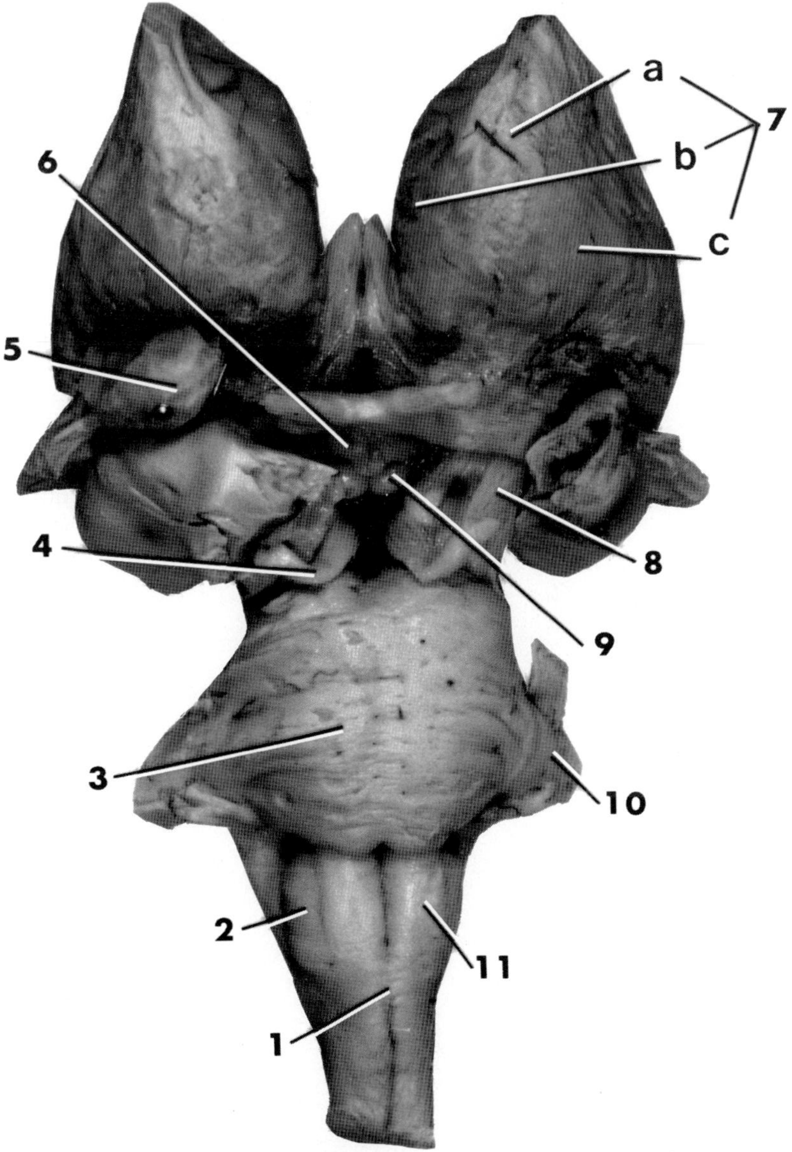

Figure 16*B* Ventral view of the brain stem, the diencephalon, and the **corpus striatum**. Most of the cerebral hemispheres were dissected away to show the corpus striatum (head of the caudate nucleus and the lentiform nucleus) and its relationship to the internal capsule.

1. **Anterior Commissure**—communicating fibers between the cortex of the left and right temporal lobes. It courses through the lentiform nucleus on each side. The term "commissure" is derived from the Latin word *commissura* meaning a joining together.
2. **Uncinate Fasciculus** (L. *uncus*, a hook)—long association fibers connecting the cortex of the inferolateral frontal lobe with the temporal lobe cortex.
3. **Internal Capsule**—projection fibers of the corona radiata coursing between the lentiform nucleus (partially removed) and the caudate nucleus and the thalamus located deep to the capsule. Examples of tracts comprising the internal capsule are the corticospinal, corticopontine, corticobulbar, and thalamocortical (see also no. **6**, Fig. 19 and nos. **8** and **9**, fig. 20).
4. **Arcuate Fibers**—short association fibers connecting the cortex of nearby gyri.
5. **Corona Radiata**—projecting fibers from the cerebral cortex coursing deep in the medullary center to become the internal capsule.
6. **Optic Radiation (Geniculocalcarine tract).** See also no. **4**, Fig. 20.
7. **Lentiform Nucleus (Small Remaining Portion)**—most of it has been removed to show the internal capsule (see also no. **2**, Fig. 14, no. **6**, Fig. 15, and no. **7**, Fig. 18).
8. **Inferior Longitudinal Fasciculus**—long association fibers connecting the inferior part of the temporal lobe with the occipital lobe.

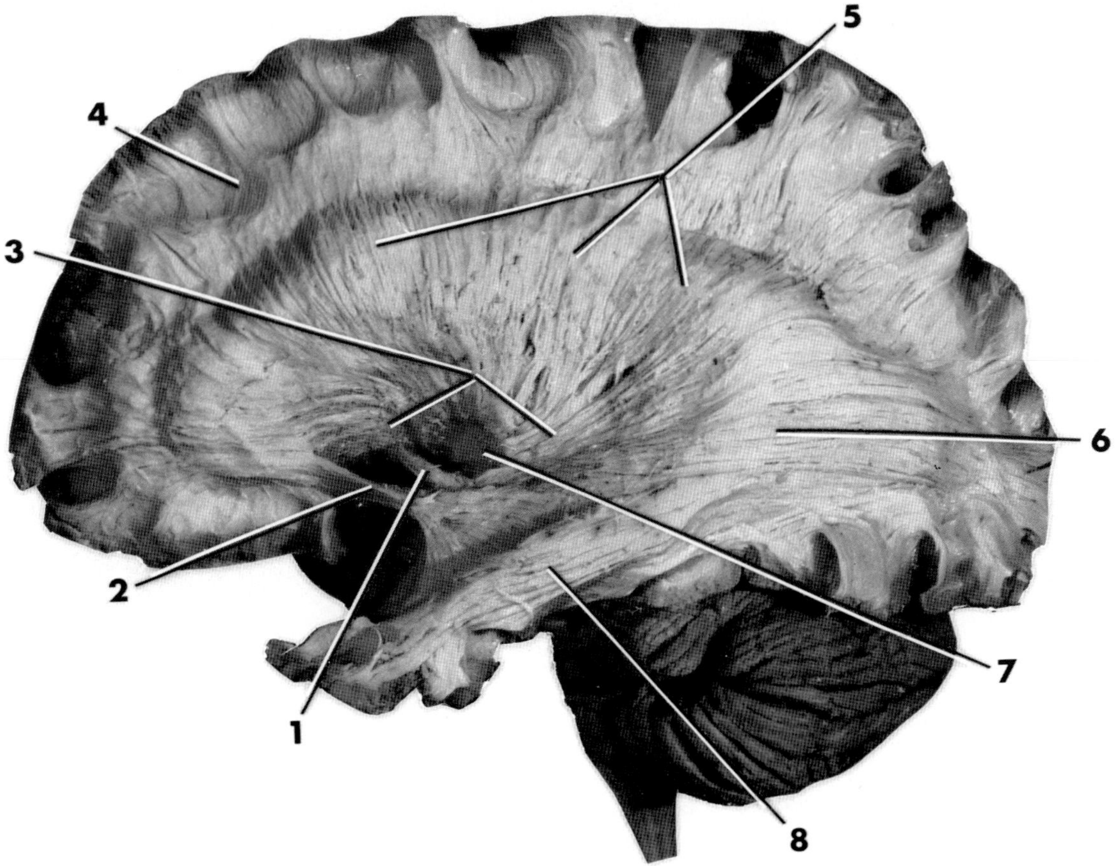

Figure 17 Mainly shows **projection fibers converging from the corona radiata** to form the internal capsule in the depths of the medullary center of the left cerebral hemisphere. This was accomplished by removing most of the long association fiber fasciculi and most of the lentiform nucleus. Note also the optic radiation fibers sweeping posterior to the occipital pole.

1. **Site of Choroid Plexus**—in the exposed body of the lateral ventricle. This structure secretes cerebrospinal fluid into the lateral ventricle.
2. **Lateral Ventricle**—exposed at the area where the body of the lateral ventricle curves downward and forward to form the inferior horn. **Note**: The entire black area is the exposed lateral ventricle.
3. **Optic Radiation (Geniculocalcarine Tract)**—part of the visual pathway. Fibers from the lateral geniculate body synapse with neurons in the visual cortex, which is located in the walls of the calcarine sulcus.
4. **Superior Longitudinal Fasciculus (Arcuate Fasciculus)**—long association fibers connecting the association cortex on the lateral surface of the frontal, parietal, occipital, and temporal lobes.
5. **Internal Capsule**—exposed projection fibers from the corona radiata (**6**) coursing medial to the lentiform nucleus (**7**) to form the internal capsule. The anterior limb of the internal capsule is located between the lentiform nucleus and the caudate nucleus, and its posterior limb is located between the lentiform nucleus and the thalamus (see also no. **3**, Fig. 17).
6. **Corona Radiata**—composed of converging projection fibers above the basal ganglia (represented here by the lentiform and caudate nuclei) and the thalamus. These fibers become the internal capsule.
7. **Lentiform Nucleus (Anterior Half)**—the posterior half of this nucleus has been removed to show the fibers of the internal capsule (**5**) which lie immediately medial to it (see also no. **2**, Fig. 14, no. **6c**, Fig. 16, and no. **7**, Fig. 17).
8. **External Capsule**—composed of projection, association, and commissural fibers. This thin layer of white matter covers the lateral surface of the lentiform nucleus.
9. **Uncinate Fasciculus**—composed of association fibers connecting the association cortex of the frontal and temporal lobes. It is called the uncinate fasciculus because it hooks (L. *uncus*, a hook) around the lateral sulcus.
10. **Inferior Occipitofrontal Fasciculus**—long association fibers connecting the cerebral cortex of the frontal, temporal, and occipital lobes (see also no. **1**, Fig. 14 and no. **7**, Fig. 15).

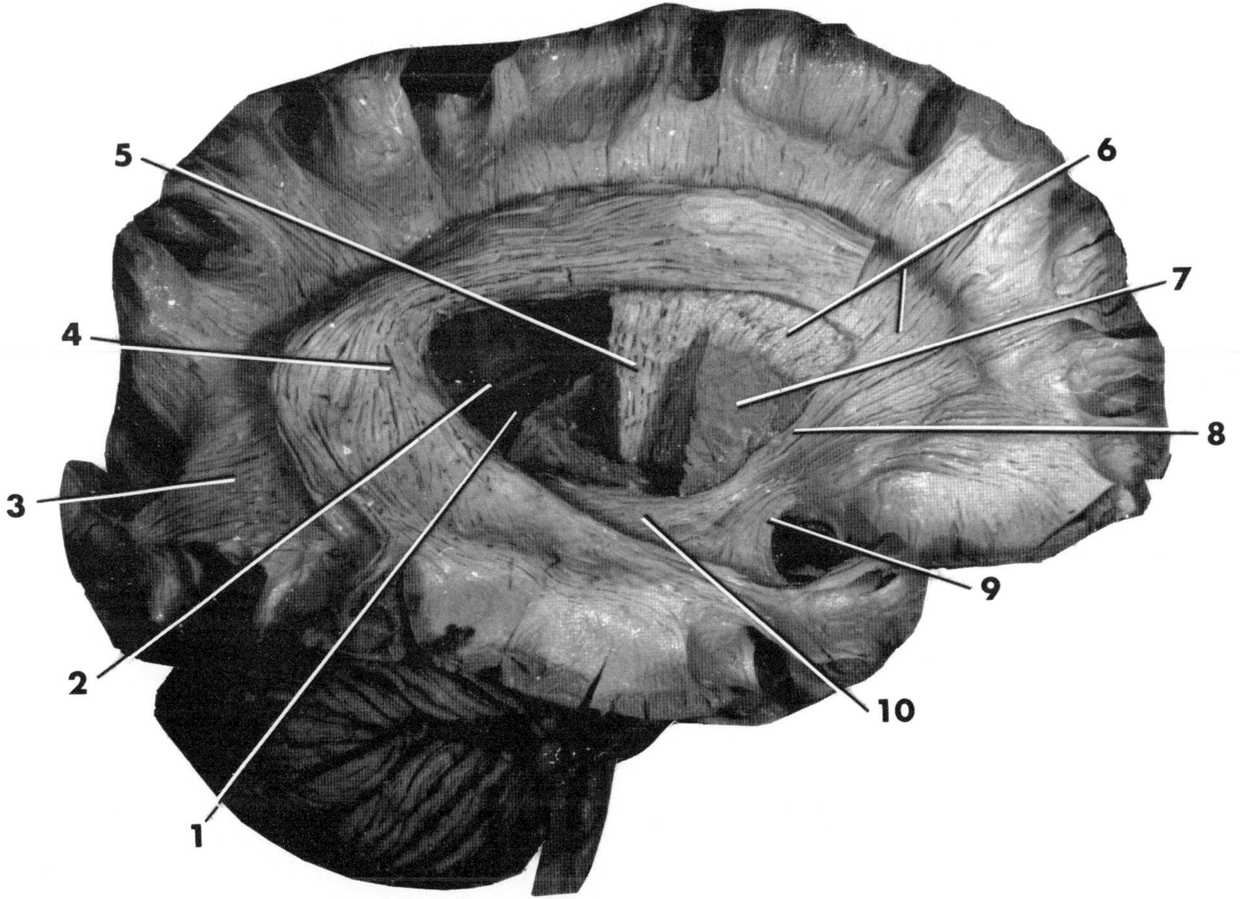

Figure 18 This dissection shows many intact association fiber fasciculi, the optic radiation, and the relationship of the lentiform nucleus to the internal capsule and to portions of the lateral ventricle. This exposure was accomplished by removing much of the external capsule, the caudal area of the lentiform nucleus, as well as the posterior part of the internal capsule which forms part of the lateral wall of the lateral ventricle.

1. **Inferior Occipitofrontal Fasciculus**—long association fibers connecting the cortex on the lateral surface of the inferior frontal lobe with the cortex of the lateral surface of the occipital lobe. Note: the posterior part of this fasciculus has been removed to show the deeper structures (see also no. **8**, Fig. 13; no. **8**, Fig. 14; and no. **10**, Fig. 18).
2. **Internal Capsule (Area of Anterior Limb)**—projecting fibers of the corona radiata course between the lentiform nucleus (removed) and the head of the caudate nucleus (anterior limb of the internal capsule is located medial to this structure).
3. **Arcuate Fibers**—short association fibers connecting the cortex of nearby gyri.
4. **Corona Radiata**—projecting fibers from the cerebral cortex coursing inferiorly between the basal ganglia (lentiform nucleus laterally and the head of the caudate nucleus and the thalamus medially) to become the internal capsule (**2** and **6**).
5. **Superior Longitudinal Fasciculus (Arcuate Fasciculus)**—long association fibers connecting the cortex of the lateral surface of the frontal, parietal, occipital, and temporal lobes.
6. **Internal Capsule (Area of Posterior Limb)**—projecting fibers of the corona radiata course between the lentiform nucleus (removed) and the thalamus. Examples of projecting fibers located here are the corticospinal, corticobulbar, and thalamocortical tracts.
7. **Optic Radiation (Geniculocalcarine Tract)**—part of the visual system connecting the lateral geniculate body with the visual cortex located around the calcarine fissure (see also no. **1**, Fig. 16; no. **3**, Fig. 18; and no. **4**, Fig. 20).

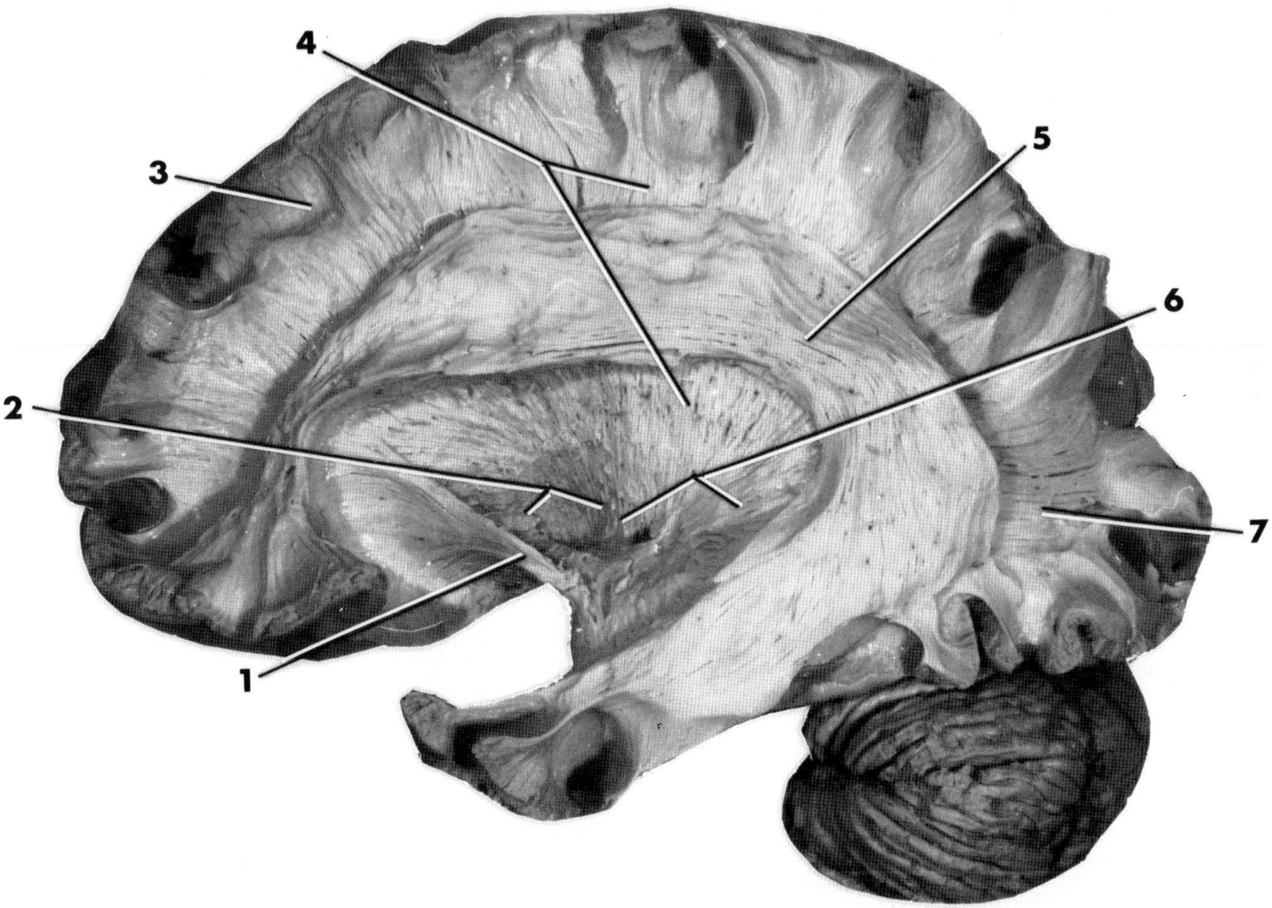

Figure 19 The external capsule and the lentiform nucleus have been removed to expose the **projection fibers in the internal capsule** of the left cerebral hemisphere.

1. **Middle Cerebellar Peduncle (Branchium Pontis)**—the origin of these fibers (contralateral basal pons) has been removed to show the projection fibers (**12**).
2. **Superior Colliculus**—dome-like eminence or mound (L. *colliculus*) on the rostral half of the dorsal surface of the midbrain.
3. **Lateral Geniculate Body**—many optic tract fibers terminate in the nucleus which forms this body.
4. **Optic Radiation (Geniculocalcarine Tract)**—part of the visual pathway (see also no. **6**, Fig. 7).
5. **Superior Longitudinal Fasciculus (Arcuate Fasciculus)**—long association fibers. A section of this fasciculus has been removed to show the fibers of the corona radiata (**7**) (see also no. **4**, Fig. 18).
6. **Arcuate Fibers**—short association fibers.
7. **Corona Radiata**—composed of projection fibers coursing inferiorly to become the internal capsule (**8**).
8. **Internal Capsule (Projection Fibers)**—area of the posterior limb (composed of corticospinal, corticobulbar, corticopontine, thalamocortical fibers, etc.) located between the lentiform nucleus (removed) and the thalamus.
9. **Internal Capsule**—area of the anterior limb (composed of corticopontine, thalamocortical fibers, etc.) located between the lentiform (removed) and caudate nuclei (see also no. **6**, Fig. 21).
10. **Optic Tract**—optic nerve fibers terminating in the lateral geniculate body (**3**) at the end of this tract (Fig. 21).
11. **Basis Pedunculi (Crus Cerebri)**—basal part of the cerebral peduncle in the midbrain containing projection fibers. Continuation of fibers from the internal capsule (**8**) (see also no. **8**, Fig. 21).
12. **Projection Fibers (Corticospinal)**—continued from the internal capsule (**8** and **9**) and the basis pedunculi (**11**) to course through the basal pons.

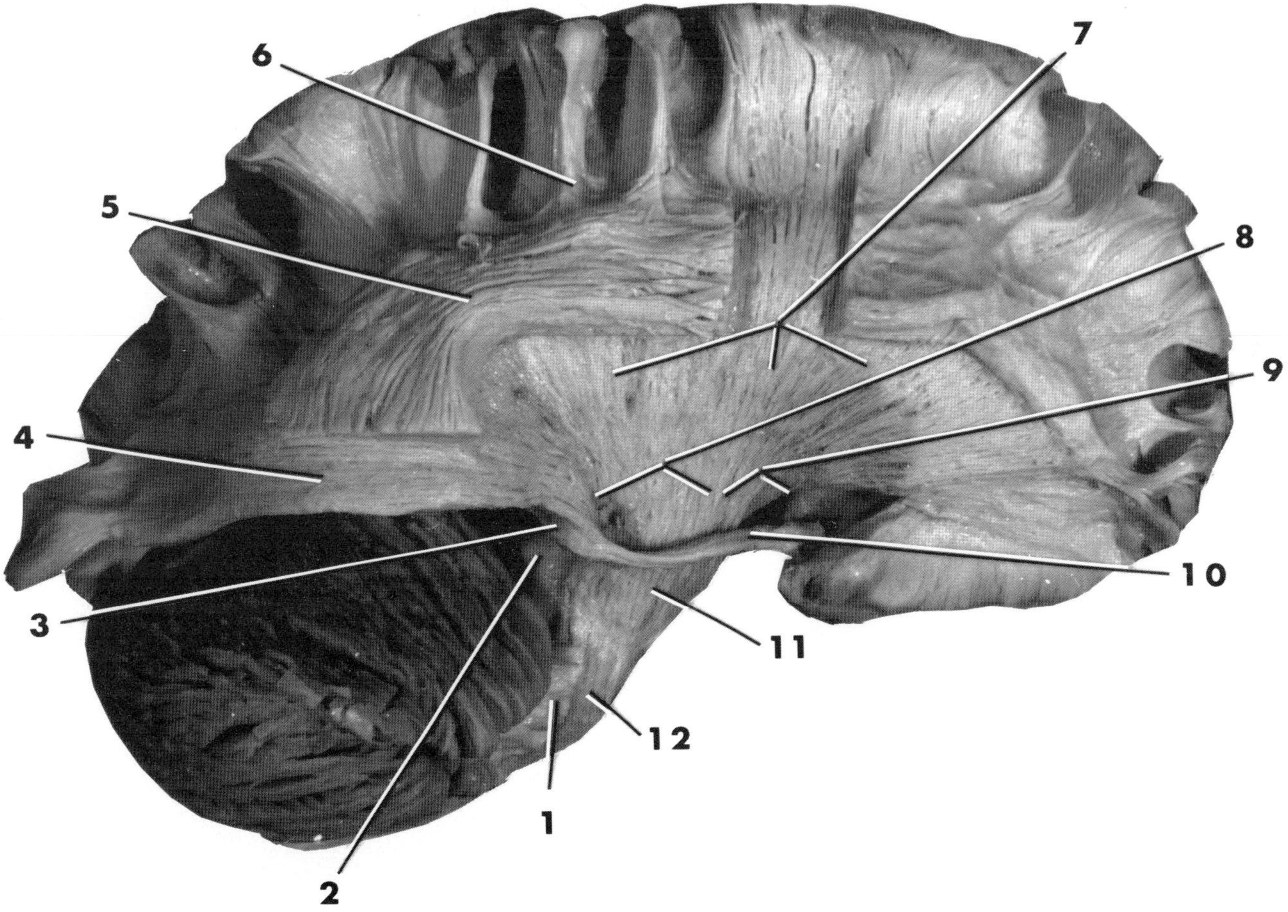

Figure 20 Many structures in the right cerebral hemisphere have been removed to show the projection fibers forming the corona radiata, the internal capsule, and the basis pedunculi.

1. **Medulla (Medulla Oblongata)**—in common usage the medulla oblongata (the caudal portion of the brain stem) is referred to as the medulla.
2. **Lateral Geniculate Body**—many fibers of the optic tract (**7**) synapse on neurons of this geniculate body.
3. **Optic Radiation (Geniculocalcarine Tract)**—composed of axons of the lateral geniculate neurons that project to the visual cortex located in the lips of the calcarine sulcus (see also no. **4**, Fig. 20).
4. **Arcuate Fibers**—short association fibers which make synaptic connections with cortical neurons in nearby gyri.
5. **Corona Radiata**—composed of converging projection fibers in the medullary center above the lentiform and caudate nuclei (two of the basal ganglia) and the thalamus. These fibers continue as the internal capsule (see also no. **7**, Fig. 20).
6. **Internal Capsule**—the lentiform nucleus has been removed to show that the projection fibers of the corona radiata are continuous with those of the internal capsule. The caudate nucleus and thalamus lie immediately medial to this capsule (see also no. **3**, Fig. 17).
7. **Optic Tract**—optic nerve fibers running between the optic chiasma and the lateral geniculate body. The optic tract fibers curve around the cerebral peduncle to synapse on neurons in the lateral geniculate body (**2**).
8. **Basis Pedunculi**—fibers of the internal capsule continue into the cerebral peduncle of the midbrain in a basal area identified as the basis pedunculi. Also called crus cerebri (L. leg of cerebrum) because the cerebral hemispheres rest on these rope-like fiber bundles (see also no. **11**, Fig. 20).
9. **Corticospinal Tract Fibers**—from the internal capsule and the basis pedunculi continuing into and through the basal pons on their way to the medulla and the spinal cord.
10. **Flocculus**—of flocculonodular lobe of cerebellum. (For a better view of this mass, see no. **3**, Fig. 53.)

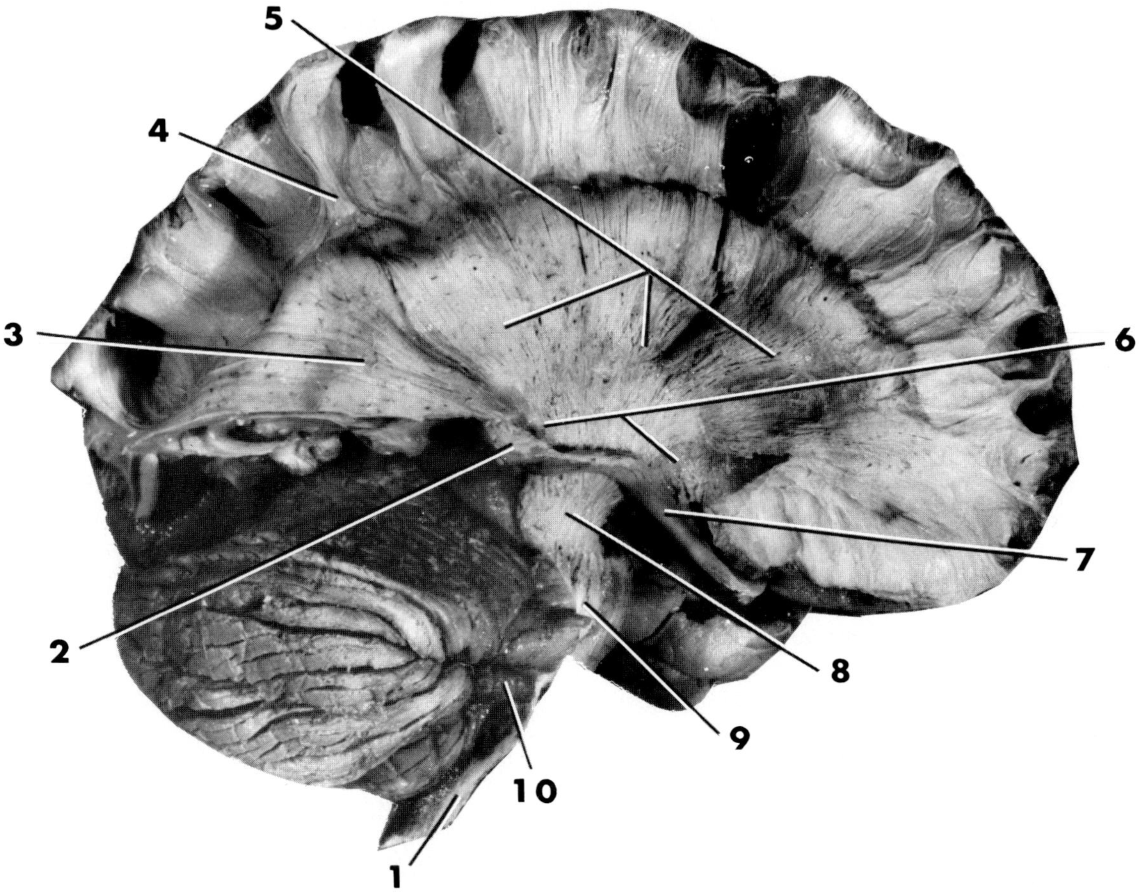

Figure 21 Dissection showing descending cortical projection fibers **(corona radiata)** converging to form the **internal capsule**, and then the basis pedunculi **(cerebral peduncle)** of the right cerebral hemisphere and midbrain. This exposure was accomplished by removing most of the cortex, medullary center, and lentiform nucleus.

1. **Mammillothalamic Tract**—part of the limbic system connecting the anterior thalamic tubercle (nucleus) with the mammillary body of the hypothalamus.
2. **Body of Fornix**—part of the limbic system connecting the hippocampus with the hypothalamic mammillary bodies.
3. **IVth Ventricle**—space between the cerebellum and the tegmentum of the pons and medulla. Most caudal of the ventricles of the brain.
4. **Superior Medullary Velum**—forms part of the roof of the IVth ventricle. Consists of a thin sheet of tissue composed of pia mater and ependyma with a few nerve fibers between them.
5. **Cerebral Aqueduct (of Sylvius)**—canal in the midbrain connecting the IIIrd and IVth ventricles. Sylvius, a Frenchman, first described this canal (see also no. **10**, Fig. 4*A* and no. **4**, Fig. 32).
6. **Superior and Inferior Colliculi (Corpora Quadrigemina)**—two of the four rounded elevations making up the roof (L. *tectum*) or dorsal surface of the midbrain (see also no. **10**, Fig. 4*B*).
7. **Forceps Major**—commissural fibers running from one occipital lobe to the other (see no. **1**, Fig. 23). Because of their U-shaped configuration, they are called "forceps" (L. a pair of tongs).
8. **Cingulate Fasciculus**—long association fibers connecting the cortex on the medial surface of the frontal, parietal, occipital, and temporal lobes (see also no. **7**, Fig. 32).
9. **Corpus Callosum**—sagittal cut showing three of its subdivisions (**a**) *genu*, (**b**) *body*, and (**c**) *splenium*. Its tapered portion, the **rostrum** (L. beak), extending from the genu toward the lamina terminalis (**11**), is not labelled.
10. **Septum Pellucidum** (L. transparent partition)—separating the posterior half of the anterior horns of lateral ventricles.
11. **Lamina Terminalis**—thin membrane forming the anterior wall of the third ventricle.
12. **Anterior Commissure**—small bundle of nerve fibers crossing the midline in the lamina terminalis (**11**).
13. **Column of Fornix**—formed by division of the body of the fornix. Most of its fibers end in the mammillary body (**15**).
14. **Optic Chiasma**—about half the fibers of each optic nerve cross the midline here.
15. **Mammillary Body**—one of two small, nipple-like swellings on the basal surface of the hypothalamus. The Latin word *mammilla* is a derivatve of the word *mamma* for the breast.
16. **Basis Pedunculi**—part of the cerebral peduncle (see also no. **8**, Fig. 38).
17. **Basal Pons.**—the distinctive part of the brain stem (see also no. **3**, Fig. 16*B*).

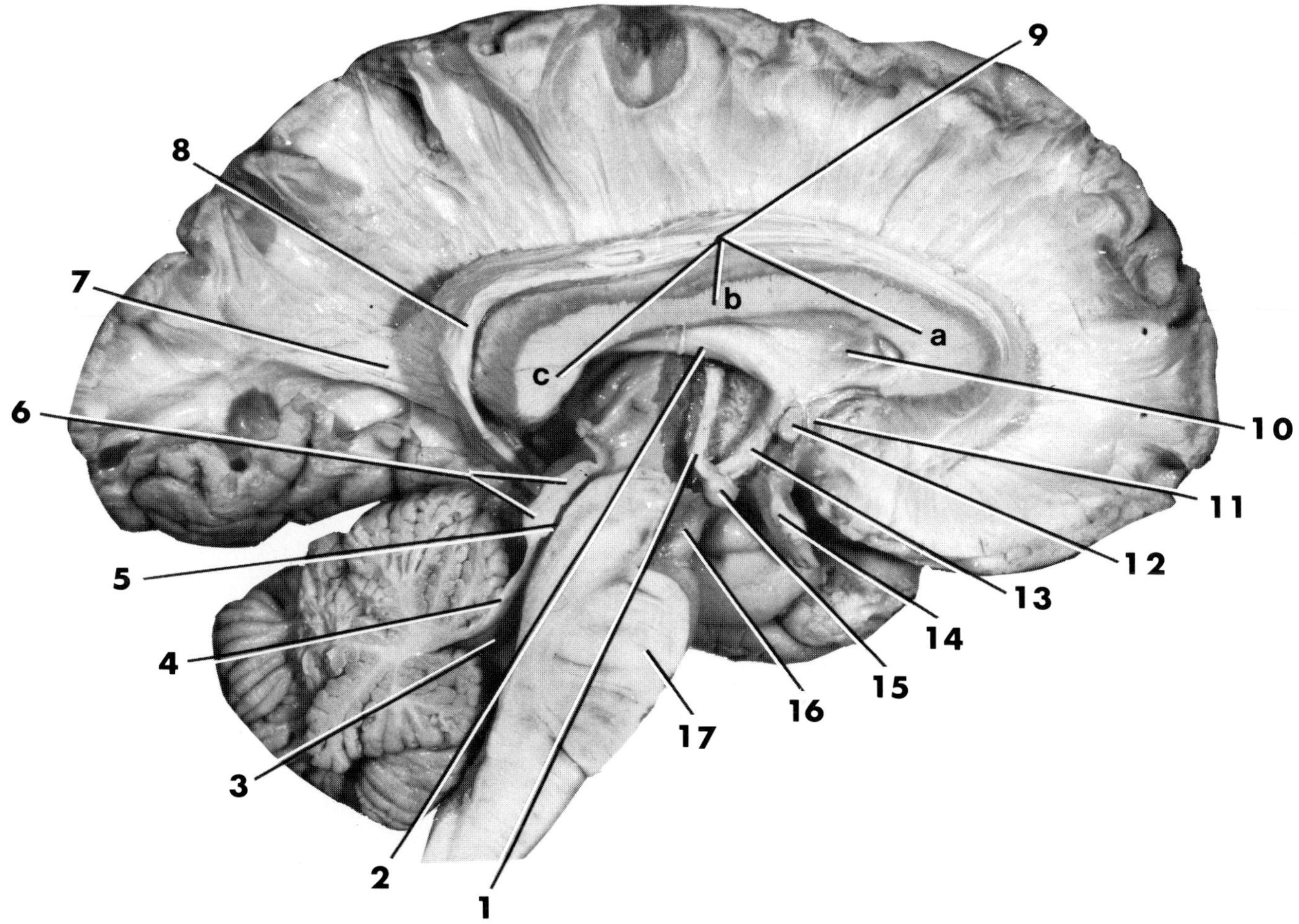

Figure 22 Left half of the brain (medial aspect), showing some midline structures as well as the relationship of the long **association fibers of the cingulate fasciculus** to the different regions of the transected corpus callosum.

1. **Splenium of Corpus Callosum**—the thickened posterior edge of the corpus callosum somewhat resembles a bandage (G. *splenion*) (see also no. **9c**, Fig. 22 and no. **10**, Fig. 24).
2. **Forceps Major**—radiating commissural fibers from each occipital lobe constitute the forceps major. These converging fibers form the splenium of the corpus callosum (see also no. **7**, Fig. 22).
3. **Tapetum**—commissural fibers of corpus callosum sweep over the lateral ventricles like a carpet (L. *tapete*) to form the lateral walls of the posterior and inferior horns (see also no. **1**, Fig. 25).
4. **Optic Radiation (Geniculocalcarine Tract)**—visual pathway fibers extending from the lateral geniculate body to the visual cortex (see also no. **4**, Fig. 20).
5. **External Capsule**—some commissural fibers extend lateral to the lenticular nucleus and mix with association and projection fibers to form the external capsule.
6. **Genu of Corpus Callosum** (L. *genu*, knee)—the anterior end of corpus callosum is knee-shaped on median section (see also no. **9a**, Fig. 22 and no. **6**, Fig. 24).
7. **Forceps Minor**—commissural fibers connecting the frontal poles constitute the forceps minor. These fibers converge to form the genu of corpus callosum. The Latin word forceps means a pair of tongs.
8. **Body of Corpus Callosum**—the portion forming the upper border of the hard (L. *callosus*), canopy-like layer of commissural fibers that extends into the medullary center of each cerebral hemisphere (see also no. **9b**, Fig. 22).

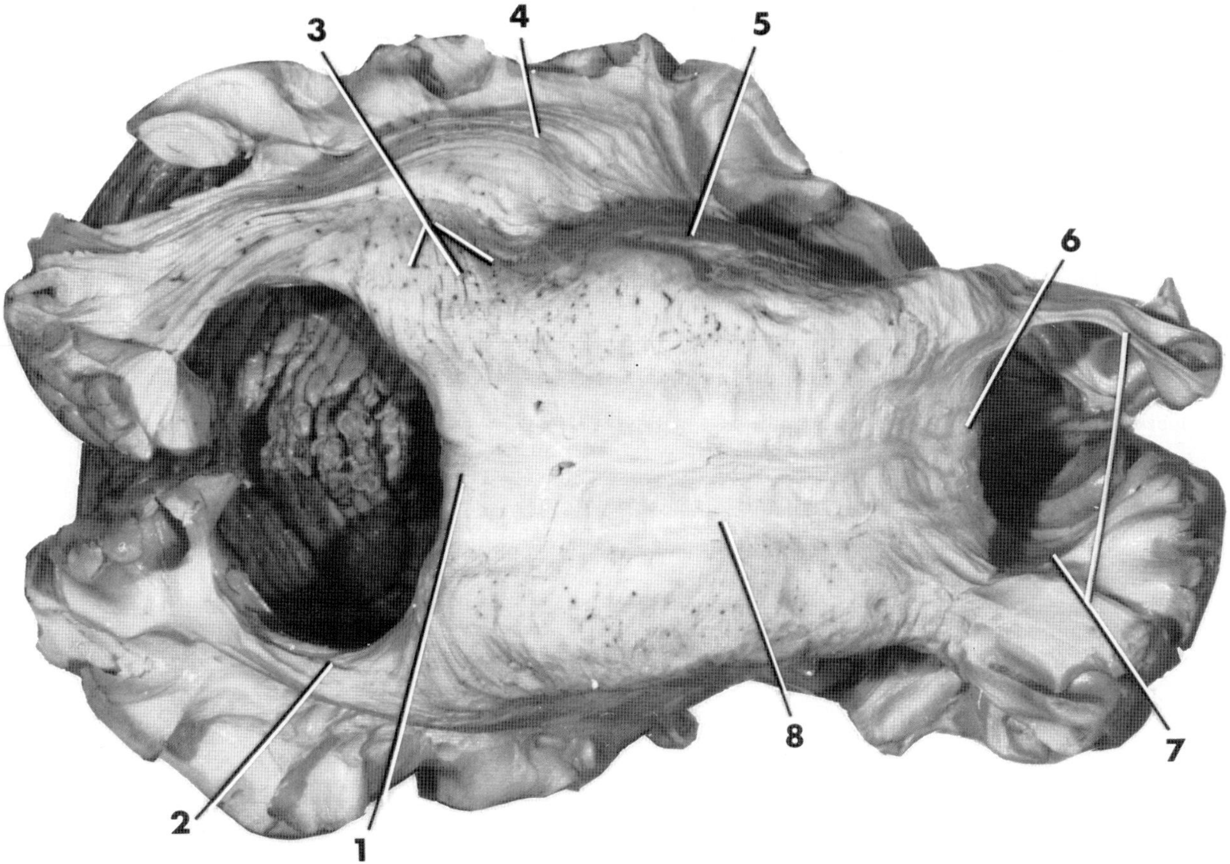

Figure 23 Superior view of the corpus callosum. Much of the cerebral hemisphere (cortex and medullary center) has been dissected away to show the **major parts of the corpus callosum** and the direction of its commissural fibers into the frontal, parietal, temporal, and occipital lobes.

1. **Thalamic Area (Cut Surface)**—the brain stem has been removed to expose the medial, lateral, and pulvinar areas of the thalamus.
2. **Third Ventricle**—is located between the left and right thalamic (and hypothalamic) areas. Its anterior wall is formed by the lamina terminalis. The anterior commissure (**3**) crosses the midline in the dorsal part of the lamina terminalis. The floor (removed) is indented by the optic chiasma and slopes upward and posteriorly to the cerebral aqueduct.
3. **Anterior Commissure**—a small bundle of reciprocal commissural fibers that cross the midline in the lamina terminalis, traverse the ventral part of the corpus striatum (**4**), and course to the anterior area of the temporal lobes. These fibers provide additional communication between the temporal lobes.
4. **Corpus Striatum (Ventral Aspect)**—consists of the head of the caudate nucleus and the putamen of the lentiform nucleus. Much of the ventral aspect of the corpus striatum has been dissected away to show the fibers of the anterior commissure (**3**) as they course through it to the temporal lobe (see also no. **7**, Fig. 16*B*).
5. **Septum Pellucidum** (L. transparent partition)—separates the posterior halves of the anterior horns (**8**) of the lateral ventricles.
6. **Genu of Corpus Callosum** (L. *genu*, knee)—it is the anterior end of the corpus callosum that bends back on itself (knee-shaped in median section). It consists of reciprocal commissural fibers which curve forwards into the frontal lobes as the forceps minor (**7**) (see also no. **6**, Fig. 23).
7. **Forceps Minor**—consists of reciprocal commissural fibers connecting the frontal poles. These fibers converge to form the genu (**6**) of the corpus callosum (see also no.**7**, Fig. 23).
8. **Anterior Horn of Lateral Ventricle**—is bounded anteriorly by the genu of corpus callosum (**6**). The rostrum of the corpus callosum lies between the anterior halves of the anterior horns, and the septum pellucidum (**5**) between the posterior halves of the anterior horns. Laterally the anterior horn is bounded by fibers making up the internal capsule. Posterior to the interventricular foramen, the anterior horn becomes the body of the lateral ventricle.
9. **Internal Capsule (Anterior Limb-Cut Surface)**—the surrounding gray matter has been dissected away to demonstrate the projection fibers of the anterior limb of the internal capsule.
10. **Splenium of Corpus Callosum** (G. *splenion*, bandage)—is the thickened posterior part of the corpus callosum composed of reciprocal commissural fibers that sweep posteriorly into the occipital lobes as the forceps major (**12**) (see also no. **1**, Fig. 23 and no. **9c**, Fig. 22).
11. **Lateral Ventricle (Collateral Trigone Area)**—at the level of the splenium (**10**). The body of the lateral ventricle widens to form the trigone which bifurcates to form the posterior and inferior horns that course posteriorly into the occipital lobe and inferiorly into the temporal lobe, respectively (see Fig. 26).
12. **Forceps Major** (L. *forceps*, tong)—consists of reciprocal radiating commissural fibers that converge from each occipital lobe to form the splenium of the corpus callosum. Note that many of the fibers of the major forceps form the medial wall of the posterior horn of the lateral ventricle (see no. **2**, Fig. 23).

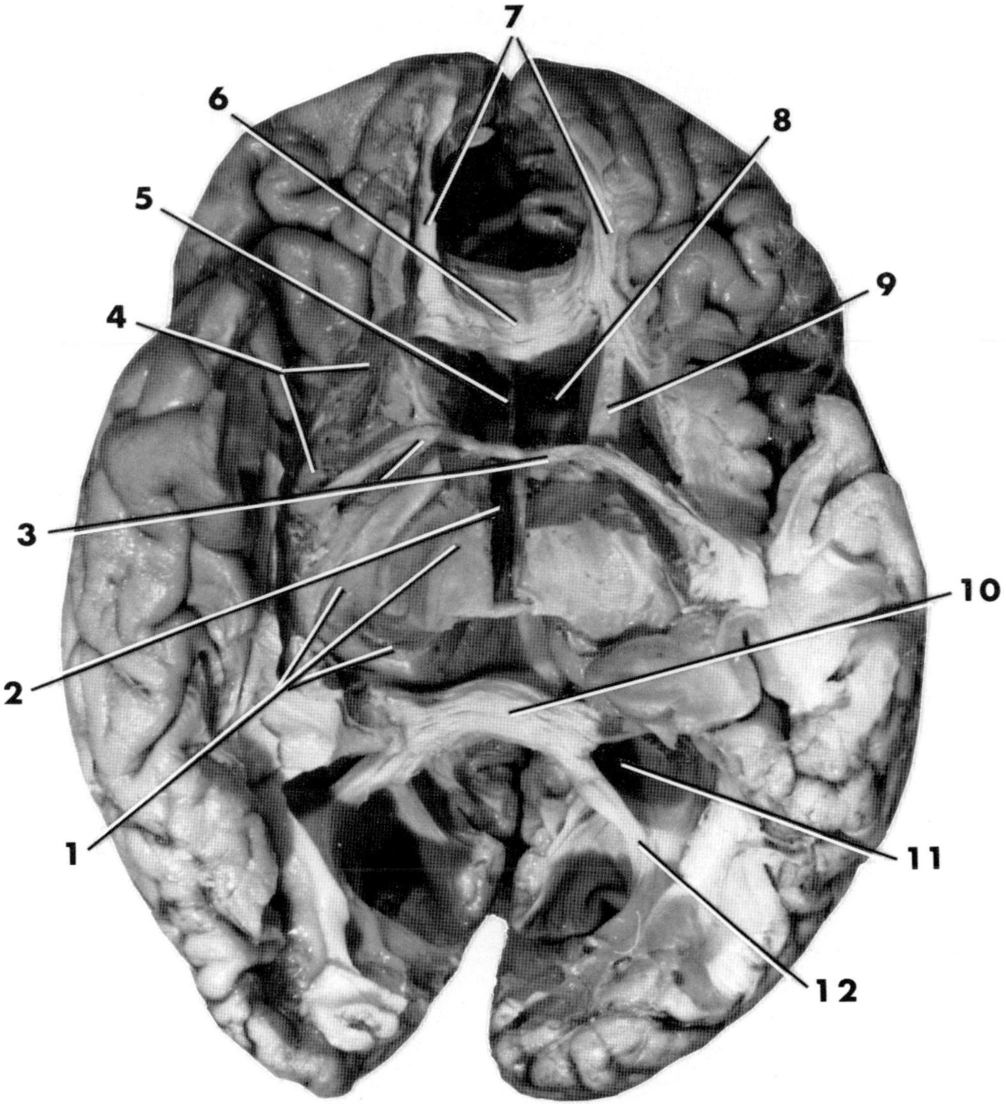

Figure 24 Inferior view of left and right halves of the cerebrum showing the extent of the commissural fibers of **anterior commissure**, and the splenium/forceps major, genu/forceps minor of the **corpus callosum**. The brain stem has been removed and much of the inferior area of the occipital, temporal, and parts of the frontal lobes have been dissected away to show these commissural fibers.

1. **Tapetum** (L. *tapete*, curtain, veil)—fibers from the corpus callosum sweep over the lateral ventricle and down into the medullary center of the occipital and temporal lobes, forming the lateral wall of parts of the posterior and inferior horns. These fibers are covered medially with ependyma lining the ventricle. The geniculocalcarine tract is immediately lateral to the tapetum (see also no. **3**, Fig. 23).
2. **Calcar Avis**—an elevation on the medial wall of the posterior horn of the lateral ventricle formed by the gray and white matter deep to the calcarine sulcus bulging into the ventricle (see also no. **7b**, Fig. 14).
3. **Corona Radiata**—cortical (afferent and efferent) projection fibers course inferiorly in the medullary center to converge and pass deep to (medial to) the lentiform nucleus (**7**). At this point the projection fiber are called the internal capsule which separates the lentiform nucleus from the thalamus and most of the head of the caudate nucleus.
4. **Superior Longitudinal Fasciculus (Arcuate Fasciculus)**—long association fibers located in the medullary center superior to the corpus callosum, connect the association cortex of the lateral surface of the frontal, parietal, occipital, and temporal lobes.
5. **Location of Internal Capsule**—here, the projection fibers that formed the area of the corona radiata that converges into the internal capsule have been removed to show that the anterior part of the internal capsule is located between and partially separates the lentiform nucleus (**7**) and the head of the caudate nucleus (**6**) (see also no. **3**, Fig. 17).
6. **Head of Caudate Nucleus**—bulges into the floor and lateral wall of the anterior horn of the lateral ventricle. It is part of the corpus striatum which is composed of the putamen of lentiform nucleus (**7**) and the head of the caudate nucleus. Inferiorly these two structures are continuous because the internal capsule does not extend inferior enough to separate them.
7. **Lentiform Nucleus**—a cerebral basal ganglion located between the external and internal capsules. It consists of a putamen (lateral portion) and a globus pallidus (medial portion). The inferior portion of this nucleus is continuous with the head of the caudate nucleus, and the two nuclei are known as the corpus striatum.
8. **Uncinate Fasciculus**—long association fibers connecting the cortex of the inferolateral frontal lobe with the temporal lobe cortex.
9. **Inferior Frontooccipital Fasciculus**—composed of reciprocal long association fibers connecting the cortex of the inferior area of the frontal lobe with the temporal and occipital lobes.
10. **Inferior Temporal Gyrus**—located on the inferior part of the lateral surface of the cerebral hemisphere. It curves onto the inferior and medial surfaces of the temporal lobe, and as it does this, it forms much of the inferior surface of the temporal lobe.
11. **Hippocampus** (G. sea horse)—a structure which constitutes an important part of the limbic system. It produces a prominent elevation on the floor of the inferior horn of the lateral ventricle. Note that the lateral wall of the ventricle has been removed to show this relationship. The lateral wall would include fibers of the tapetum (**1**), as well as the inferior frontooccipital fasciculus (**9**) (see also no. **1**, Fig. 34).

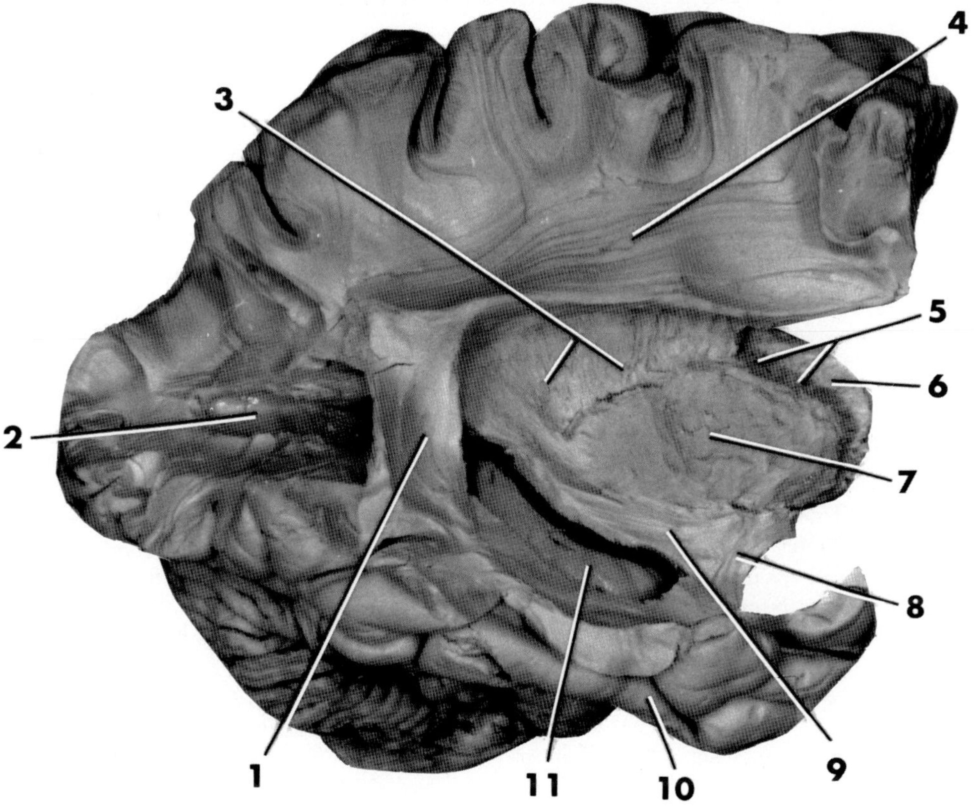

Figure 25 Lateral view of the parieto-occipito-temporal area of the right cerebral hemisphere, showing how the **commissural fibers of the tapetum** make up the lateral wall of the posterior and inferior horns of the lateral ventricle.

4

The Ventricles of the Brain

1. **Temporal Lobe**—is limited superiorly by the lateral sulcus and its imaginary posterior projection and posteriorly by the lower half of the imaginary line joining the parietooccipital sulcus with the preoccipital notch (see Fig. 5). The inferior horn (**a**) and the collateral trigone (**c**) of the lateral ventricle are located in this lobe.
2. **Occipital Lobe**—is limited anteriorly and separated from the parietal (**3**) and temporal (**1**) lobes by an imaginary line which joins the parietooccipital sulcus with the preoccipital notch (see Fig. 5). The posterior horn (**b**) of the lateral ventricle extends a variable distance into the occipital lobe.
3. **Parietal Lobe**—is limited anteriorly by the central sulcus, inferiorly by the lateral sulcus and its posterior imaginary projection, and posteriorly by the upper half of the imaginary line extending from the parietooccipital sulcus to the preoccipital notch (see Fig. 5). Much of the body (**d**) the lateral ventricle is located in this lobe.
4. **Frontal Lobe**—is limited posteriorly by the central sulcus and its imaginary projection to the lateral sulcus, and inferiorly by the lateral sulcus (see Fig. 5). The anterior horn (**e**) and the rostral portion of the body (**d**) of the lateral ventricle are located in the frontal lobe.

Regions of Lateral Ventricle

a. **Inferior Horn of Lateral Ventricle**—begins at the collateral trigone (**c**) and extends rostrally into the medial part of the temporal lobe.

b. **Posterior Horn of Lateral Ventricle**—extends a variable distance into the occipital lobe from the collateral trigone (**c**).

c. **Collateral Trigone**—is formed by the junction of the posterior horn (**b**) and inferior horn (**a**) into a triangular enlarged space. Anteriorly this cavity continues as the body (**d**) of the lateral ventricle.

d. **Body of Lateral Ventricle**—the central portion (body) of the lateral ventricle extends from the collateral trigone as far rostrally as the interventricular foramen, connecting the lateral ventricle with the third ventricle. The body of the lateral ventricle is located in the rostral parietal and caudal frontal lobes.

e. **Anterior Horn of Lateral Ventricle**—is the rostral extension of the lateral ventricle beyond the interventricular foramen and into the frontal lobe. The septum pellucidum is the common medial wall for the anterior horn of each lateral ventricle.

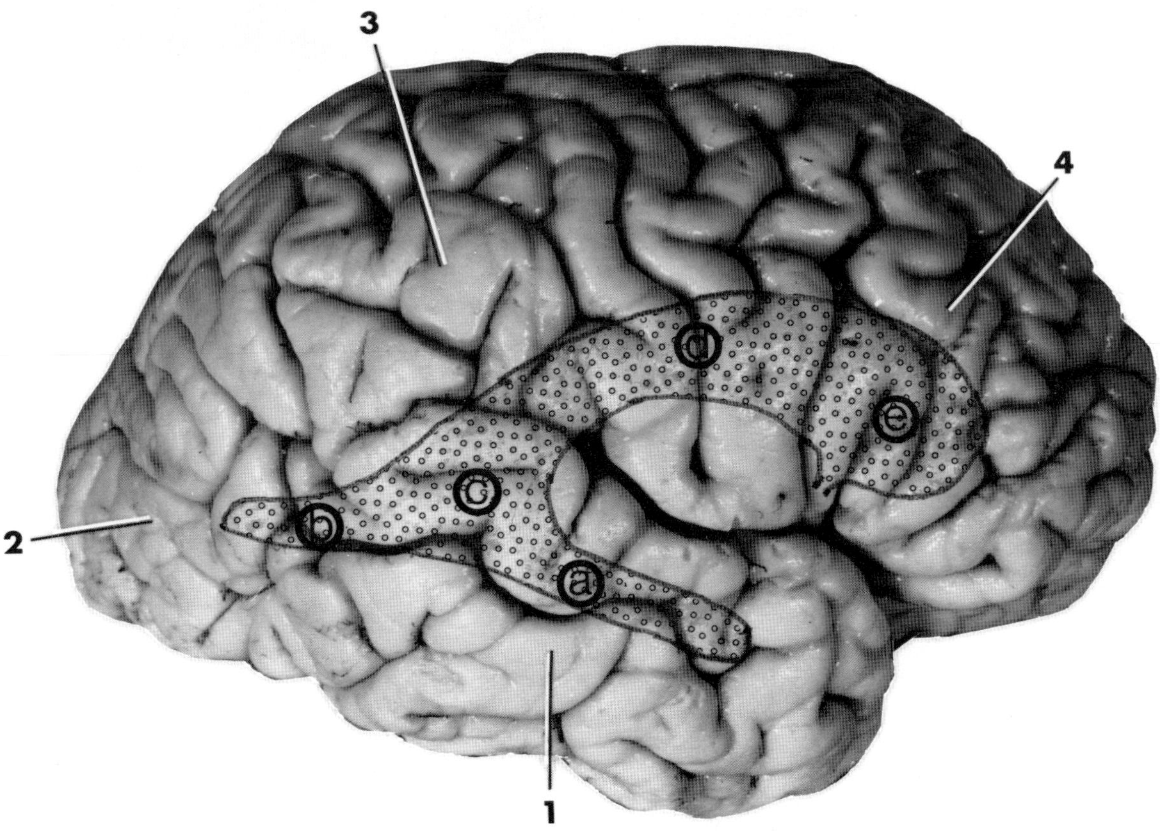

Figure 26 Lateral view of the right cerebral hemisphere showing the relative position, shape, and size of the **lateral ventricle** within it.

1. **Medulla**—the caudal portion of the brain stem (midbrain, pons, and medulla). As the rostral portion of the spinal cord passes into the skull through the foramen magnum, it enlarges into the medulla oblongata in the posterior cranial fossa.
2. **Pons**—the middle portion of the brain stem. It has an enlarged basal portion, which is connected with the cerebellum through the middle cerebellar peduncle, and a tegmental portion. The dorsal surface of the tegmental pons forms part of the floor of the fourth ventricle (**C**).
3. **Midbrain**—the rostral portion of the brain stem connects the diencephalon and the pons. The cerebral aqueduct (**6**) connects the third and fourth ventricles.
4. **Area of the Diencephalon**—the interbrain consists of the thalamus, the epithalamus, the hypothalamus, and the subthalamus. The left and right thalami and hypothalami form the lateral walls of the midline space, the third ventricle (**B**).
5. **Cerebral Hemisphere** (right)—the large expanded portion of the secondary brain vesicle, the telencephalon, occupies most of the right side of the interior of the skull. It consists of the frontal, parietal, occipital, and temporal lobes, and the lateral ventricles which are the derivatives of the neural canal of the developing neural tube.
6. **Cerebral Aqueduct (of Sylvius)**—connects the third and fourth ventricles. The aqueduct passes through the midbrain in the central area of gray matter, immediately inferior to the tectum.
7. **Cerebellum ("the Little Brain")**—located posterior to the tegmental area of both the pons and the open portion of the medulla. The fourth ventricle (**C**) intervenes between the cerebellum and the pons and medulla.

Ventricles

A. **Lateral Ventricle of Right Cereberal Hemisphere**—a C-shaped cavity deep in the cerebral hemisphere. Its shape results from the direction of growth of the embryonic brain—first anteriorly, then posteriorly, then anteriorly again to form the temporal lobes. The lateral ventricle has an anterior horn extending into the frontal lobe, a body contained in the caudal portion of the frontal lobe, and the rostral portion of the parietal lobe; a horn extending posteriorly into the occipital lobe, and an inferior horn extending inferiorly and anteriorly into the temporal lobe. The lateral ventricle communicates with the third ventricle through the interventricular foramen.

B. **Third Ventricle**—a narrow vertical space between the left and right thalami and hypothalami of the diencephalon. The anterior wall is the lamina terminalis. The lateral wall is formed by the thalamus and the hypothalamus. The roof is a thin membrane attached to the stria medullaris thalamicus on each side. The floor is indented by the optic chiasma, and an infundibular recess dips into the pituitary stalk. The floor then slopes posteriorly and superiorly to the cerebral aqueduct through which cerebrospinal fluid flows into the fourth ventricle.

C. **Fourth Ventricle**—the dorsal surface of the open portions of the medulla and the pons contributes to its floor. It converges caudally into the central canal of the closed part of the medulla and into the cerebral aqueduct of the midbrain rostrally. The roof is shaped like a tent protruding into the medullary center of the cerebellum. The rostral part of the roof is formed by the superior medullary velum and the superior cerebellar peduncles. The posterior part is membranous and is covered by the vermis. The lateral walls include the fibers of the inferior and the middle cerebellar peduncles as they curve into the cerebellum.

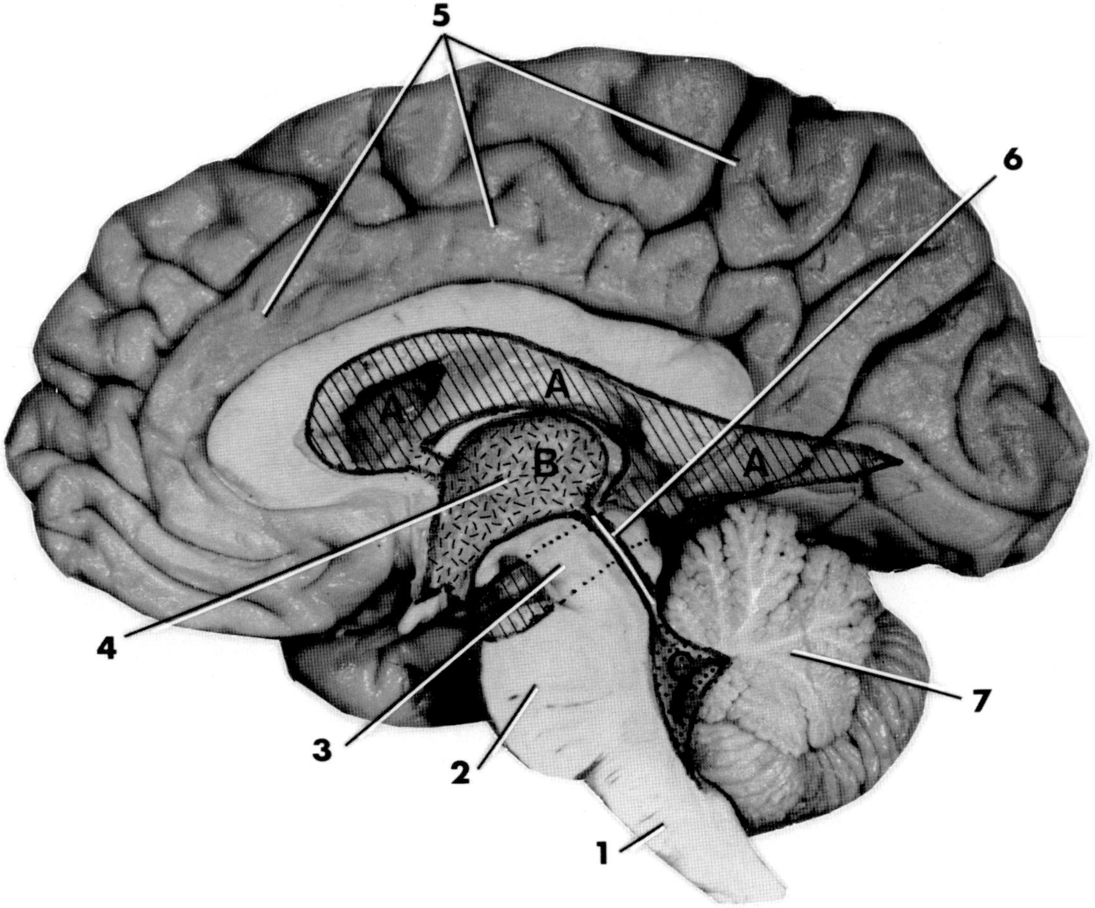

Figure 27 Medial view of the right half of the brain sectioned in the median (midsagittal) plane. Sketches have been added to show the relative positions, shapes, and sizes of the lateral (**A**), the third (**B**), and the fourth ventricles (**C**) of the brain.

1. **Inferior Horn of Lateral Ventricle**—begins at the collateral trigone (**3**), curves inferiorly around the pulvinar of the thalamus, and extends rostrally into the medial part of the temporal lobe to end approximately 2.5 cm from the temporal pole. The roof and lateral walls of the ventricle are largely formed by the tapetum (commissural fibers, see no. **1**, Fig. 25) and optic radiations (geniculocalcarine tract).
2. **Middle Temporal Gyrus**—located between the superior (removed in this dissection) and inferior temporal gyri. Note how far rostrally the inferior horn (**1**) extends into the temporal lobe.
3. **Collateral Trigone**—formed in the region of the splenium of the corpus callosum when the body of the lateral ventricle enlarges and separates to form the posterior and inferior horns of the lateral ventricle (**1**).
4. **Projection Fibers**—from the cerebral cortex course inferiorly in the medullary center and assist in forming the lateral wall of the body of the lateral ventricle (**5**). Above the lentiform nucleus (**8**), these radiating fibers may be seen converging to form the corona radiata.
5. **Body of Lateral Ventricle**—the central portion of the lateral ventricle extends from the interventricular foramen to the splenium of the corpus callosum, where it enlarges to form the collateral trigone (**3**). Its roof is formed by the corpus callosum. Laterally it is bounded by projection fibers of the internal capsule. The superior surface of the thalamus forms most of its floor.
6. **Corona Radiata**—projection fibers from the cerebral cortex (like **4**) course inferiorly in the medullary center. Superior to the lentiform nucleus, these converging fibers from the corona radiata. Most of these fibers descend medial to the lentiform nucleus to form the internal capsule. Some fibers of the corona radiata pass lateral to the lentiform nucleus, forming the external capsule.
7. **Anterior Horn of Lateral Ventricle**—the lateral ventricle extends anteriorly beyond the interventricular foramen into the frontal lobe as the anterior horn. Its roof and rostral wall are formed by the corpus callosum. The anterior part of the septum pellucidum lies between the posterior parts of the anterior horns of the lateral ventricles. The inferior parts of the medial portion of the corpus callosum (rostrum and part of the genu) lie between the anterior parts of the lateral ventricles. The medial wall of the anterior horn is formed mainly by the head of the caudate nucleus.
8. **External Capsule and Lentiform Nucleus**—projection and association fibers of the medullary center pass lateral to the lentiform nucleus, a cerebral basal ganglion consisting of the putamen (outer lateral part) and the globus pallidus (inner medial part). The internal capsule lies medial to and separates this nucleus from the thalamus and the head of the caudate nucleus.
9. **Uncinate Fasciculus**—composed of association fibers connecting the association cortex of the frontal and temporal lobes.

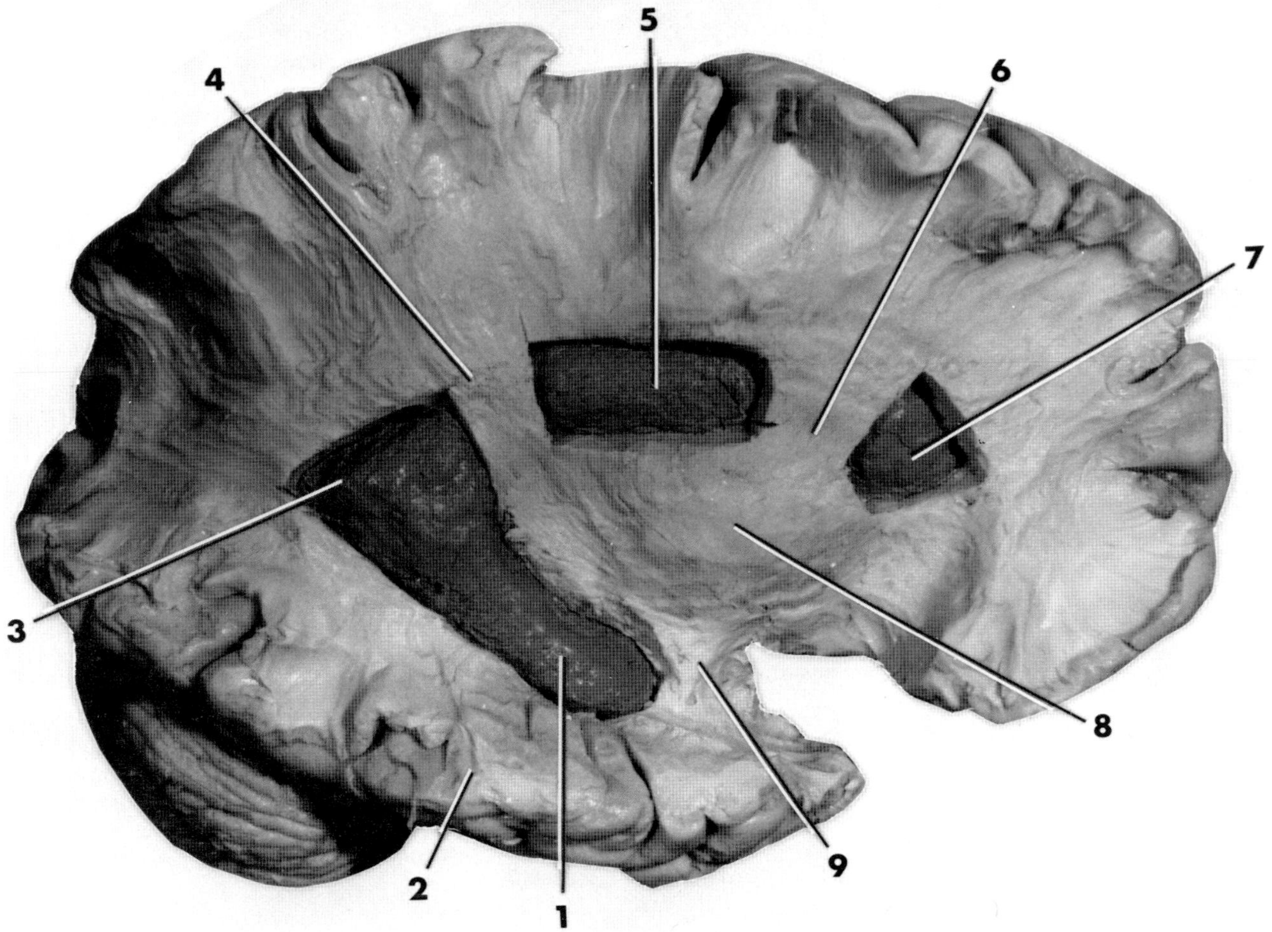

Figure 28 Lateral view of the right cerebral hemisphere showing the position of the **lateral ventricle**. For this demonstration, the ventricle was injected with liquid latex which hardened *in situ*. The cerebral cortex was removed as well as much of the medullary center as far as the external capsule and the lentiform nucleus. ''Windows'' were cut in the remaining white matter to show the shape and position of the lateral ventricle.

1. **Left Lateral Ventricle**—roughly a C-shaped cavity that is lined by ependymal cells and was filled with ventricular fluid in the left cerebral hemisphere. Each ventricle consists of a body (**b**), from which anterior (**a**), posterior (**e**), and inferior (**c**) horns extend into the frontal, occipital, and temporal lobes, respectively.
   a. **Anterior Horn**—the rostral extension of the lateral ventricle beyond the interventricular foramen and into the frontal lobe is called the anterior horn. The ventricle is limited rostrally and superiorly by the genu and body of the corpus callosum, respectively. The septum pellucidum is the common medial wall for the anterior horn of each lateral ventricle (see also no. **7**, Fig. 28).
   b. **Body of Lateral Ventricle**—the central portion (body) of the lateral ventricle extends from the collateral trigone (**d**) as far rostrally as the interventricular foramen, connecting the ventricle with the third ventricle. The roof is formed by the body of the corpus callosum (**2**) and the lateral wall is bounded by the internal capsule (see also no. **5**, Fig. 28).
   c. **Inferior Horn**—begins at the collateral trigone (**d**), curves inferiorly around the posterior portion of the thalamus, and extends rostrally into the medial part of the temporal lobe. Its roof and lateral wall are mainly formed by fibers of the optic radiations (geniculocalcarine tract) and the tapetum (commissural fibers) (see also no. **1**, Fig. 28).
   d. **Collateral Trigone**—is formed at the region of the splenium of the corpus callosum by the junction of the posterior (**e**) and inferior (**c**) horns into a triangular enlarged area. Anteriorly this cavity continues as the body (**b**) of the lateral ventricle (see also no. **3**, Fig. 28).
   e. **Posterior Horn**—extends a variable distance into the occipital lobe from the collateral trigone (**d**). Most of the posterior horn is not seen in this dissection because the roof and lateral wall, which is formed by the tapetum of the corpus callosum, has not been dissected away. On its medial wall is a prominence, the calcar avis, which is produced by the deep intrusion of the calcarine fissure.
2. **Corpus Callosum**—this superior view shows the positions of three of its subdivisions (**a**) genu, (**b**) body, and (**c**) splenium. Its body and genu form the roof and rostral limit of the body and anterior horn of the lateral ventricle, respectively. Compact communicating fibers pass from each cerebral hemisphere and cross the midline in the region of the genu, body, and splenium of the corpus callosum.
3. **Internal Capsule**—the projection fibers from the corona radiata that course inferiorly to pass medial to the lentiform nucleus (**4**) as the internal capsule have been transected and removed just superior to the lentiform nucleus. When intact, these fibers form the lateral wall of the lateral ventricle.
4. **Lentiform Nucleus**—a horizontal cut has been made in this nucleus, and its superior portion has been removed to show the fibers of the internal capsule (**3**) coursing medial to it. The lentiform nucleus is situated between the external and internal capsules and consists of an outer part, the putamen, and an inner part, the globus pallidus.
5. **Optic Radiation and Tapetum**—consist of projection fibers from the lateral geniculate body (geniculocalcarine tract) that extend to the visual cortex of the occipital lobe, and commissural fibers that extend from the splenium of the corpus callosum inferiorly into the medullary center of the temporal and occipital lobes. Note that these fibers form the lateral wall of the posterior horn of the lateral ventricle.

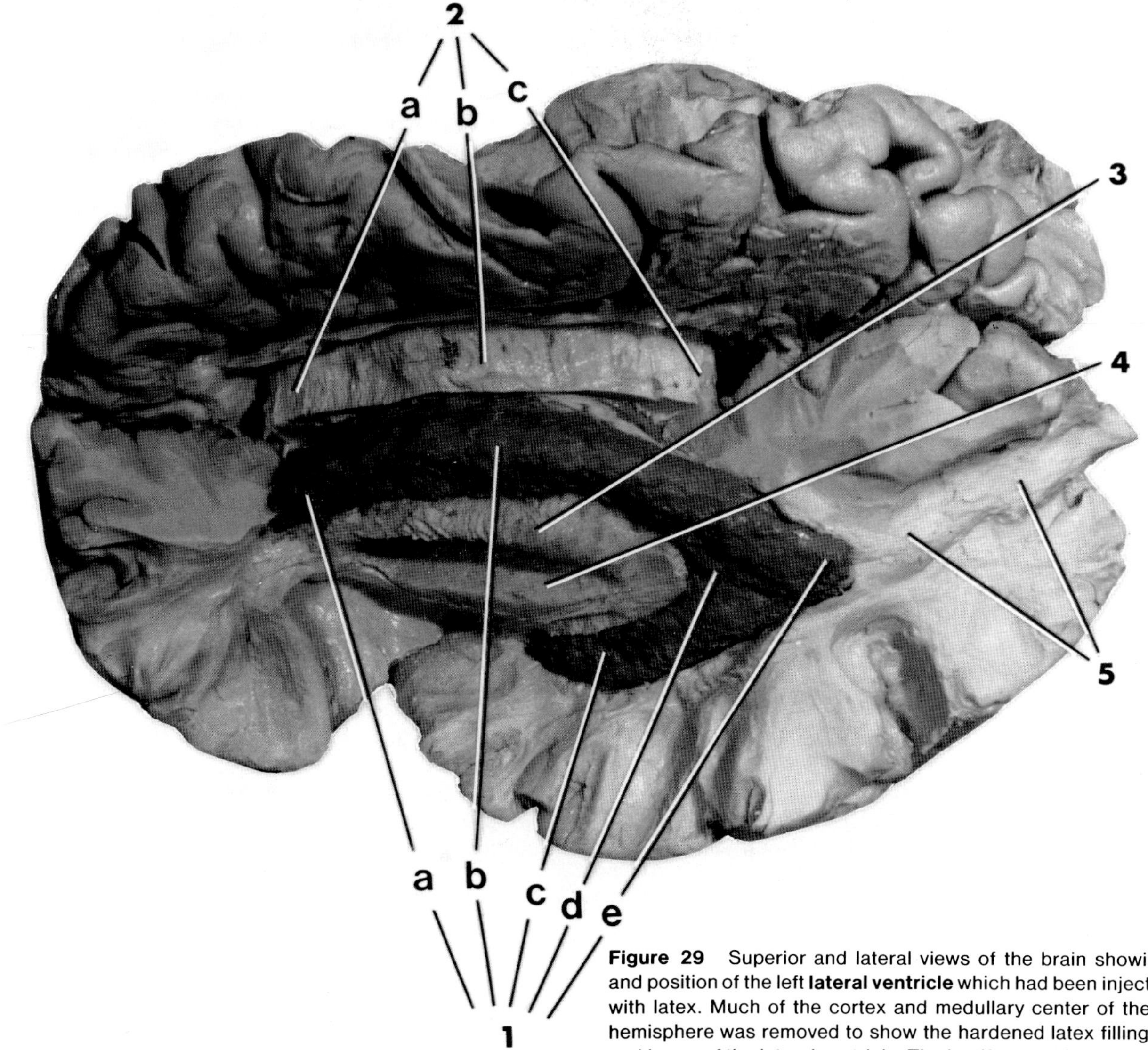

Figure 29 Superior and lateral views of the brain showing the shape and position of the left **lateral ventricle** which had been injected previously with latex. Much of the cortex and medullary center of the left cerebral hemisphere was removed to show the hardened latex filling the contours and horns of the lateral ventricle. The lentiform nucleus was exposed, and the superior half of it was removed to show the angle of the fibers that form the internal capsule.

1. **Posterior Horn of Lateral Ventricle**—begins at the collateral trigone (the area where the body of the lateral ventricle bifurcates to form the posterior and inferior horns) and extends a variable distance into the occipital lobe. The medial wall of this space shows a prominent bulge, the calcar avis, formed by the white matter deep to the gray matter of the deeply penetrating calcarine sulcus (see also no. **1e**, Fig. 29).
2. **Body of Lateral Ventricle**—extends from the area of the interventricular foramen posteriorly to the area of the splenium of the corpus callosum, where it bifurcates to form the posterior horn (**1**) and the inferior horn. Its roof is the body of the corpus callosum (removed to show this part of the ventricle), and its floor is the dorsal surface of the thalamus. The choroid plexus (**10**) is located in the ventricle. The septum pellucidum (no. **3** Fig. 4*A*) is hidden by the body of the corpus callosum in this view) (see also no. **5**, Fig. 28).
3. **Lentiform Nucleus (Cut Surface)**—the superior portion of the lentiform nucleus was removed. The internal capsule (**5**) lies medial to the lentiform nucleus. This cerebral basal ganglion consists of the putamen (lateral part) shown here and the globus pallidus (medial part) not shown here, because the horizontal cut was made superior to the globus pallidus.
4. **Postcentral Gyrus (Cut Surface)**—is located between the central and postcentral sulci. Its cortex is concerned with general somesthetic sensations.
5. **Internal Capsule (Cut Surface)**—consists of bundles of projection fibers (cortical afferents and efferents) which separate the caudate nucleus (**7**) and thalamus from the lentiform nucleus (**3**) (see also no. **7b**, Fig. 36).
6. **Anterior Horn of Lateral Ventricle**—the lateral ventricle extends anteriorly beyond the interventricular foramen into the frontal lobe as the anterior horn. The body and genu of the corpus callosum form its roof (removed) and anterior limit. The head of the caudate nucleus (**7**) bulges into its floor and lateral wall (see also no. **1a**, Fig. 29).
7. **Head of Caudate Nucleus**—bulges into the floor and lateral wall of the anterior horn of the lateral ventricle (**6**). It rapidly tapers into a slender tail which lies on the dorsal surface of the thalamus along the lateral margin of the body of the lateral ventricle.
8. **Vena Terminalis (Thalamostriate Vein)**—begins in the region of the amygdaloid nucleus in the temporal pole and follows the curve of the tail of the caudate nucleus around onto the dorsal surface of the thalamus. The vena terminalis courses anteriorly to the interventricular foramen where it unites with the choroidal vein to form the internal cerebral vein (see also no. **10**, Fig. 35).
9. **Stria Terminalis**—a slender bundle of fibers originating in the amygdaloid nucleus and following the curvature of the tail of the caudate nucleus onto the dorsal surface of the thalamus in the floor of the body of the lateral ventricle. The fibers terminate in the hypothalamus and the medial olfactory area (see also no. **12**, Fig. 35).
10. **Choroid Plexus**—visible here in the body of the lateral ventricle. It begins in the inferior horn, follows the contour of the lateral ventricle anteriorly and through the interventricular foramen. It is supplied by the anterior choroidal artery. Its cells secrete cerebrospinal fluid which flows into the third ventricle through the interventricular foramen.
11. **Splenium of Corpus Callosum**—the thickened posterior area of the corpus callosum is composed of commissural fibers connecting the association cortex of each occipital lobe. The commissural fibers arch backwards from the splenium into the occipital lobes in a bundle known as the forceps major.

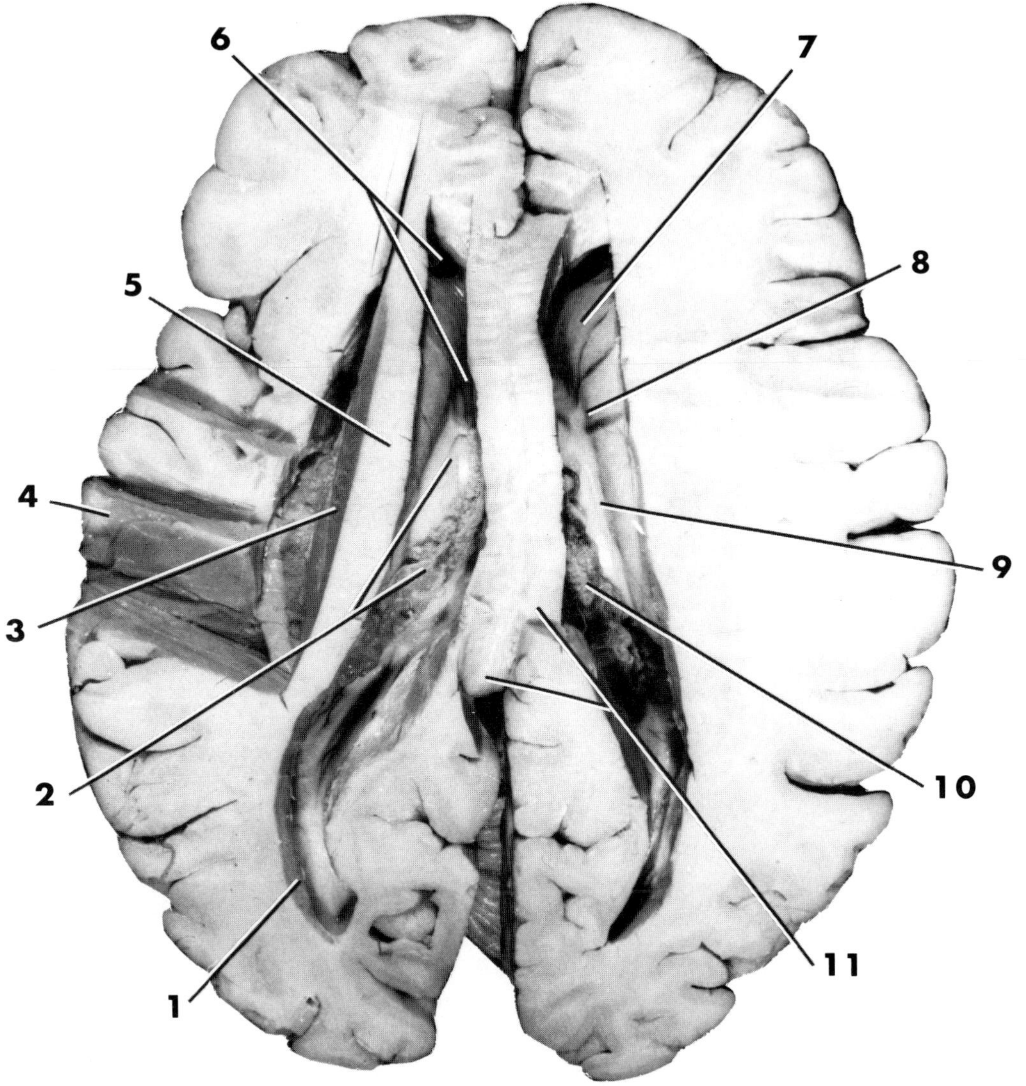

Figure 30 Superior view of a horizontal section of the brain showing the position of the **lateral ventricles** and some of their internal features. On the right side, a horizontal slice was made through the cerebrum into the lateral ventricle at the level of the body of the corpus callosum. The piece of cerebrum was then removed. On the left side, a horizontal slice was made at a slightly lower level then on the right. The lentiform nucleus was partially exposed in the medullary center.

5

The Limbic System

The **limbic lobe** consists of the following three areas:

A. **Parahippocampal Gyrus**—located between the hippocampal sulcus (**3**) and the collateral sulcus. This convolution extends almost as far anteriorly as the temporal pole, where it hooks sharply backward as the uncus (see no. **12**, Fig. 9*B*). At the hippocampal sulcus, the parahippocampal gyrus is continuous with the hippocampus, which occupies the floor of the inferior horn of the lateral ventricle (see also no. **2**, Fig. 9*B*).

B. **Isthmus**—a narrow cortical area inferior to the splenium of the corpus callosum that connects the cingulate gyrus (**C**) with the parahippocampal gyrus (**A**). These three structures form the limbic lobe which includes the upper brain stem.

C. **Cingulate Gyrus**—begins inferior to the genu of the corpos callosum and parallels the corpus callosum as far as the splenium, where the isthmus (**C**) connects it with the parahippocampal gyrus. It is limited by the cingulate sulcus (**5**) superiorly and the callosal sulcus (**7**) inferiorly.

Featured Structures

1. **Hypothalamus**—located inferior to the thalamus. The left and right hypothalami form the inferior half of the lateral wall and the floor of the third ventricle. In the limibic system there are connections of the hypothalamus with other limbic structures (*i.e.*, hippocampus, amygdaloid nucleus, anterior tubercle of the thalamus, etc.).
2. **Mammillary Body** (left)—one of a pair of hypothalamic nuclei lying on the basal surface of the diencephalon. It has extensive connections with the hippocampus via the fornix and with the anterior tubercle of the thalamus via the mammillothalamic tract.
3. **Hippocampal Sulcus**—a deep sulcus on the medial side of the temporal lobe which separates the parahippocampal gyrus from the dentate gyrus.
4. **Corpus Callosum (Midline Cut)**—consists of reciprocal commissural fibers that extend into the frontal, parietal, occipital, and temporal lobe cortices. Three regions, the body, the genu, and the splenium are easily identified. The superior part of the limbic lobe is located above it.
5. **Cingulate Sulcus**—demarcates the cingulate gyrus (superior portion of the limbic lobe) from the medial surface of the superior frontal gyrus and the paracentral lobule.
6. **Fornix**—an important group of fibers in the limbic system that connects the hippocampus with the mammillary body. It consists of the **crus fornix** (**a**) emerging from the inferior horn of the lateral ventricle, the **body** (**b**) that lies on the dorsomedial surface of the thalamus, and the **column of the fornix** (**c**), the part of the fornix curving inferiorly in front of the thalamus and the interventricular foramen to course through the hypothalamic nuclear areas to the mammillary body.
7. **Callosal Sulcus (Sulcus of Corpus Callosum)**—separates the corpus callosum from the cingulate gyrus (superior half of the limbic lobe). It curves around the splenium and continues as the hippocampal sulcus.
8. **Septum Pellucidum**—this triangular, sometimes double membrane, separates the anterior horns of the lateral ventricles.
9. **Olfactory Tract**—consists of fibers that connect the olfactory bulb with the brain (olfactory trigone, **10**) anterior to the anterior perforated substance.
10. **Olfactory Trigone**—a noticeable triangular area on the ventromedial surface of the frontal lobe, directly anterior to the anterior perforated substance. The medial and lateral olfactory striae extend from the trigone to the respective olfactory cortices. There are connections between this part of the olfactory system and the limbic system.

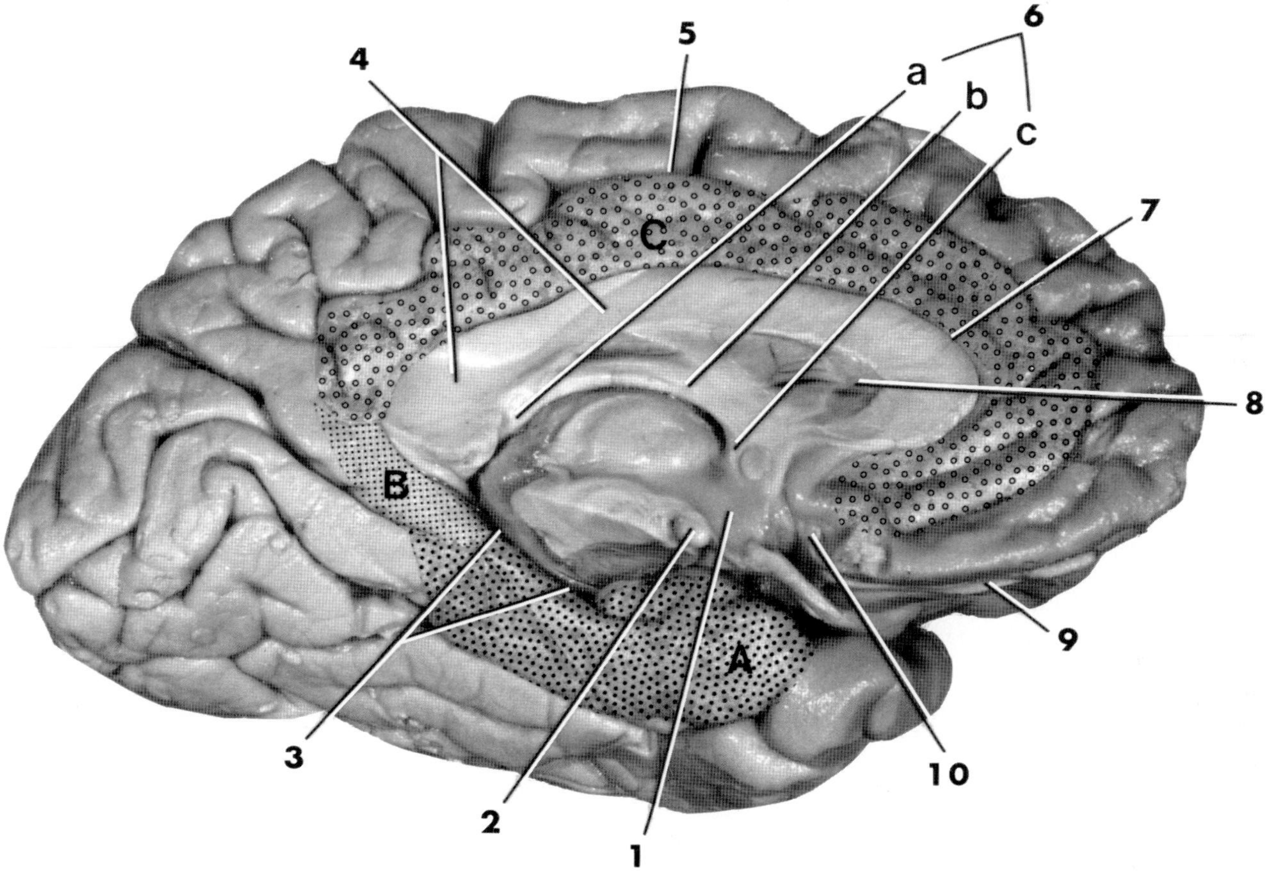

Figure 31 A view of the medial and inferior surfaces of the left cerebral hemisphere to show the components of the **limbic lobe and related structures**.

1. **Mammillothalamic Tract**—part of the limbic system connecting the mammillary body of the hypothalamus with the anterior thalamic nucleus (see also no. **6**, Fig. 33).
2. **Body of the Fornix**—fibers from the left and right hippocampi and dentate gyri form the left and right crura (L. legs) of the fornix, which curve superiorly and anteriorly to merge on the dorsomedial surface of the thalamus to form the body of the fornix. The body of the fornix is in contact with the inferior surface of the body of the corpus callosum (see also no. **6**, Fig. 35).
3. **IVth Ventricle**—the space between the cerebellum and the tegmentum of pons and medulla, forming part of the ventricular system of the brain.
4. **Cerebral Aqueduct (of Sylvius)**—the canal in the midbrain connecting the IIIrd and IVth ventricles (see also no. **10**, Fig. 4*A*).
5. **Tectum**—roof of the midbrain composed of the two superior and the two inferior colliculi (also called the corpora quadrigemina). *Tectum* is a Latin word meaning roof.
6. **Pineal Body**—a gland that is shaped like a pine cone (L. *pineus*, relating to pine). It serves as a useful neuroradiological and neurosurgical landmark when calcified.
7. **Cingulate Fasciculus**—consists of long association fibers connecting much of the limbic cortex on the medial surface of the frontal, parietal, and occipital lobes with the limbic cortex on the inferior and medial surfaces of the temporal lobe (see also no. **8**, Fig. 22).
8. **Corpus Callosum (Midline Cut)**—showing three of its parts: (**a**) genu, (**b**) body, and (**c**) splenium. The rostrum (L. beak) of the corpus callosum, passing posteriorly from the genu to the lamina terminalis, is not labelled.
9. **Head of Caudate Nucleus**—the septum pellucidum has been removed to show its position in the left anterior horn of the lateral ventricle (see also no. 7, Fig. 30).
10. **Lamina Terminalis**—a thin membrane stretching from the inferior part of the front of the optic chiasma to the anterior commissure. It forms part of the anterior wall of the third ventricle (see also no. **4**, Fig. 4*B*).
11. **Anterior Commissure**—a compact bundle of reciprocal commissural fibers crossing the midline in the lamina terminalis. It provides communication between the temporal lobes (see also no. **5**, Fig. 4*B*). At the midline, this commissure lies anterior to the column of the fornix which lies anterior to the interventricular foramen.
12. **Column of Fornix**—fibers from the body of the fornix (**2**) separate into two columns that turn ventrally away from the corpus callosum and pass between the anterior tubercle of the thalamus and the anterior commissure. The fibers pass posteriorly in the substance of the hypothalamic nuclei to reach the mammillary bodies (see also no. **6c**, Fig. 31).
13. **Mammillary Body** (left)—the mammillary bodies are posterior hypothalamic nuclei lying on the basal surface of the diencephalon, immediately anterior to the midbrain. They are connected with the hippocampus by the fibers of the fornix, and with the anterior thalamic tubercle by the mammillothalamic tract fibers. They have an important function in the limbic system.
14. **Oculomotor Nerve (C.N. III)**—given its name because it supplies most of the eye (L. *oculus*) muscles.

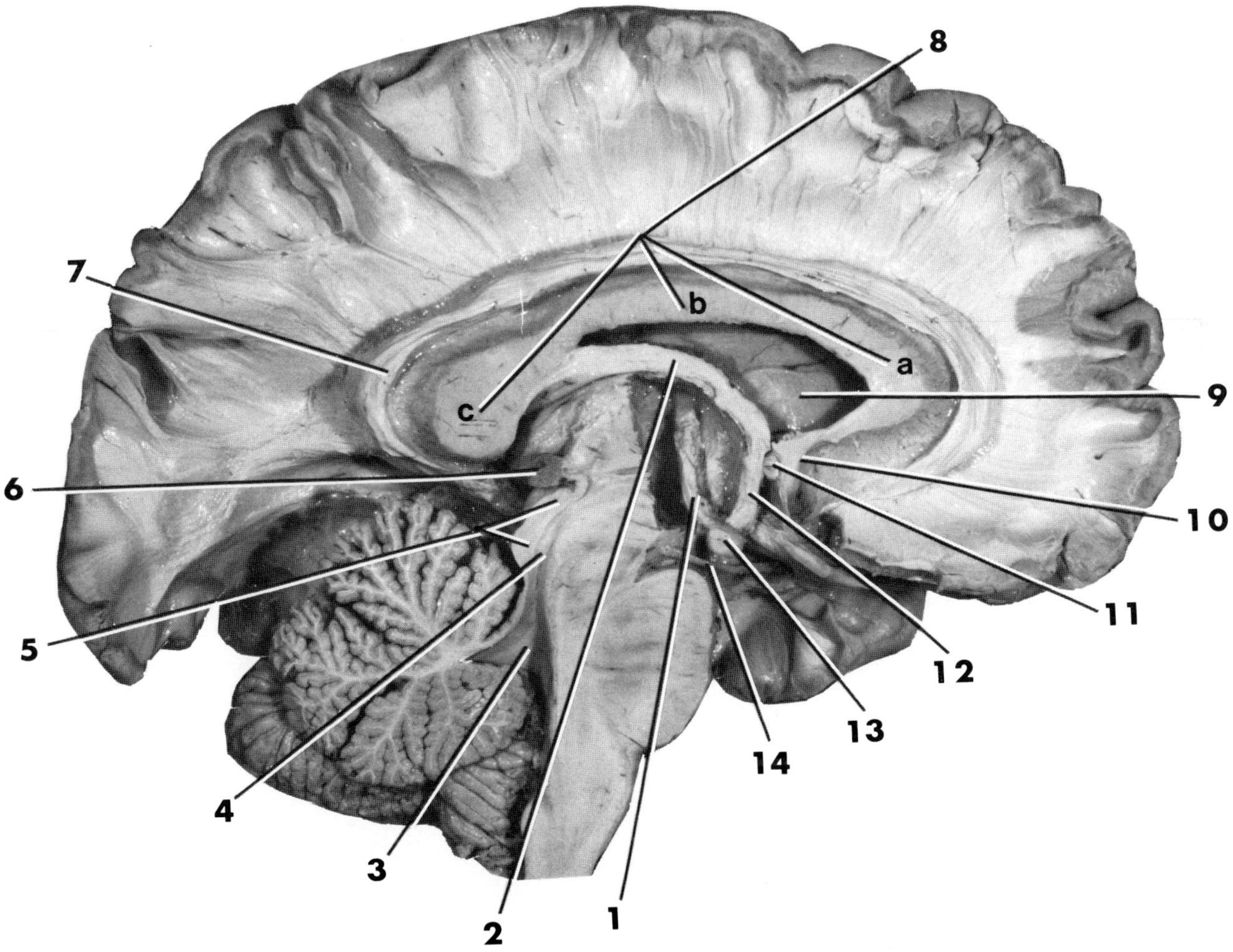

Figure 32 Dissection of the medial surface of the left half of the brain, showing the **fiber bundles of the limbic system**: the cingulate fasciculus superior to the corpus callosum, and the column of the fornix and mammillothalamic tract coursing through the diencephalon.

1. **IVth Ventricle**—located between the cerebellum, the pons, and the medulla. Note its tent-shaped roof.
2. **Cerebral Aqueduct (of Sylvius)**—courses through the midbrain, connecting the IIIrd and IVth ventricles.
3. **Colliculi (Corpora Quadrigemina)**—composed of left and right superior and inferior colliculi (L. *colliculus*, a small elevation or mound) (see also no. **10a** and **b**, Fig. 37*A* and no. **10**, Fig. 4*B*).
4. **Pineal Body** (L. *pineus*, relating to the pine)—part of the epithalamus. Pine cone-shaped gland attached to the diencephalon by the pineal stalk.
5. **Pulvinar of Thalamus**—the caudal thalamus projects posteriorly, forming a cushion-like prominence which overhangs the midbrain. The Latin word *pulvinus* means a cushion.
6. **Mammillothalamic Tract (Fasciculus)**—courses through the thalamus and the hypothalamus. It is part of the limbic system connecting the mammillary body with the anterior thalamic nucleus (see also no. **1**, Fig. 22).
7. **Cingulate Fasciculus**—consists of long association reciprocal fibers, connecting much of the limbic cortex on the medial surface of the frontal, parietal, and occipital lobes with the limbic cortex on the inferior and medial surfaces of the temporal lobe (see also no. **8**, Fig. 22).
8. **Body of Fornix** (L. arch)—efferent tract of the hippocampus which adheres to the inferior surface of the corpus callosum (see also no. **2**, Fig. 22 and no. **2**, Fig. 32).
9. **Corpus Callosum (Midline Cut)**—Names are assigned to the regions of the body of this large commissure. The enlarged posterior portion of the body is called the splenium (Gr. *splenion*, bandage). The anterior portion or genu thins out to form the rostrum (L. beak). Note that the fibers of the cingulate fasciculus parallel the contour of the corpus callosum. The septum pellucidum, which is attached to the fornix and the inferior surface of the corpus callosum, has been removed to show the head of the caudate nucleus in the anterior horn of the lateral ventricle.
10. **Anterior Commissure**—located in the lamina terminalis (no. **10**, Fig. 32), anterior to the column of the fornix (**11**).
11. **Column of Fornix**—the body of the fornix (**8**) divides into two columns, each of which curves ventrally through the hypothalamus to reach the mammillary body (**13**) (see also no. **12**, Fig. 32).
12. **Optic Chiasma**—the point of crossing or decussation of the optic nerve fibers. *Chiasma* is a Greek word meaning two crossing lines.
13. **Mammillary Body**—one of two small swellings on the basal surface of the hypothalamus (see also no. **15**, Fig. 22).
14. **Oculomotor Nerve (C.N. III)**—(see also no. **11**, Fig. 38).

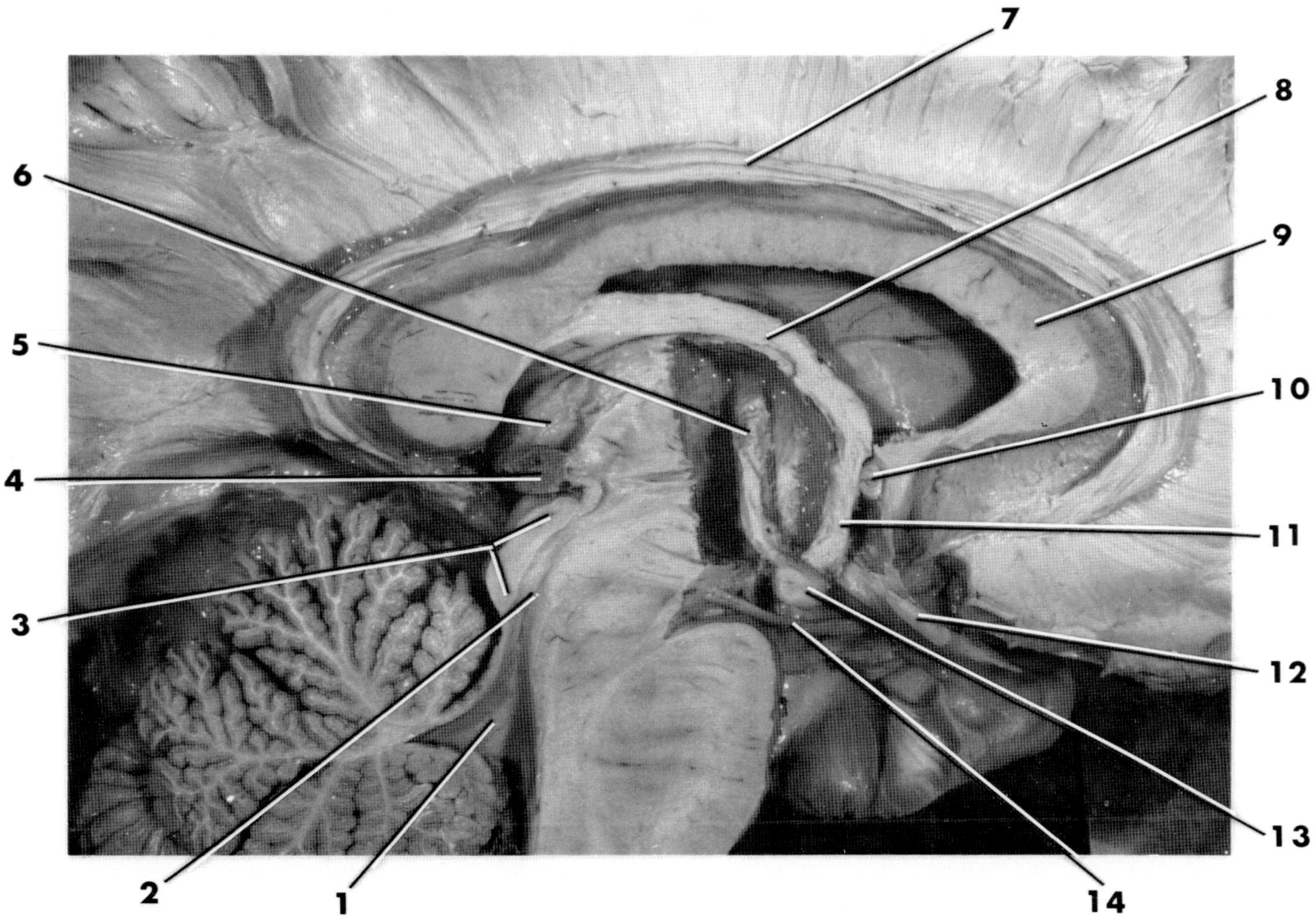

Figure 33 Midsagittal cut through the inferior area of the right cerebral hemisphere, diencephalon, and rostral part of the brain stem. The medial surface has been dissected to show the **components and tracts of the limbic system**.

1. **Hippocampus** (Gr. *hippocampus*, seahorse)—an important limbic structure produced by infolding of the cortex from the parahippocampal gyrus to form an elevation in the floor and medial wall of the inferior horn of the lateral ventricle (see also no. **2**, Fig. 35).
2. **Inferior Horn of Lateral Ventricle**—extends rostrally in the medial part of the temporal lobe from the collateral trigone. The hippocampus is located in the floor and the tail of the caudate nucleus, and the striae terminalis are located in the roof of the inferior horn (see also no. **1**, Fig. 28).
3. **Bulb of Posterior Horn**—a prominent bulge on the medial wall of the posterior horn, formed by commissural fibers in the forceps major.
4. **Geniculocalcarine Tract (Optic Radiation)**—the long projection fibers from the lateral geniculate body to the visual cortex surrounding the calcarine sulcus were removed rostrally to expose part of the posterior and inferior horns of the lateral ventricle.
5. **Posterior Horn of Lateral Ventricle**—begins at the expanded posterior part of the body of the lateral ventricle, known as the collateral trigone of the lateral ventricle, and extends a variable distance posteriorly into the occipital lobe (see also no. **1**, Fig. 30).
6. **Fimbria of the Hippocampus**—fibers originating in the hippocampus proceed posteriorly as the fimbria of the hippocampus which constitutes the crus of the fornix beneath the splenium of the corpus callosum.
7. **Cut Fibers of Corpus Callosum**—a longitudinal portion of the body of the corpus callosum, consisting of a compact mass of commissural fibers which formed the roof of the body of the lateral ventricle, was cut and removed. Note that the fibers of the fimbria (**6**) form the crus fornix which curves around the pulvinar of the thalamus onto the dorsal surface of the thalamus.
8. **Internal Capsule (Cut Surface)**—the projection fibers that converged in the corona radiata to course inferiorly and medially to the lentiform nucleus as the internal capsule, were cut and removed. This exposed the lateral ventricle as these fibers formed its lateral wall.
9. **External Capsule**—thin layer of white matter composed of projecting, commissural, and association fibers. It is located lateral to the lentiform nucleus (see also no. **7**, Fig. 13).
10. **Inferior Occipitofrontal Fasciculus**—composed of long reciprocal association fibers connecting the cortex of the lateral surface of the occipital lobe with the cortex of the inferior and lateral surfaces of the frontal lobe and vice versa.
11. **Uncinate Fasciculus**—hook-like bundle of long reciprocal association fibers connecting the cortex of the frontal lobe with the temporal lobe (see also no. **7**, Fig. 15).

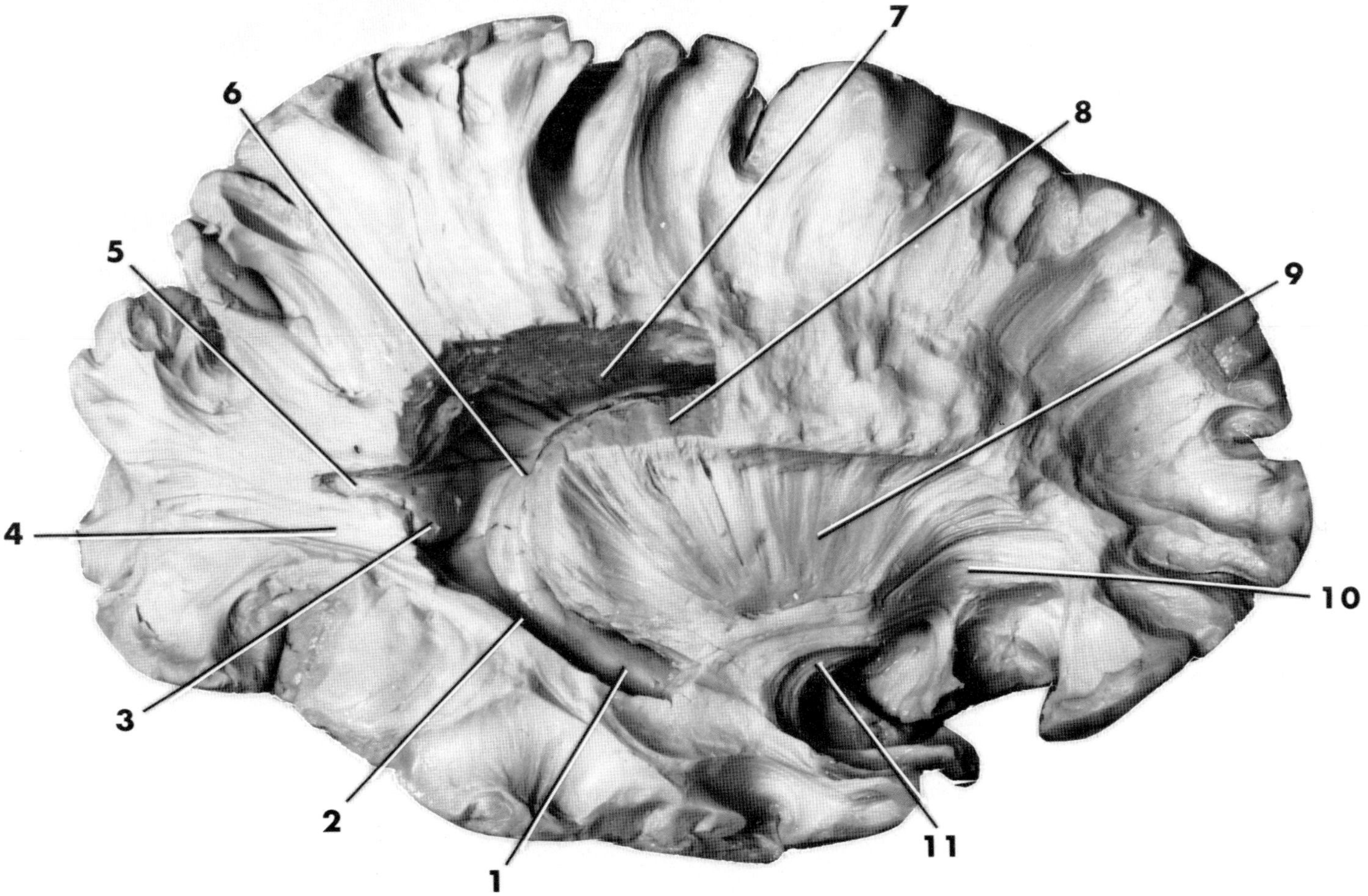

Figure 34 Lateral view of the inferior horn and the body of the lateral ventricle to show the **hippocampus, the fimbria, and the crux fornix of the limbic system.** To illustrate this, much of the medullary center was dissected, and the lateral wall of this portion of the lateral ventricle was removed.

1. **Superior Cerebellar Peduncle**—consists of fibers coursing from the dentate, emboliform, and globose cerebellar nuclei into the tegmentum of the midbrain where they decussate enroute to the red nucleus and ventral lateral nucleus of the thalamus (see also no. **4**, Fig. 55).
2. **Hippocampus** (Gr. *hippocampus*, seahorse)—the lateral wall of the inferior horn of the lateral ventricle has been removed. This gyrus forms an important part of the limbic system. It produces an elevation in the inferomedial wall of the inferior horn of the lateral ventricle (see also no. **1**, Fig. 34).
3. **Pulvinar of Thalamus**—the projecting posterior part of the thalamus, formed by the posterior nuclei of the lateral thalamus. Fibers of the fornix and the stria terminalis and the terminal vein course around it from the inferior horn to the body of the lateral ventricle.
4. **Crus Fornix**—fibers emerge from the hippocampus (**2**) as the fimbria and then arch over the pulvinar of the thalamus as the crus onto the dorsomedial surface of the thalamus to form the body of the fornix (**6**) (see also no. **6**, Fig. 34).
5. **Tail of Caudate Nucleus**—extends from the head of the caudate nucleus to the amygdaloid nucleus. In the floor of the body of the lateral ventricle, it is located on the dorsolateral surface of the thalamus, medial to the internal capsule.
6. **Body of the Fornix**—fibers from the hippocampus form the fimbria which converge and curve over the pulvinar of the thalamus as the crus (**4**). This robust bundle of fibers joins with fibers from the opposite crus in the dorsomedial surface of the thalamus to form the body of the fornix, which largely conceals that part of the thalamus (see also no. **8**, Fig. 33).
7. **Anterior Tubercle of the Thalamus (Anterior Nucleus)**—the anterior pole of the thalamus is situated dorsal and posterior to the interventricular foramen. It is an important nucleus of the limbic system which has reciprocal connections with the mammillary bodies and the cingulate cortex.
8. **Head of Caudate Nucleus**—bulges into the floor and the lateral wall of the anterior horn of the lateral ventricle. It is an important extrapyramidal nuclear area and is part of the corpus striatum.
9. **Column of Fornix**—fibers from the body of the fornix (**6**) arch over the anterior pole of the thalamus anterior to the interventricular foramen and pass inferiorly into the hypothalamus as two columns to end in the mammillary bodies (see also no. **11**, Fig. 33).
10. **Terminal Vein (Vena Terminalis)**—courses on the dorsolateral surface of the thalamus medial to the tail of the caudate nucleus. It drains the caudate nucleus, the thalamus, the internal capsule, and other structures (see also no. **8**, Fig. 30).
11. **Thalamus (Dorsal Surface)**—forms the floor of the body of the lateral ventricle. Medially it is largely concealed by fibers of the fornix. Laterally the stria terminalis (**12**), the terminal vein (**10**), and the tail of the caudate nucleus (**5**) lie next to the internal capsule which forms the lateral wall of the thalamus.
12. **Stria Terminalis**—a slender bundle of fibers that originates in the amygdaloid nucleus and courses in the roof of the inferior horn of the lateral ventricle around the pulvinar and onto the dorsolateral surface of the thalamus. In the floor of the body of the lateral ventricle, this stria lies medial to the terminal vein which is medial to the tail of the caudate nucleus. Fibers of the stria terminalis end in the anterior portion of the hypothalamus (see also no. **9**, Fig. 30).
13. **Transverse Fissure (Anterior Portion)**—this triangular space is bounded by the fornices as they converge and pass forward between the thalamus and the corpus callosum. It contains vascular connective tissue which blends with the coverings (removed) and choroid plexus in the roof of the third ventricle.
14. **Tectum of Midbrain**—consists of the left and right superior and inferior colliculi that are collectively called the corpora quadrigemina.
15. **Middle Cerebellar Peduncle**—consists of a large compact bundle of pontocerebellar fibers that extend from the contralateral side of the basal pons to the cortex of the cerebellar hemisphere.

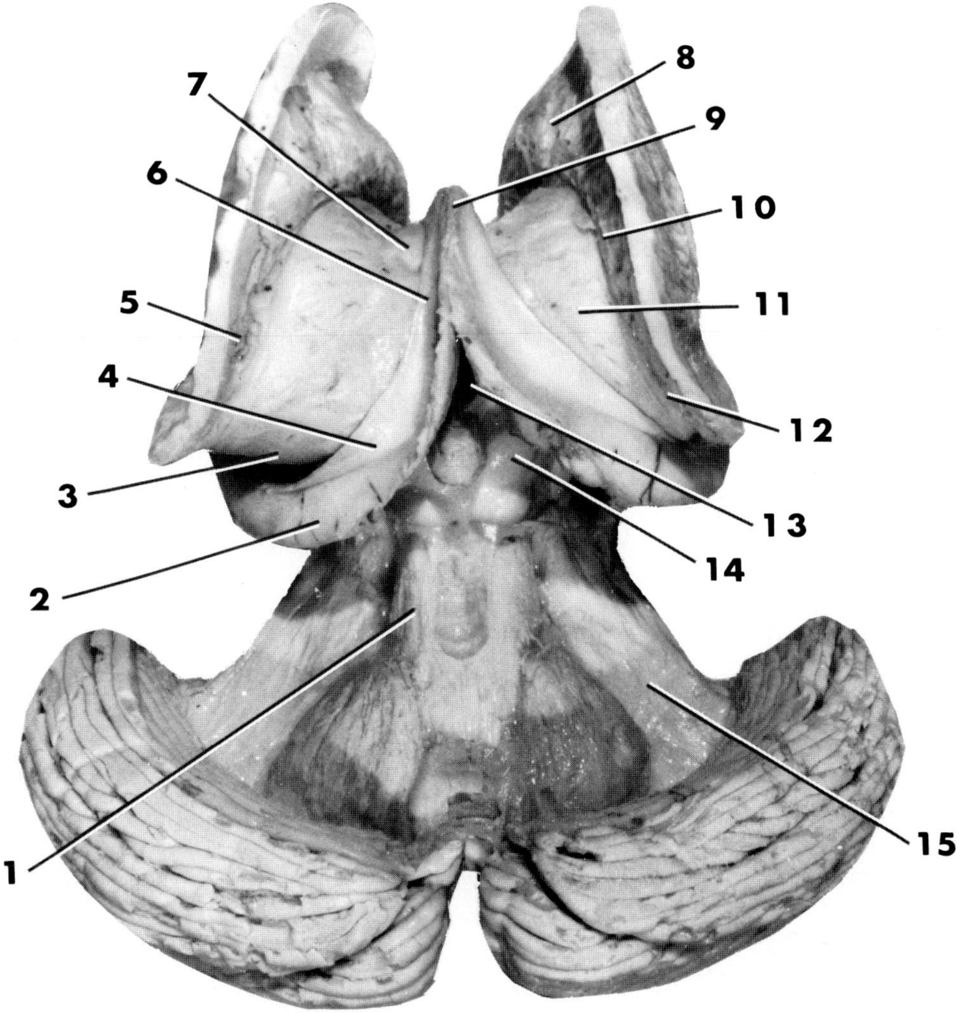

Figure 35 Dorsal view of the diencephalon, the caudate nucleus, and the midbrain showing **the relationship of some components of the limbic system** (hippocampus, fornices, and stria terminalis) with the thalamus. Most of the cerebral hemispheres was removed to show the caudate nucleus and the internal capsule. The dorsal aspect of the cerebellum was also dissected away to show the dentate nucleus and the superior cerebellar peduncle.

6

The Brain Stem and Cranial Nerves

The Brain Stem (Figs. 36 to 44)

1. **Clava (Nucleus Gracilis)**—the clava (L. club) is a club-shaped swelling on the dorsal surface of the caudal part of the medulla produced by the nucleus gracilis (see also no. **4**, Fig. 37*A*).
2. **Cuneate Tubercle (Nucleus Cuneatus)**—a wedge-shaped swelling (L. *cuneus*, wedge) produced by the nucleus cuneatus in the medulla (see also no. **12**, Fig. 37*A*).
3. **Middle Cerebellar Peduncle (Brachium Pontis)**—largest of the three cerebellar peduncles. It carries fibers from the nuclei pontis of the opposite side.
4. **Colliculi (Corpora Quadrigemina)**—composed of two superior and two inferior colliculi.
5. **Pulvinar of Thalamus**—posterior projection of the thalamus formed by the posterior nuclei of the lateral thalamus.
6. **Dorsolateral Surface of Thalamus**—the thalamus makes up about four-fifths of the diencephalon.
7. **Corpus Striatum**—composed of the putamen of the lentiform nucleus (**a**), the anterior limb of the internal capsule (**b**), and the head of the caudate nucleus (**c**). Inferiorly the head of the caudate nucleus and the lentiform nucleus form a continuous mass of gray matter (see also no. **7**, Fig. 16*B*).
   a. **Lentiform Nucleus (Putamen)**—the (lentiform) lenticular nucleus consists of the globus pallidus and the putamen. The globus pallidus (L. pale body) forms the medial portion of the lentiform nucleus.
   b. **Internal Capsule (Anterior Limb)**—compact band of projection fibers partially separating the caudate nucleus (**c**) and the putamen (**a**).
   c. **Head of Caudate Nucleus**—enlarged anterior portion of the caudate nucleus lying rostral to the thalamus, and bulging into the anterior horn of the lateral ventricle.
8. **Column of Fornix**—the body of the fornix (**10**) separates into two columns, each of which curves ventrally and runs forward in the wall of the temporal horn.
9. **Thalamic Tubercle (Anterior Thalamic Nucleus)**—cone-shaped mass or tubercle formed by a group of nerve cells which is called a nucleus in neurological terminology.
10. **Body of Fornix**—the crura of the fornix converge to form the body of the fornix (L. arch). This part of the fornix lies on the floor of the body of the lateral ventricle (see also no. **8**, Fig. 33).
11. **Crus Fornix**—the crura (L. legs) of the fornix (L. arch) arch over the thalamus and join to form the body of the fornix (see also no. **4**, Fig. 35).
12. **Hippocampus**—the hippocampal gyrus constitutes an important part of the limbic system.
13. **Inferior Brachium**—connecting the inferior colliculus with the medial geniculate body (part of the auditory pathway).
14. **Superior Cerebellar Peduncle (Brachium Conjunctivum)**—consists mainly of cerebellar efferent fibers passing rostrally.
15. **Medial Eminence**—located in the floor of the IVth ventricle. It contains the medial longitudinal fasciculus and some motor nuclei of the cranial nerves (see also no. **11**, Fig. 37*B*).

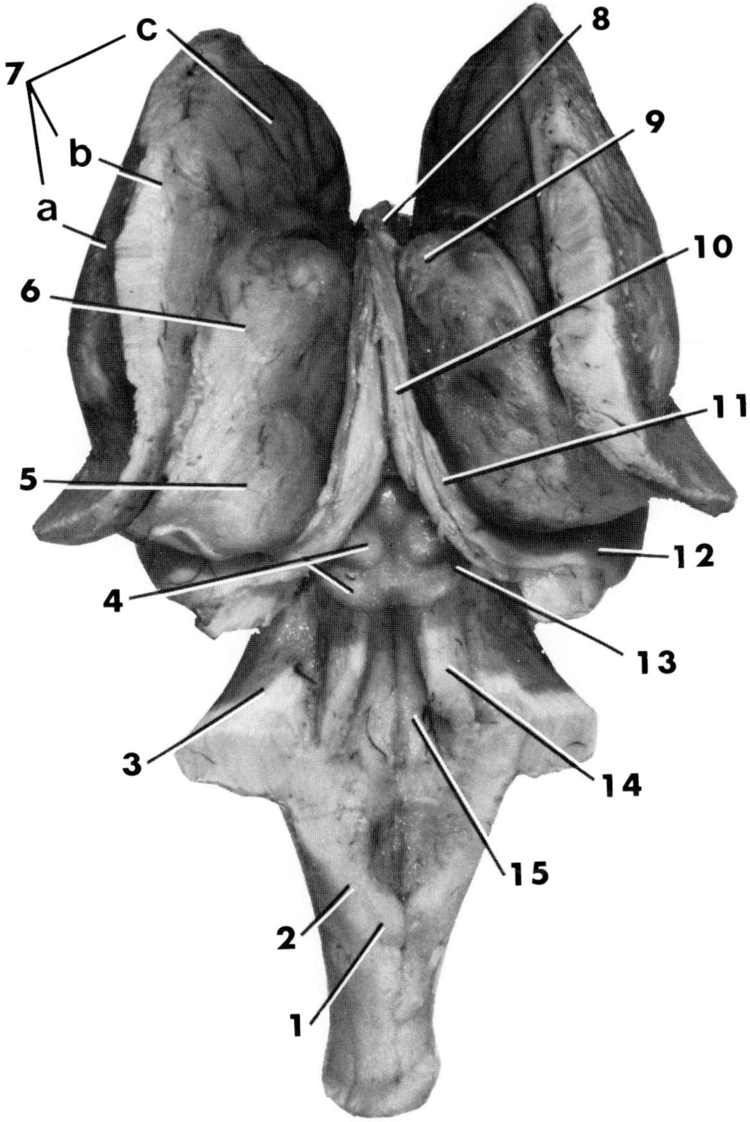

Figure 36 Dorsal view of the brain stem, diencephalon, and corpus striatum. The cerebellum has been removed by transecting the cerebellar peduncles to show the **features on the floor of the fourth ventricle.**

1. **Fasciculus Gracilis**—this uncrossed tract extends the entire length of the spinal cord and ends in the nucleus gracilis. It is composed of axons from the spinal (dorsal root) ganglia (T6 through S5).
2. **Dorsal Median Sulcus**—a furrow on the dorsal surface of the spinal cord that extends into the caudal medulla. It separates the left dorsal column of white matter from the right column of white matter.
3. **Dorsal Intermediate Sulcus**—it is located between the dorsal median sulcus (**2**) and the dorsolateral sulcus (**14**). It separates the fasciculus gracilis (**1**) from the fasciculus cuneatus (**13**).
4. **Clava (Nucleus Gracilis)**—the clava (L. club) is a club-shaped swelling on the dorsal surface of the caudal (closed) part of the medulla produced by the nucleus gracilis (see also no. **1**, Fig. 36).
5. **Middle Cerebellar Peduncle (Brachium Pontis)**—the largest of the three cerebellar peduncles, it consists of fibers from the nuclei pontis of the opposite side.
6. **Median Sulcus**—courses the length of the floor of the fourth ventricle, and divides the floor into two symmetrical halves. On each side is the median eminence.
7. **Inferior Brachium**—part of the auditory pathway that connects the inferior collicular nucleus with the medial geniculate nucleus.
8. **Pulvinar of Thalamus**—the posterior projection of the thalamus formed by its posterior nuclei. The metathalamus (medial and lateral geniculate bodies) lies inferior to the pulvinar (see also no. **5**, Fig. 36).
9. **Medial Geniculate Body**—this nuclear relay area of the auditory system receives connections from the nucleus of the inferior colliculus. Fibers from the medial geniculate nucleus pass to the auditory cortex of the transverse temporal gyrus.
10. **Tectum** (L. roof)—consists of four rounded elevations, the corpora quadrigemina. The paired superior colliculi (**a**) and the inferior colliculi (**b**) function in the visual and auditory pathways, respectively (see also no. **4**, Fig. 36).
11. **Inferior Cerebellar Peduncle**—is on the medial aspect of the middle cerebellar peduncle. Fibers from the spinal cord and the brain stem enter the cerebellum from the caudal part of the pons. It helps to form the lateral wall of the fourth ventricle.
12. **Cuneate Tubercle (Nucleus Cuneatus)**—a wedge-shaped swelling (L. *cuneus*, wedge) produced by the nucleus cuneatus in the medulla.
13. **Fasciculus Cuneatus**—consists of heavily myelinated axons of neurons from the spinal (dorsal root) ganglia (from C1 to T5). This uncrossed tract is located in the superior half of the dorsal white column and ends on the nucleus cuneatus in the caudal medulla.
14. **Dorsolateral Sulcus**—a shallow groove on the dorsolateral side of the spinal cord that extends into the medulla. It marks the line of entry of the dorsal root fibers.

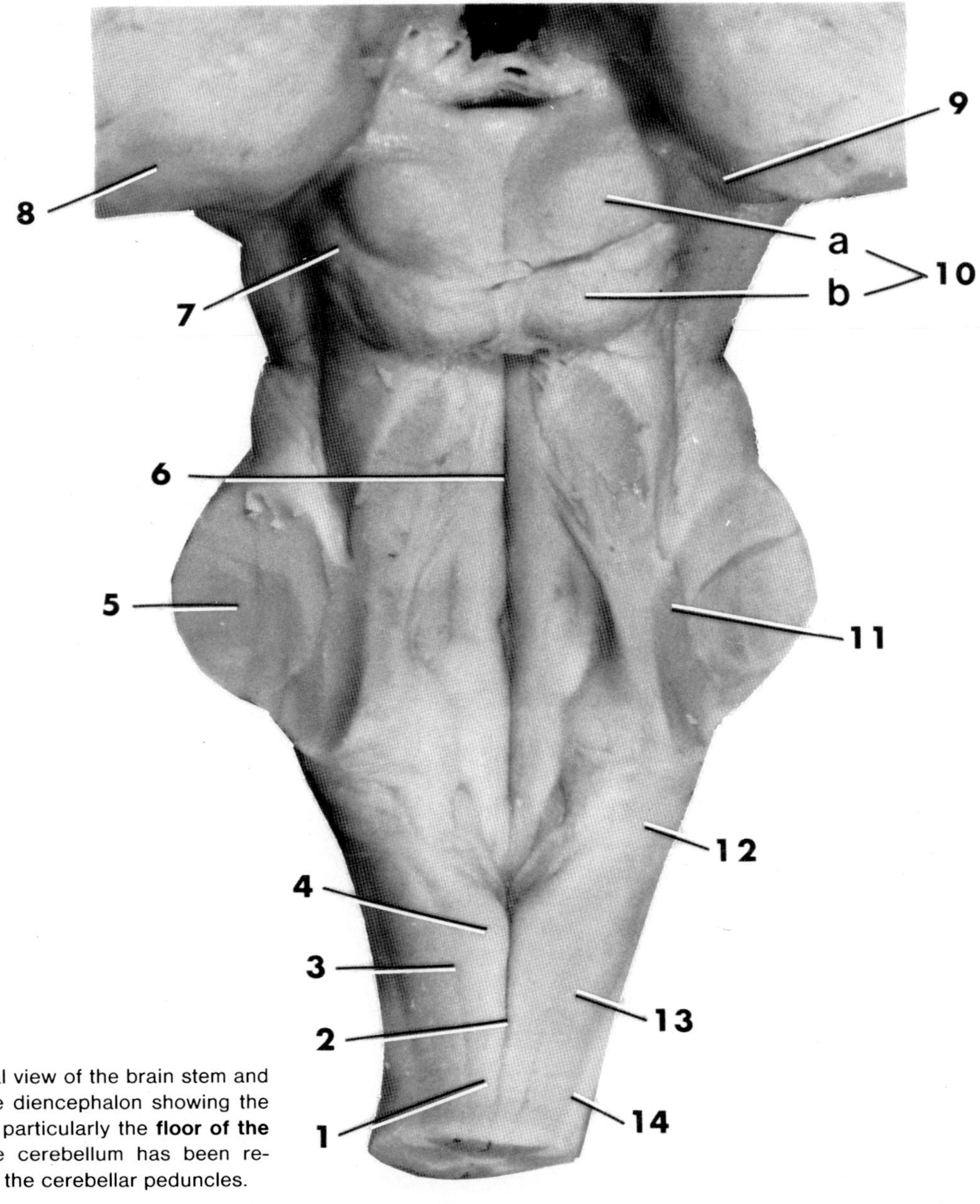

Figure 37 *A*. Dorsal view of the brain stem and the caudal end of the diencephalon showing the features of this area, particularly the **floor of the fourth ventricle.** The cerebellum has been removed by transecting the cerebellar peduncles.

1. **Hypoglossal Triangle**—situated on each side of the median sulcus (no. **6**, Fig. 37*A*) in the caudal end of the floor of the fourth ventricle. The vagal triangle (**13**) lies immediately lateral to it. The rostral end of the hypoglossal nucleus lies beneath this triangle.
2. **Dorsal Cochlear Nucleus**—lies on the restiform body, at the base of the inferior cerebellar peduncle, in the region of the lateral aperture (recess connecting the fourth ventricle with subarachnoid space).
3. **Vestibular Area**—lies beneath most of the lateral area of the fourth ventricle (lateral to the sulcus limitans, **12**). It consists of four vestibular nuclei (medial, lateral, superior, and inferior).
4. **Facial Colliculus**—a slight swelling of the median eminence near the caudal end of the pons. It is formed by fibers of the facial nerve looping over the abducens nucleus.
5. **Superior Cerebellar Peduncle**—consists mainly of cerebellar efferent fibers from the dentate nucleus which pass rostrally to decussate in the midbrain en route to the ventral lateral nucleus of the thalamus (see also no. **14**, Fig. 36).
6. **Superior Brachium**—functions in the visual pathways. It contains fibers from the retina and the cortex of the occipital lobe proceeding to the superior colliculus.
7. **Habenular Trigone**—part of the epithalamus. It is the small triangular area on each side of the roof of the third ventricle, just anterior to the midbrain. It contains the habenular nucleus.
8. **Habenular Commissure**—contained in the dorsal wall of the pineal stalk and consists of fibers of the stria medullaris thalami (olfactory function) that terminate in the opposite habenular nucleus. Note that the pineal body has been removed and that its recess (**9**) is showing.
9. **Pineal Recess**—part of the posterior area of the third ventricle that extends into the stalk of the pineal body (removed). The habenular and posterior commissures lie superior and inferior to this recess.
10. **Lateral Lemniscus**—part of the auditory pathway. It is located in the lateral wall of the midbrain tegmentum. The fibers of this tract originate in the cochlear and the superior olivary nuclei and end in the nucleus of the inferior colliculus.
11. **Median Eminence**—lies adjacent to the median sulcus and is separated from the vestibular area (**3**) by the sulcus limitans (**12**). The medial longitudinal fasciculus is contained in this elevated area (see also no. **15**, Fig. 36).
12. **Sulcus Limitans**—divides each half of the floor of the fourth ventricle into medial and lateral areas. It is an embryological remnant that divided each side of the neural tube into alar and basal plates.
13. **Vagal Triangle (Ala Cinerea)**—located in the caudal end of the floor of the fourth ventricle, lateral to the hypoglossal triangle (**1**). The rostral end of the dorsal vagal nucleus lies beneath it.
14. **Obex** (L. barrier)—the apex of the V-shaped boundary of the caudal portion of the fourth ventricle. At this region a small transverse fold (removed) overhangs the opening of the fourth ventricle into the central canal of the closed portion of the medulla.

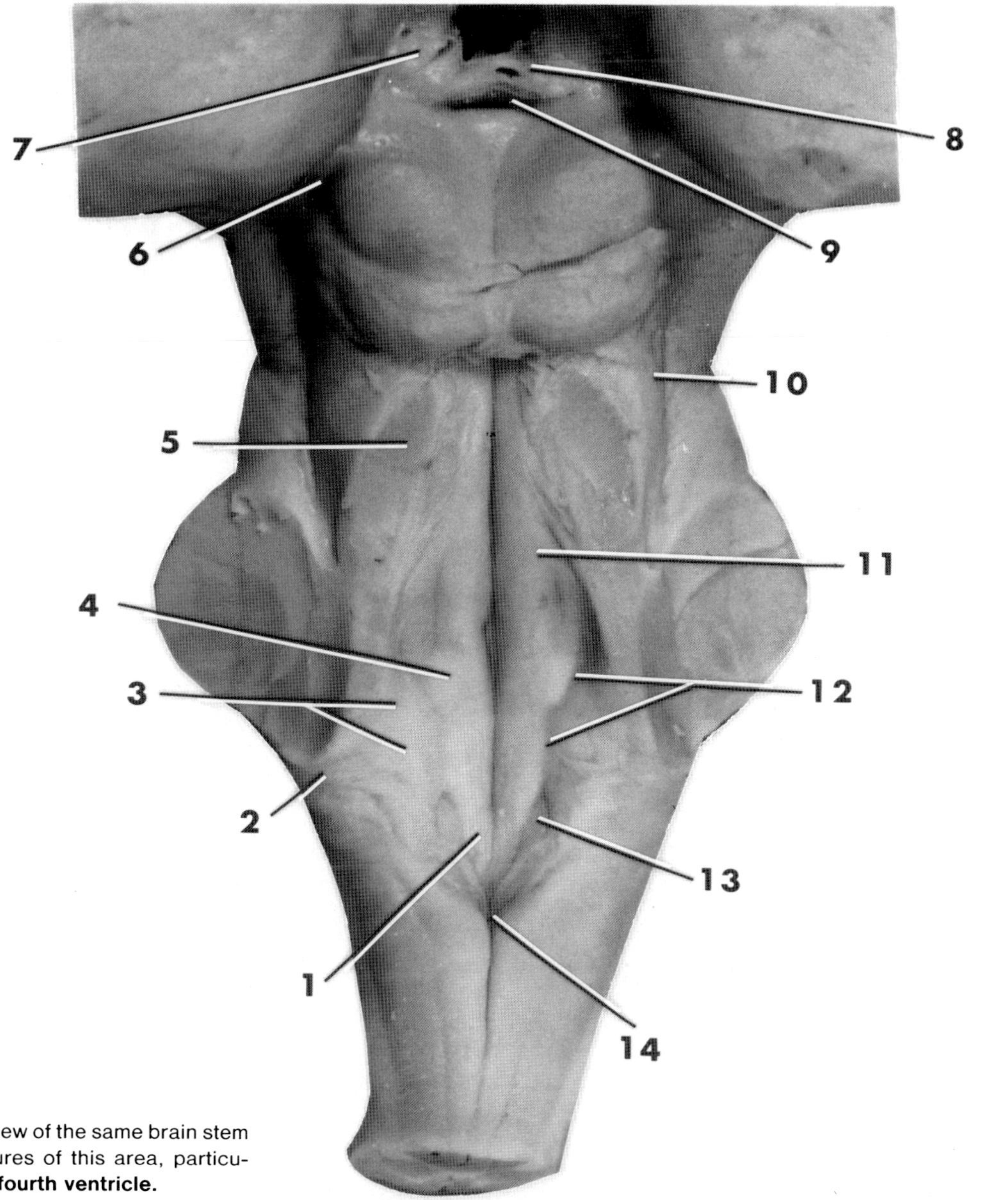

Figure 37 *B*. Dorsal view of the same brain stem showing additional features of this area, particularly on the **floor of the fourth ventricle.**

1. **Hypoglossal Nerve (C.N. XII)**—emerges between the pyramid (**16**) and the olive (**2**).
2. **Olive**—located between the pyramid (**16**) and the dorsolateral sulcus. It contains the inferior olivary nucleus of the extrapyramidal motor system.
3. **Spinal Accessory Nerve (C.N. XI)**—the cranial root fibers of this nerve emerge with C.N. IX (**15**) and C.N. X (**4**) between the olive (**2**) and the tuberculum cinereum.
4. **Vagus Nerve (C.N. X)**—emerges with C.N. IX (**15**) and C.N. XI (**3**).
5. **Abducens Nerve (C.N. VI)**—emerges from the anteroinferior border of the pons.
6. **Middle Cerebellar Peduncle (Brachium Pontis)**—the transverse pontocerebellar fibers from the basal pons course laterally and posteriorly into the cerebellum. This compact bundle of fibers is the middle cerebellar peduncle.
7. **Basal Pons (L. bridge)**—the distinct rostral and caudal border of the pons demarcate it from the midbrain and medulla. The axons of pontine neurons in the basal pons course to the contralateral side in a transverse direction, then posteriorly and laterally into the cerebellar hemispheres. Note that groups of these fibers make transverse ridges on the basal pons.
8. **Basis Pedunculi (Crus Cerebri)**—the ventral part of the cerebral peduncle of the midbrain. It is separated from the dorsal tegmental portion by the substantia nigra (see no. **13**, Fig. 43).
9. **Interpeduncular Fossa**—the deep space between the left and right basis pedunculi is the interpeduncular fossa. Many small blood vessels penetrate the floor of this fossa which is known as the posterior perforated substance.
10. **Corticospinal, Corticobulbar, and Corticopontine Fibers**—constitute the basis pedunculi. The corticospinal and corticobulbar tracts, as they pass through the basis pedunculi, occupy the middle three-fifths and the corticopontine fibers, the medial and lateral one-fifth of the peduncle (see nos. **1** to **3**, Fig. 44).
11. **Oculomotor Nerve (C.N. III)**—emerges at the rostral border of the pons in the interpeduncular fossa.
12. **Trigeminal Nerve (C.N. V)**—sensory fibers enter at the junction of the basal pons and the middle cerebellar peduncle.
13. **Facial Nerve (C.N. VII)**—fibers enter and emerge with C.N. VIII at the caudal border of the pons on the lateral side of the brain stem.
14. **Vestibulocochlear Nerve (C.N. VIII)**—enters with C.N. VII. Consists of vestibular and cochlear (auditory) parts.
15. **Glossopharyngeal Nerve (C.N. IX)**—emerges with C.N. X (**4**) and C.N. XI (**3**) in the dorsolateral sulcus superior to the olive.
16. **Pyramid**—occupies the ventral area on each side of the medulla between the ventral median fissure and the ventrolateral sulcus. It consists of corticospinal fibers of the pyramidal tract pathway.
17. **Decussation of Pyramids**—at the caudal end of the medulla, approximately 85% of the corticospinal fibers in each pyramid cross the midline in the ventral median fissure to the contralateral column of white matter in the spinal cord. The fibers from each side interdigitate at this level (see no. **9d**, Fig. 39).

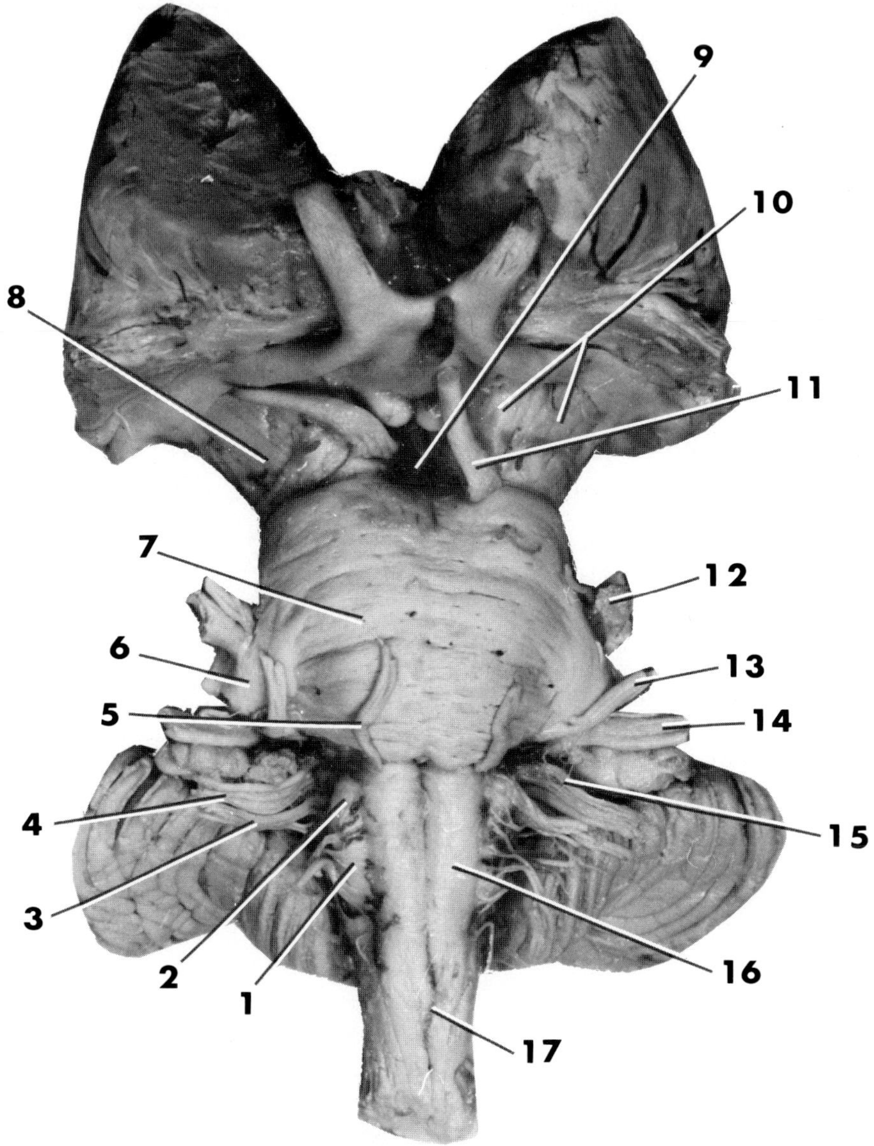

Figure 38 Ventral view of the brain stem with the attached cerebellum and the corpus striatum. It shows some of the features of the ventral brain stem and the location of the emergence (or entrance) of some of the **cranial nerves.**

1. **Medulla Oblongata**—located in the posterior cranial fossa. As the spinal cord passes through the foramen magnum it expands into a wedge-shaped structure called the medulla (medulla oblongata), which is the caudal portion of the brain stem. Part of the pyramidal pathway (**9c** and **d**) is shown on the ventral aspect of the dissected medulla.
2. **Olive**—an oval swelling formed by the inferior olivary nucleus on the ventrolateral surface of the medulla. The olive lies lateral to the pyramid and the fibers of the C.N. XII emerge between the pyramid and the olive.
3. **Right Cerebellar Hemisphere**—ventral surface of the posterior lobe of the right cerebellar hemisphere shows the many parallel folia. About 85% of the cortex is concealed.
4. **Flocculus** (right)—part of the flocculonodular lobe. Phylogenetically this is the oldest part of the cerebellum (called the archicerebellum). It functions for equilibrium (see also no. **10,** Fig. 21).
5. **Middle Cerebellar Peduncle (Beginning Portion)**—horizontal fibers (featured in **8**) in the basal part of the pons (**6**) coursing posteriorly and laterally to and from the cerebellar hemispheres via the middle cerebellar peduncles (see also no. **8,** Fig. 53).
6. **Basal Pons**—located in the posterior cranial fossa, the pons is the midportion of the brain stem (midbrain, pons, and medulla). Its basal (ventral) area is featured here and consists of descending tract fibers (**9b**), horizontal (pontocerebellar) fibers, and pontine nuclei.
7. **Midbrain (Basis Pedunculi)**—the cephalic end of the brain stem (midbrain, pons, and medulla) lies caudal to the diencephalon. Its basal area consists of the left and right cerebral peduncles and the interpeduncular fossa. The ventral area of the cerebral peduncle, called the basis pedunculi, is made up of descending cortical (motor) fibers that pass into the brain stem and the spinal cord.
8. **Pons (Deep Basal Area)**—much of the basal aspect of the pons has been dissected to show: (1) the horizontal fibers (axons of contralateral pontine neurons) that are identified as pontocerebellar fibers and course into the cerebellar hemispheres via the middle cerebellar peduncle; and (2) the descending bundles of pyramidal tract fibers (**9b**) that course uninterrupted into the medulla.
9. **Pyramidal Tract**—consists of corticospinal and corticobulbar tracts that course into and/or through the basal part of the brain stem and into the spinal cord. These fibers mainly originate in the motor cortex and descend into the cerebral medullary center as part of the corona radiata and the internal capsule. In the midbrain they form the central three-fifths of the basis pedunculi (**a**) and pass into and through the basal pons (**b**) and on into the pyramids of the medulla (**c**) as corticospinal fibers. At the caudal end of the medulla 85 to 90% of these fibers cross (decussate) in the anterior median fissure as the decussation of the pyramidal tract (**d**). These fibers descend into the lateral column of white matter of the spinal cord (**e**) as the lateral corticospinal tract. Throughout the brain stem the descending corticobulbar fibers, which are part of the pyramidal tract fibers (**a, b,** and **c**), leave this pathway and terminate on motor cranial nerve nuclei in the tegmental area of the brain stem (see also nos. **11** and **12,** Fig. 20 and no. **8,** Fig. 21).

Figure 39 Ventral aspect of the brain stem showing the position of **pyramidal tract fibers** in the midbrain, pons, and medulla. Parts of the basis pedunculi, basal portion of the pons, and the pyramids were dissected away to show the location and direction of these fibers.

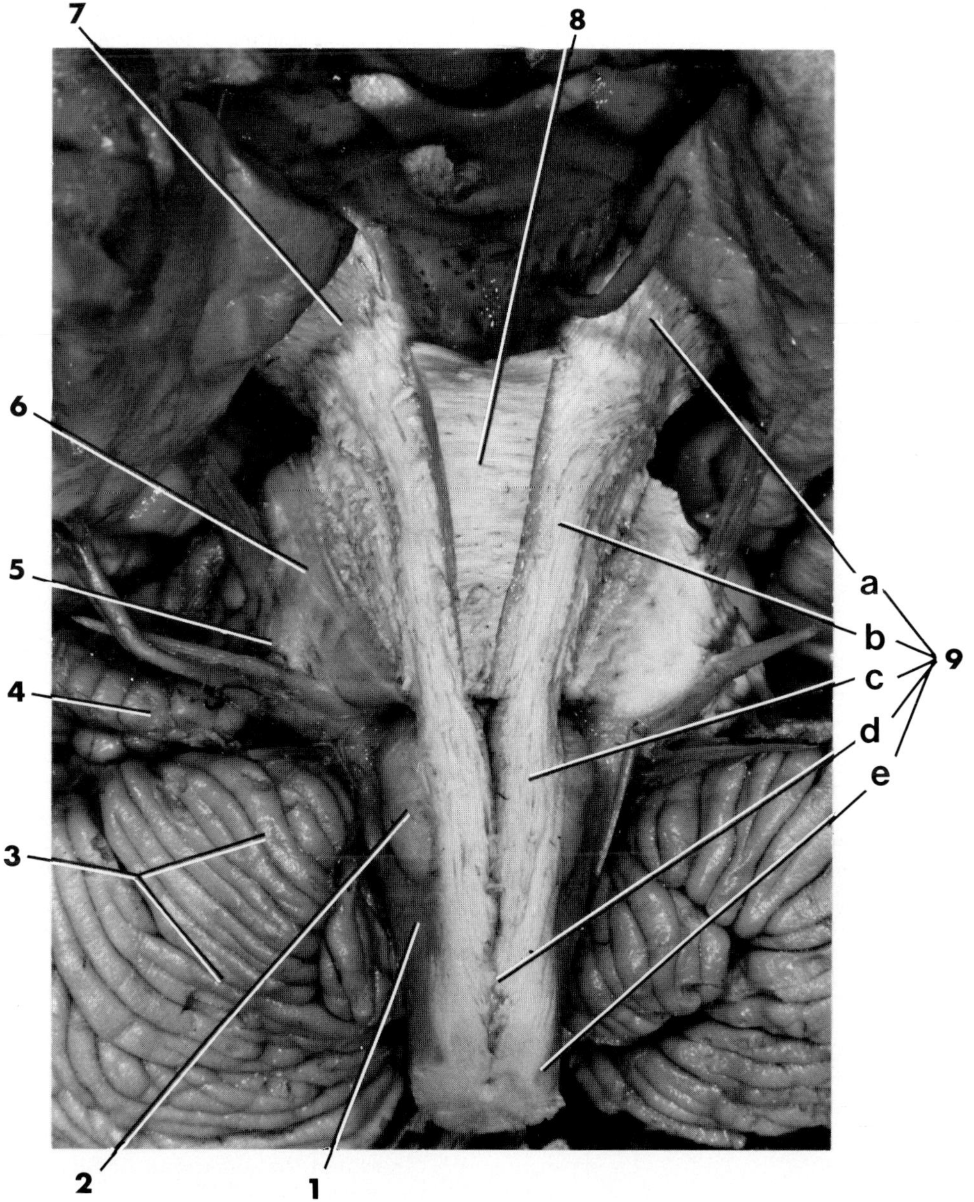

Figure 39

Medulla—Caudal Portion

1. **Pyramid**—cross-section of a bundle of corticospinal fibers on each side, located between the ventral median fissure and the ventrolateral sulcus. It is called a pyramid because of its shape on the surface of the brain stem.
2. **Decussation of Medial Lemniscus**—myelinated fibers from the nucleus gracilis (**9**) and the nucleus cuneatus (**10**) pursue a curved course to the median raphe as the internal arcuate fibers (**3**). They decussate (cross) in the midline and form right and left medial lemnisci.
3. **Internal Arcuate Fibers**—myelinated fibers from the nucleus gracilis (**9**) and the nucleus cuneatus (**10**) curve inferiorly and medially, where they decussate and form the medial lemnisci. These fibers conduct proprioceptive, discriminative touch, and vibration sense to the ventral posterolateral nucleus of the thalamus.
4. **Nucleus Ambiguus (Caudal Tip)**—an elongated oval nucleus situated dorsal to the inferior olivary complex (**14**). This nucleus supplies the muscles of the larynx, pharynx, and soft palate through the glossopharyngeal, the vagus, and the cranial root of the accessory cranial nerve.
5. **Dorsal Spinocerebellar Tract**—this uncrossed tract of the lateral white column of the spinal cord traverses the medulla in the periphery of the lateral area. Its fibers course to the cerebellar cortex via the restiform body of the inferior cerebellar peduncle.
6. **Spinal Tract of Trigeminal Nerve (C.N. V)**—many fibers from the trigeminal ganglion turn caudally on entering the pons to pass through the dorsolateral medulla and the rostral spinal cord as far as the third cervical segment. In the caudal medulla and rostral spinal cord, this tract is located between the fasciculus cuneatus and the dorsal spinocerebellar tract. The tract transmits pain, temperature, light touch, and pressure for the head region.
7. **Fasciculus Cuneatus**—the heavily myelinated dorsal root fibers from C1 through T5 occupy the lateral area of the dorsal white column of the rostral half of the spinal cord. They reach the nucleus cuneatus (**10**) *on the same side* in the dorsolateral area of the medulla. This tract is concerned with proprioception, discriminative touch, and vibration impulses from the upper trunk, upper limb, and neck regions.
8. **Fasciculus Gracilis**—the dorsal root fibers from T6 through S5 occupy the medial area of the dorsal white column of the spinal cord and extend into the dorsal area of the medulla to end on the nucleus gracilis (**9**). This uncrossed tract conducts the same sensory data as the fasciculus cuneatus, but from the lower limb and lower trunk.
9. **Nucleus Gracilis**—is present throughout the closed portion of the middorsal area of the medulla. Fibers from the fasciculus gracilis (**8**) terminate in this oblong-shaped nucleus which in turn gives rise to internal arcuate fibers that become the medial lemnisci.
10. **Nucleus Cuneatus**—is located lateral to the nucleus gracilis. This enlongated nucleus appears slightly rostral to the beginning of the nucleus gracilis and continues caudal to this nucleus in the dorsal area of the medulla. Fibers of the fasciculus cuneatus terminate in the nucleus cuneatus. Fibers from this nucleus and the nucleus gracilis form the internal arcuate fibers and the medial lemnisci.
11. **Nucleus of the Trigeminal Spinal Tract**—lies immediately medial to the spinal tract of the trigeminal nerve (**6**). It extends from the caudal portion of the pons through to the third cervical segment of the spinal cord. Fibers from this nucleus give rise to the trigeminothalamic tract which terminates in the contralateral posteroventral medial thalamic nucleus. It is a relay pathway for pain, temperature, and touch sensations for the head region.
12. **Dorsal Nucleus of the Vagus Nerve (Caudal Tip)**—this large parasympathetic nucleus lies dorsolateral to the hypoglossal nucleus (**13**) and extends from the vagal trigone in the floor of the fourth ventricle caudally and into the gray matter surrounding the central canal of the spinal cord. It contains the cell bodies of preganglionic neurons for smooth muscle and gland tissue of thoracic and abdominal viscera, including the heart.
13. **Hypoglossal Nucleus (Caudal Tip)**—this elongated motor nucleus is located near the midline of the medulla. It is coextensive with the inferior olivary complex and extends from the hypoglossal trigone in the floor of the fourth ventricle down into the central gray matter in the closed part of the medulla. Its fibers innervate the muscles of the tongue.
14. **Inferior Olivary Nucleus**—situated within the olive (no. **2**, Fig. 38) in the ventrolateral area of the medulla. The medial lemniscus lies medial to it and the pyramids ventral to it. It receives sensory input from the spinal cord and its efferent fibers project to the contralateral cerebellum.

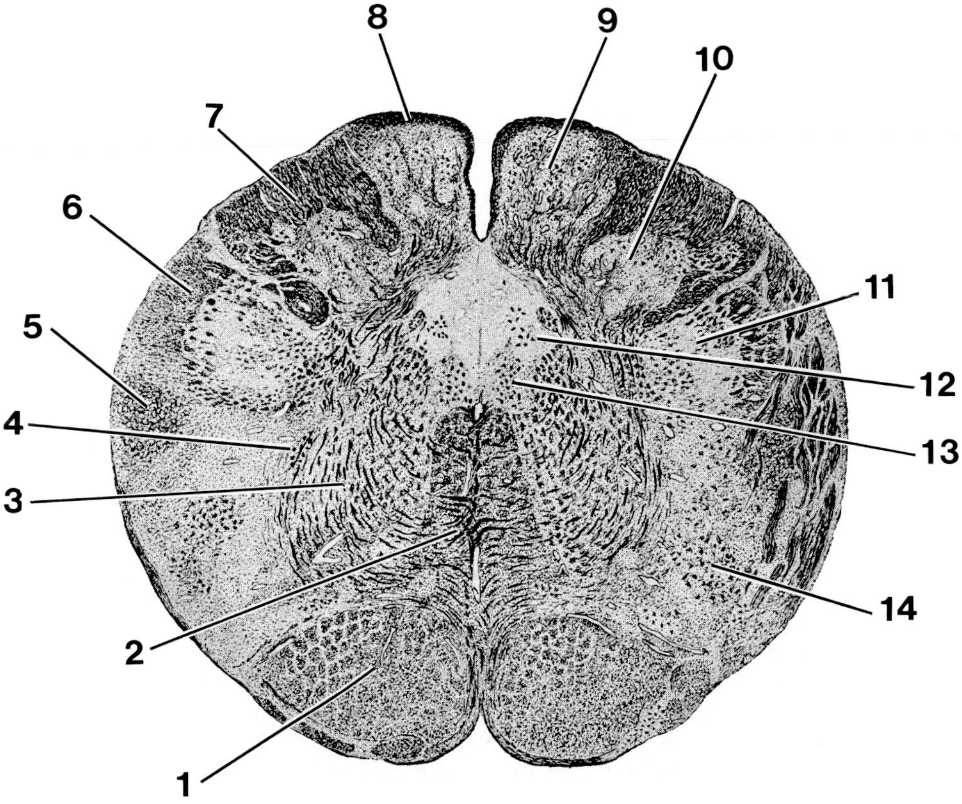

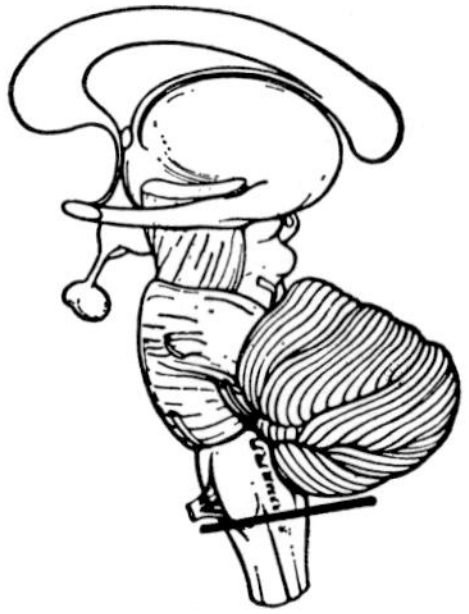

Figure 40 Modified photograph of a drawing of a transverse section of the medulla at the level of the decussation of the medial lemniscus showing some nuclear areas, fiber tracts, and the course of the internal arcuate fibers. ×8. (Modified from M. B. Carpenter: *Human Neuroanatomy*, 7th ed. Courtesy of Williams & Wilkins.)

Medulla—Open Portion

1. **Pyramid**—the pyramid-shaped area on the ventral surface of the medulla consists of corticospinal fibers. On each side it is located between the ventral median fissure and the ventrolateral sulcus. At the caudal end of the medulla, 85 to 90% of its fibers decussate in the ventral median fissure and cross into the lateral white column of the spinal cord on the opposite side (see also no. **1**, Fig. 40).
2. **Medial Lemniscus**—internal arcuate fibers from the nucleus gracilis and nucleus cuneatus decussate in the midline of the caudal portion of the medulla to form the medial lemnisci. In the medulla the medial lemniscus is a vertical column of fibers located on each side between the median raphe and the inferior olivary complex. These fibers conduct proprioceptive, discriminative touch, and vibration sensations to the ventral posterolateral nucleus of the thalamus.
3. **Nucleus Ambiguus**—this elongated motor nucleus is situated dorsal to the inferior olivary complex. Fibers from its rostral to caudal end give rise to the motor fibers of C.N. IX, C.N. X, and C.N. XI, which supply the muscles of the larynx, pharynx, and soft palate (see also no. **4**, Fig. 40).
4. **Vagus Nerve (C.N. X)**—fibers from the nucleus ambiguus (**3**) and the dorsal nucleus of the vagus nerve (**9**) emerge from the lateral side of the medulla, dorsal to the olive and the tuberculum cinereum (spinal tract and nucleus of the trigeminal nerve). The motor fibers supply most of the pharyngeal muscles, and the visceromotor fibers supply smooth muscles in the viscera of the thorax and abdomen.
5. **Spinal Tract and Nucleus of Trigeminal Nerve**—axons of neurons from the trigeminal sensory ganglion turn caudally upon entering the pons and pass through the dorsolateral caudal pons, medulla, and the rostral part of the spinal cord as far as the third cervical segment. Its fibers terminate in the spinal tract nucleus. These two structures create a ridge of tissue dorsal to the olive on the lateral surface of the medulla which is identified as the tuberculum cinereum. This tract and nucleus function in transmitting sensory data for pain, touch, and temperature from the head area to the thalamus and sensory cortex.
6. **Restiform Body (of Inferior Cerebellar Peduncle)**—in the dorsolateral portion of the open portion of the medulla, fibers from the dorsal spinocerebellar tract and the inferior olivary complex (olivocerebellar fibers) converge to form the restiform body, which courses into the cerebellum at the caudal part of the pons and medial to the middle cerebellar peduncle as part of the inferior cerebellar peduncle. The small juxtarestiform body forms the remainder of this peduncle.
7. **Medial Longitudinal Fasciculus**—fibers from the vestibular nuclei, some crossed and some uncrossed, ascend in the brain stem on each side of the midline in the floor of the fourth ventricle, and in the central area of gray matter in the midbrain. The fibers terminate in the abducens, trochlear, and oculomotor nuclei. This fasciculus functions in coordinating eye movements with head movements.
8. **Hypoglossal Nucleus**—this elongated motor nucleus is located near the midline of the medulla. It is coextensive with the inferior olivary complex and extends from the hypoglossal trigone in the floor of the fourth ventricle caudally into the central gray matter in the closed part of the medulla. Its fibers pass through the central part of the medulla and emerge between the pyramid and the olive to supply the tongue musculature (see also no. **13**, Fig. 40).

Note: Legends for nos. **9–16** are found on page 96.

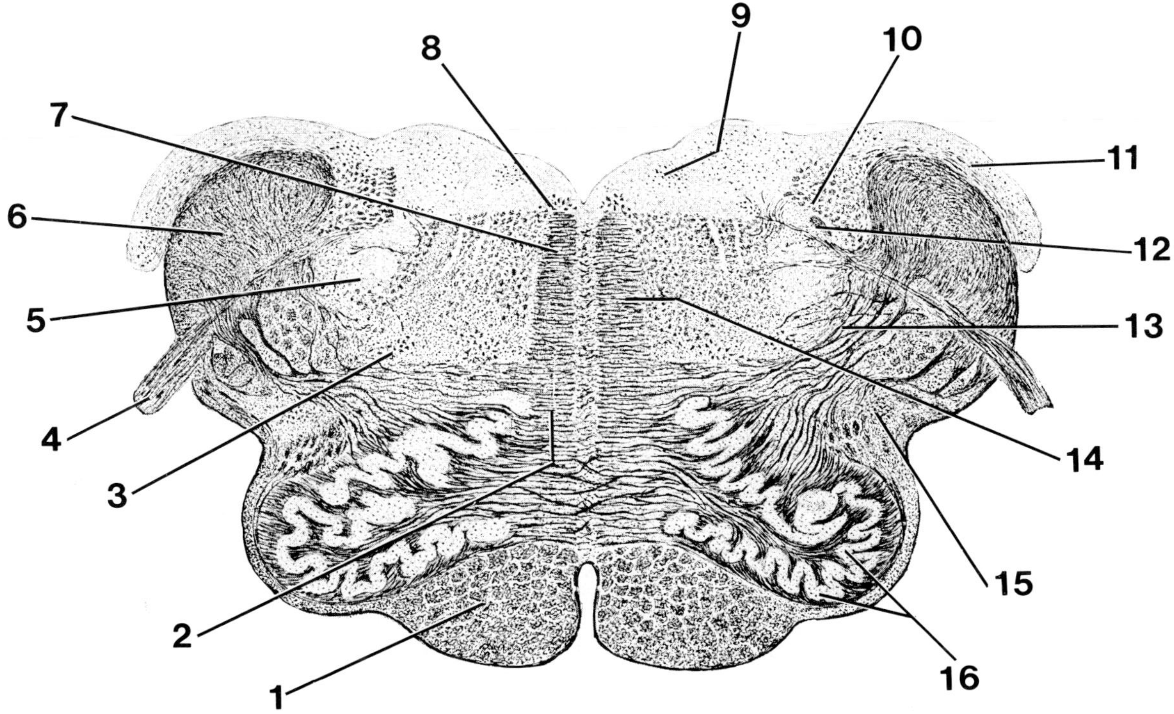

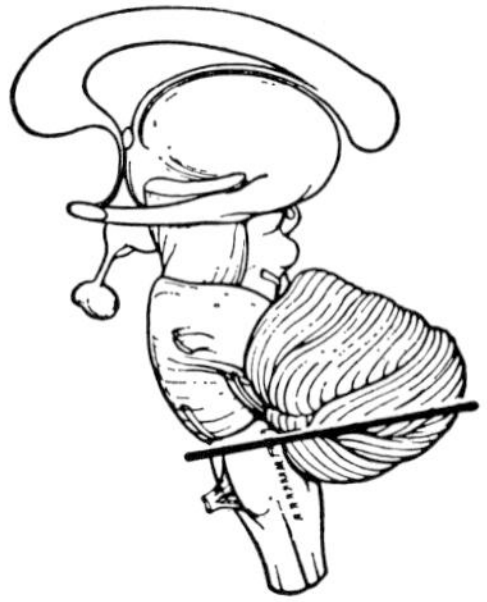

Figure 41 Modified photograph of a drawing of a transverse section of the rostral (open) medulla showing some nuclear areas, ascending and descending fiber tracts. ×6.5 (Modified from M. B. Carpenter: *Human Neuroanatomy*, 7th ed. Courtesy of Williams & Wilkins.)

Medulla—Open Portion (*continued*)

9. **Dorsal Nucleus of Vagus Nerve**—this large parasympathetic nucleus lies lateral to the hypoglossal nucleus (**8**) and extends from the vagal trigone in the floor of the fourth ventricle caudally and into the gray matter surrounding the central canal of the spinal cord. It contains the cell bodies of preganglionic neurons for smooth muscle and gland tissue of thoracic and abdominal viscera, including the heart (see also no. **12**, Fig. 40).
10. **Inferior Vestibular Nuclei**—situated beneath the area vestibuli in the lateral area of the floor of the fourth ventricle, at the rostral end of the medulla. Axons (vestibular nerve fibers) from vestibular ganglion cells of the internal ear terminate in the vestibular nuclei. Fibers from the lateral vestibular nucleus give rise to the descending vestibulospinal tract. Other fibers from the lateral vestibular nucleus, along with fibers from the remaining vestibular nuclei, form the medial longitudinal fasciculus.
11. **Dorsal Cochlear Nucleus**—lies (rests) on the restiform body (base of inferior cerebellar peduncle) in the area caudal to the middle cerebellar peduncle, where the fourth ventricle communicates with the subarachnoid space (lateral aperture, foramen of Luschka). Axons (cochlear nerve fibers) from the cochlear ganglion of the internal ear terminate in this nucleus and the ventral cochlear nucleus. Fibers from the dorsal cochlear nucleus give rise to the crossed and uncrossed lateral lemniscus (part of the auditory pathway).
12. **Tractus Solitarius**—these visceral afferent fibers, from the ganglia of the facial, glossopharyngeal, and vagus nerves, are located lateral to the dorsal nucleus of the vagus nerve (**9**) and ventral to the vestibular complex. The fibers in this tract are directed caudally and terminate in the nucleus solitarius, a column of cells that lies adjacent to and partially surrounds this tract. It transmits taste impulses to higher centers.
13. **Olivocerebellar Fibers**—from the inferior olivary complex decussate in the median raphe of the medulla, curve in a dorsolateral direction to project to the cerebellum via the contralateral restiform body of the inferior cerebellar peduncle. It relays impulses from the olivary complex which are important to ensure efficiency of voluntary movements.
14. **Tectospinal Tract**—in the medulla on each side located in the midline between the column of fibers of the medial longitudinal fasciculus (dorsal) and the medial lemniscus. It originates in the contralateral superior colliculus of the midbrain, and the fibers descend throughout the brain stem into the superior half of the ventral white column of the spinal cord. Its fibers terminate on ventral horn cells and function for head and upper limb movements in response to visual and auditory stimuli.
15. **Lateral Reticular Nucleus**—is located dorsal to the inferior olivary nucleus near the lateral surface of the medulla. It extends from a point caudal to the inferior olivary nucleus to the mid-olivary level. It receives general sensory data from the spinal cord and relays sensory data to the cerebellum.
16. **Inferior Olivary Nucleus**—in cross-section it is shaped like a crumpled bag, with its hilum facing medially. It is situated within the olive in the ventrolateral area of the medulla. The medial lemniscus lies medial to it and the pyramids ventral to it. It receives sensory input from the spinal cord, and its efferent fibers project to the contralateral cerebellum.

Note: Legends for nos. **1-8** are found on page 94.

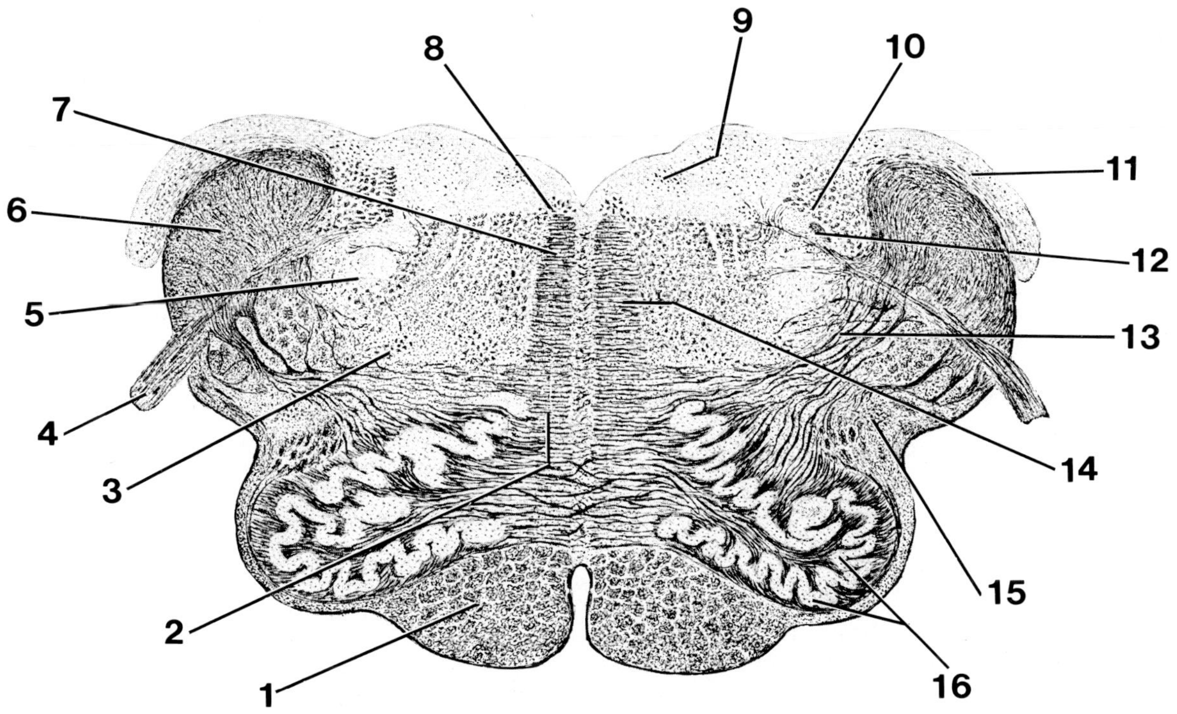

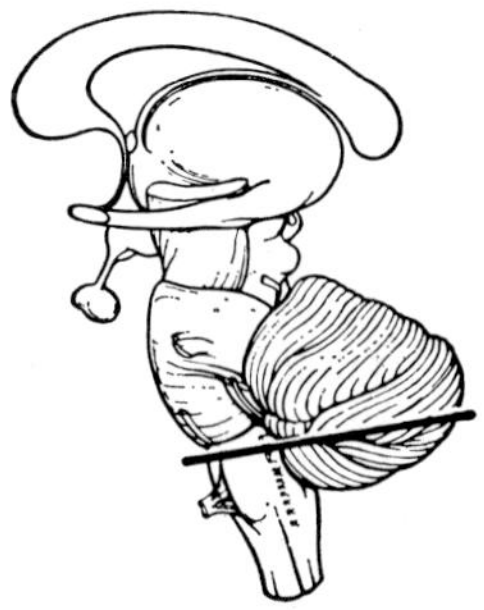

Figure 41 Modified photograph of a drawing of a transverse section of the rostral (open) medulla showing some nuclear areas, ascending and descending fiber tracts. ×6.5 (Modified from M. B. Carpenter: *Human Neuroanatomy*, 7th ed. Courtesy of Williams & Wilkins.)

Pons

1. **Trapezoid Body**—located in the ventral tegmental portion of the pons, lying ventral to the medial lemniscus (**13**). It consists of transverse strands of acoustic fibers, some of which intersect the medial lemniscus.
2. **Middle Cerebellar Peduncle**—a lateral continuation of the basal pons. It consists of pontocerebellar fibers which originate from contralateral pontine nuclei in the basal pons and terminate on neurons in the cortex of the cerebellar hemispheres.
3. **Facial Nucleus (Motor)**—located in the ventrolateral part of the pons tegmentum. Fibers from this nucleus course in a dorsomedial direction to loop over the abducens nucleus (**5**), forming the facial colliculus in the floor of the fourth ventricle. They then pass ventrolaterally between their nucleus of origin and the trigeminal spinal nucleus (**9**) to emerge laterally at the junction of the pons and medulla. It supplies the muscles of facial expression.
4. **Medial Longitudinal Fasciculus**—fibers from the vestibular nuclei, some crossed and some uncrossed, ascend in the brain stem on each side of the midline in the floor of the fourth ventricle, and in the central area of gray matter in the midbrain. The fibers terminate in the abducens, trochlear, and oculomotor nuclei. It functions in coordinating eye movements with head movements (see also no. **7**, Fig. 41).
5. **Abducens Nucleus (C.N. VI)**—located beneath the facial colliculus, consisting of the abducens nucleus and fibers of the facial nerve in the floor of the fourth ventricle. The axons of the abducens neurons course in a ventral and caudal direction through the tegmentum to emerge at the posterior border of the pons near the midline as the abducens nerve. This nerve innervates the lateral rectus muscle of the eye.
6. **Inferior Cerebellar Peduncle**—in the pons it is located medial to the caudal portion of the middle cerebellar peduncle. These structures form the lateral wall of the fourth ventricle. The inferior peduncle consists of a lateral portion (restiform body) and a medial portion (juxtarestiform body).
7. **Superior Vestibular Nucleus**—situated beneath the rostral end of the area vestibuli, which is in the lateral area of the floor of the fourth ventricle at the caudal end of the pons. Fibers from this vestibular nucleus contribute to the ipsilateral medial longitudinal fasciculus, as well as projecting to the cortex of the flocculonodular lobe of the cerebellum via the juxtarestiform body of the inferior cerebellar peduncle.
8. **Central Tegmental Tract**—consists of fibers from the red nucleus and other gray areas in the midbrain that course through the pons and into the medulla to the inferior olivary complex. In the pons these fibers are located in the central tegmental area, dorsal to the medial lemniscus (**13**).
9. **Spinal Nucleus and Tract of Trigeminal Nerve**—axons of neurons from the trigeminal sensory ganglion turn caudally upon entering the pons and pass through the dorsolateral caudal pons, medulla, and the rostral part of the spinal cord as far as the third cervical segment. Its fibers terminate in the spinal nucleus. The tract and nucleus function in transmitting sensory data for pain, touch, and temperature from the head area to the thalamus and the sensory cortex (see also no. **5**, Fig. 41).
10. **Spinal Lemniscus**—consists of the lateral and ventral spinothalamic tracts and the spinotectal tract. In the medulla dorsal to the olive, these spinal tracts converge to form the spinal lemniscus. In the pons the spinal lemniscus is situated near the lateral edge of the medial lemniscus.
11. **Superior Olivary Nucleus**—located dorsal to the lateral portion of the trapezoid body. Some fibers from the cochlear nuclei that traverse the trapezoid body end in this nucleus. Fibers from this nucleus pass into the lateral lemniscus of the auditory pathway and to the abducens nucleus.
12. **Pontine Nuclei**—in the basal pons masses of cell bodies of pontine neurons are clustered together to form the pontine nuclei. They are found among the pontine fibers of the corticopontine, corticospinal, and pontocerebellar tracts. Fibers from these nuclei form the pontocerebellar tract fibers which course transversely to the opposite middle cerebellar peduncle. Corticopontine fibers end on the cells in these nuclei.
13. **Medial Lemniscus**—internal arcuate fibers from the nucleus gracilis and the nucleus cuneatus decussate in the midline of the caudal medulla to form the medial lemniscus. In the ventral tegmental pons, dorsal to the trapezoid body, the ascending fibers of the medial lemniscus are arranged in a horizontal plane (unlike the vertical columns in the medulla). These fibers conduct proprioceptive, discriminative touch, and vibration sensations to the ventral posterolateral nucleus of the thalamus (see also no. **2**, Fig. 41).

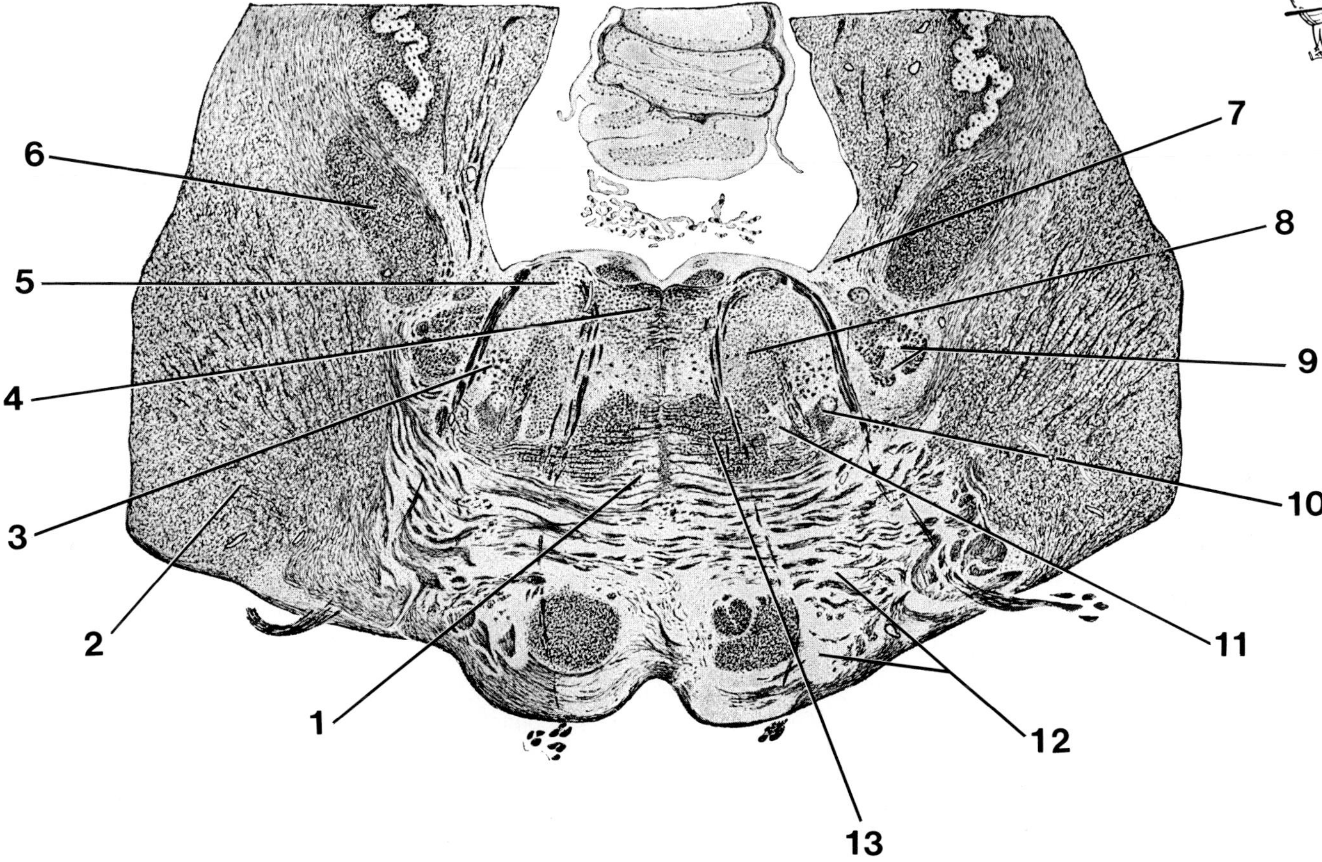

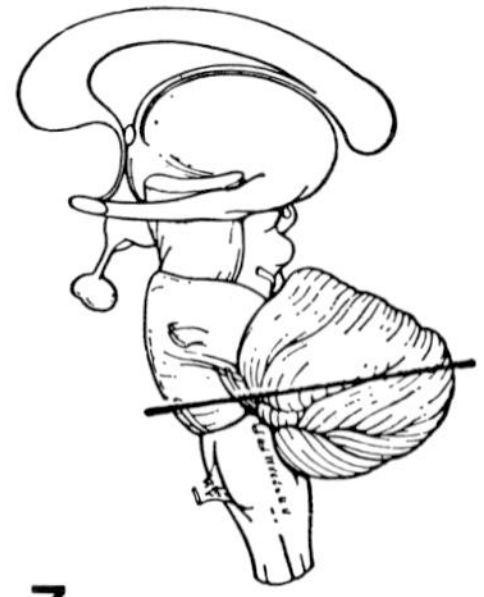

Figure 42 Modified photograph of a drawing of a transverse section through the pons at the level abducens nucleus (facial colliculus) showing some nuclear areas, ascending and descending fiber tracts, and the course of fibers of C.N. VII. The middle cerebellar peduncle, massive at this level, is seen entering the cerebellum. ×4.5 (Modified from M. B. Carpenter: *Human Neuroanatomy*, 7th ed. Courtesy of Williams & Wilkins.)

Midbrain—Caudal Portion

1. **Basis Pedunculi (Crus Cerebri)**—the ventral part of the cerebral peduncle of the midbrain. It is separated from the dorsal tegmental part by the substantia nigra and consists of fibers of the pyramidal motor system and corticopontine fibers (see also no. **8,** Fig. 38).
2. **Decussation of Superior Cerebellar Peduncles (Brachia Conjunctiva)**—the fibers of the superior cerebellar peduncle cross the midline of the midbrain in this decussation at the level of the inferior colliculus to continue forward in the tegmentum to the ventral lateral thalamic nucleus and the red nucleus.
3. **Lateral Lemniscus**—fibers from the trapezoid body that originated from the right and left cochlear and the superior olivary nuclei turn rostrally at the lateral edge of the medial lemniscus in the dorsolateral midbrain tegmentum to end in the inferior colliculus. This is part of the auditory pathway to the auditory cortex.
4. **Inferior Brachium**—located on the dorsolateral surface of the midbrain. It consists of fibers connecting the nucleus of the inferior colliculus to the medial geniculate nucleus of the thalamus, which in turn project to the auditory area of the cortex in the temporal lobe.
5. **Medial Longitudinal Fasciculus**—fibers from the vestibular nuclei, some crossed and some uncrossed, ascend in the brain stem on each side of the midline in the floor of the fourth ventricle, and in the central area of gray matter in the midbrain. The fibers terminate in the abducens, trochlear, and oculomotor nuclei. It functions in coordinating eye movements with head movements (see also no. **4,** Fig. 42).
6. **Cerebral Aqueduct (of Sylvius)**—this midline canal, surrounded by an area of gray matter, lies between the tectal (roof) and tegmental areas of the midbrain. Cerebrospinal fluid flows from the third to the fourth ventricle through this aqueduct of the midbrain.
7. **Dorsal Tegmental Nucleus**—located in the central gray matter between the oculomotor and the trochlear nuclei. It has connections with the hypothalmus and nuclei in the olfactory and limbic systems.
8. **Trochlear Nucleus (C.N. IV—motor)**—in the central gray matter at the level of the inferior colliculus, where it lies dorsal to the medial longitudinal fasciculus (**5**). Fibers from this nucleus leave the dorsal surface of the midbrain immediately behind the inferior colliculus to innervate the superior oblique muscle of the eye.
9. **Inferior Colliculus**—inferior part of the tectum (roof) of the midbrain. The tectum consists of paired superior and inferior colliculi. In the auditory pathway, fibers of the lateral lemniscus (**3**) end on cells of the inferior colliculuar nucleus, the axons of which in turn project to the medial geniculate body via the inferior brachium (**4**).
10. **Central Tegmental Tract**—consists of fibers from the red nucleus and other gray areas in the midbrain that course through the pons and into the medulla to the inferior olivary complex. In the pons these fibers are located in the central tegmental area dorsal to the medial lemniscus (see also no. **8,** Fig. 42).
11. **Spinal Lemniscus**—consists of the lateral and ventral spinothalamic tracts and the spinotectal tract. In the medulla dorsal to the olive, these spinal tracts converge to form the spinal lemniscus. In the midbrain the spinal lemniscus is dorsolateral to the medial lemniscus. Spinotectal fibers leave the lemniscus to enter the superior colliculus (see also no. **10,** Fig. 42).
12. **Medial Lemniscus**—in the medulla fibers conducting proprioception, discriminative touch, and vibration sense from the nucleus gracilis and nucleus cuneatus decussated to form the medial lemniscus. It forms a vertical column on each side of the midline. In the pons the fibers form a horizontal plane, and in the midbrain they diverge laterally dorsal to the substantia nigra in the lateral tegmentum to form a compact bundle (see also no. **2,** Fig. 41).
13. **Substantia Nigra**—a prominent extrapyramidal pigmented motor nucleus located immediately dorsal to the basis pedunculi (**1**) throughout the midbrain and extending into the subthalamic region of the diencephalon.

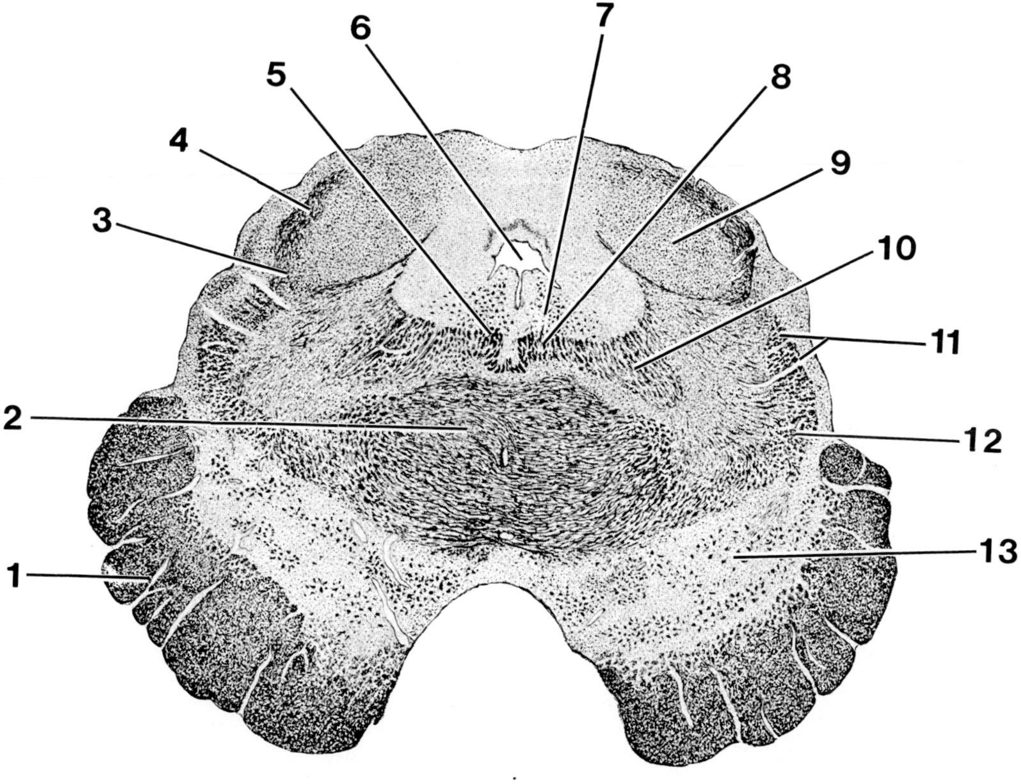

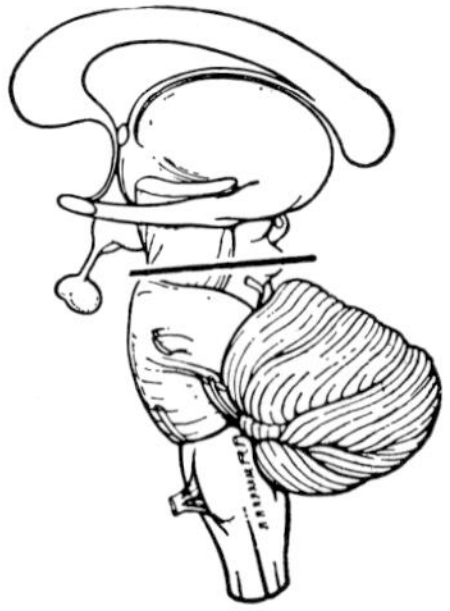

Figure 43 Modified photograph of a drawing of a transverse section through the midbrain at the level of the inferior colliculus to show nuclear areas, ascending and descending fiber tracts, and the decussation of the superior cerebellar peduncle and the basis pedunculi. ×4.5 (Modified from M. B. Carpenter: *Human Neuroanatomy*, 7th ed. Courtesy of Williams & Wilkins.)

Midbrain—Rostral Portion

1. **Frontopontine Tract**—its fibers extend from the frontal lobe cortex to the pontine nuclei in the basal pons. They course through the anterior limb of the internal capsule and the medial one-fifth of the basis pedunculi.
2. **Corticospinal and Corticobulbar Tracts**—extend from the motor cortex through the posterior limb of the internal capsule and the middle three-fifths of the basis pedunculi. The somatotopic arrangement is that of fibers for the neck, upper limb, trunk, and lower limb in a medial to lateral direction in the basis pedunculi (see also no. **9,** Fig. 39).
3. **Temporoparietal and Occipitopontine Tract**—fibers from the cortex of the temporal, parietal, and occipital lobes pass to the pontine nuclei in the basal pons. They course through the posterior limb of the internal capsule and the lateral one-fifth of the basis pedunculi.
4. **Medial Lemniscus**—in the medulla fibers conducting proprioception, discriminative touch, and vibration sense from the nucleus gracilis and the nucleus cuneatus decussated to form the medial lemniscus which formed a vertical column on each side of the midline. In the pons the fibers formed a horizontal plane, and in the midbrain they diverge laterally dorsal to the substantia nigra in the lateral tegmentum to form a compact bundle (see also no. **13,** Fig. 42).
5. **Central Tegmental Tract**—consists of fibers from the red nucleus and other gray areas in the midbrain that course through the pons and into the medulla to the inferior olivary complex. In the pons these fibers are located in the central tegmental area dorsal to the medial lemniscus (see also no. **8,** Fig. 42).
6. **Inferior Brachium**—located on the dorsolateral surface of the midbrain. Consists of fibers connecting the nucleus of the inferior colliculus to the medial geniculate nucleus of the thalamus, which in turn projects to the auditory area of the cortex in the temporal lobe (see also no. **4,** Fig. 43).
7. **Spinal Lemniscus**—consists of the lateral and ventral spinothalamic tracts and the spinotectal tract. In the medulla dorsal to the olive, these spinal tracts converge to form the spinal lemniscus. In the midbrain the spinal lemniscus is dorsolateral to the medial lemniscus. Spinotectal fibers leave the spinal lemniscus to enter the superior colliculus (see also no. **11,** Fig. 43).
8. **Superior Colliculus**—superior part of the tectum (roof) of the midbrain. The tectum consists of the paired superior and inferior colliculi. The nuclear part of the superior colliculus recieves connections from the retina and the visual cortex and functions in reflexes of the visual system. The extrapyramidal tectospinal and tectobulbar tracts originate in this collicular area.
9. **Cerebral Aqueduct (of Sylvius)**—this midline canal, surrounded by an area of gray matter, lies between the tectal (roof) and tegmental areas of the midbrain. Cerebrospinal fluid flows from the third to the fourth ventricle through this aqueduct of the midbrain (see also no. **6,** Fig. 43).
10. **Central Gray Matter**—a thick layer of gray matter throughout the midbrain surrounding the cerebral aqueduct. It contains scattered small nerve cells and some nuclear areas. The motor nuclei of C.N. III and C.N. IV are located in its ventral area.
11. **Dorsal Tegmental Nucleus**—located in the central gray matter between the oculomotor and the trochlear nuclei. It has connections with the hypothalamus and nuclei in the olfactory and limbic systems.

Note: Legends for nos. **12–18** are found on page 104.

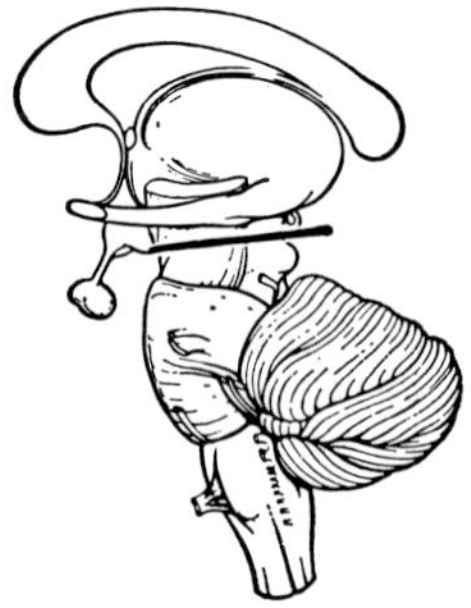

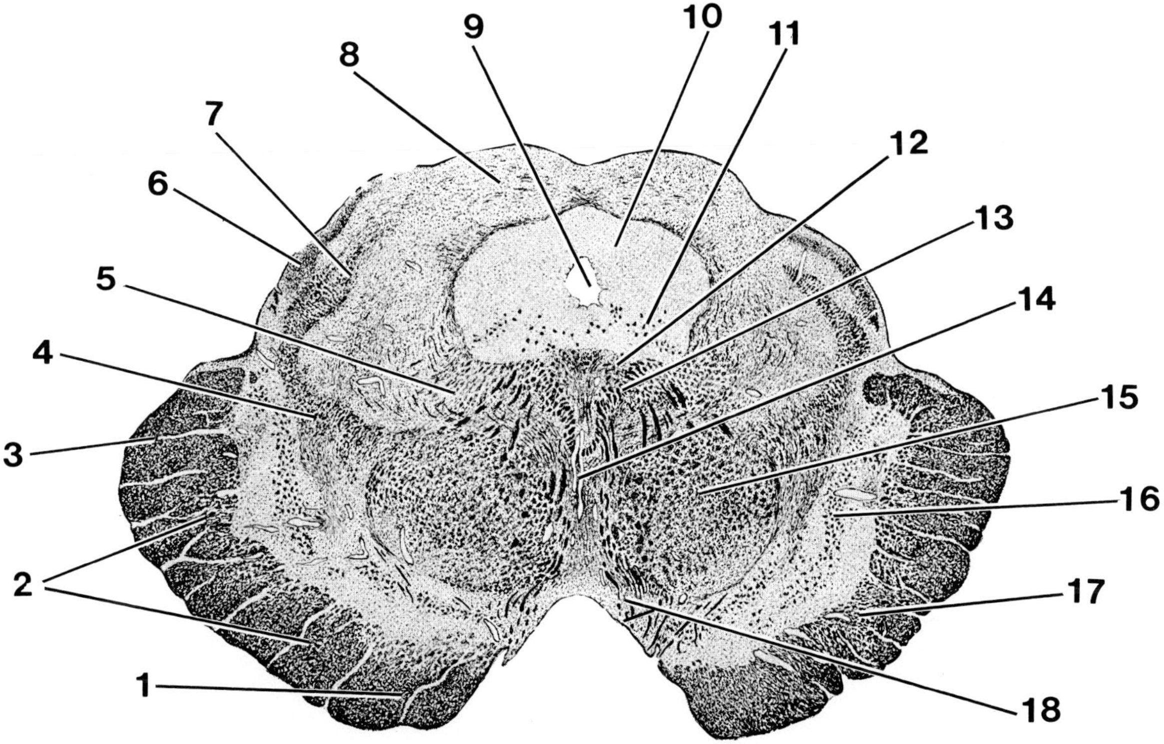

Figure 44 Modified photograph of a drawing of a transverse section through the midbrain at the level of the superior colliculus to show some nuclear areas, ascending and descending fiber tracts, and the course of the root fibers of C.N. III. ×4.5 (Modified from M. B. Carpenter: *Human Neuroanatomy*, 7th ed. Courtesy of Williams & Wilkins.)

12. Oculomotor Nucleus (C.N. III)—this elongated motor nucleus is in the central gray matter at the level of the superior colliculus. Its fibers traverse the tegmental area of the midbrain to emerge in the interpeduncular fossa. It supplies all the extraocular muscles except the superior oblique and the lateral rectus. It also contains parasympathetic cells for the ciliary muscles of the eye.

13. Medial Longitudinal Fasiculus—fibers from the vestibular nuclei, some crossed and some uncrossed, ascend in the brain stem on each side of the midline in the floor of the fourth ventricle, and in the central area of gray matter in the midbrain. The fibers terminate in the abducens, trochlear, and oculomotor nuclei. It functions in coordinating eye movements with head movements (see also no. **4,** Fig. 42 and no. **5,** Fig. 43).

14. Dorsal Tegmental Decussation—fibers from the superior colliculi are distributed to the spinal cord and the nuclei of the brain stem. They curve around the periaqueductal (central) gray matter (**10**) in the midbrain. The fibers terminate in the abducens, trochlear, and oculomotor nuclei. It functions in coordinating eye movements with head movements.

Note: Legends for nos. **1-11** are found on page 102.

15. Red Nucleus—this prominent extrapyramidal motor nucleus is located in the midbrain tegmentum, dorsal to the substantia nigra at the level of the superior colliculus. It receives connections from the cerebellum (via the superior cerebellar peduncle). Fibers from the red nucleus project to the ventral lateral nucleus of the thalamus into the spinal cord (rubrospinal tract), and into the recticular formation (rubroreticular tract).

16. Substantia Nigra—a prominent extrapyramidal pigmented motor nucleus located immediately dorsal to the basis pedunculi throughout the midbrain, and extending into the subthalamic region of the diencephalon.

17. Basis Pedunculi (Crus Cerebri)—the ventral part of the cerebral peduncle. It is separated from the tegmentum by the substantia nigra. It consists of corticospinal and corticobulbar tracts (**2**) and corticopontine fibers (**1** and **3**).

18. Oculomotor Nerve Fibers—course from the oculomotor nucleus (**12**) through structures (red nucleus and substantia nigra) of the midbrain tegmentum to emerge in the interpeduncular fossa

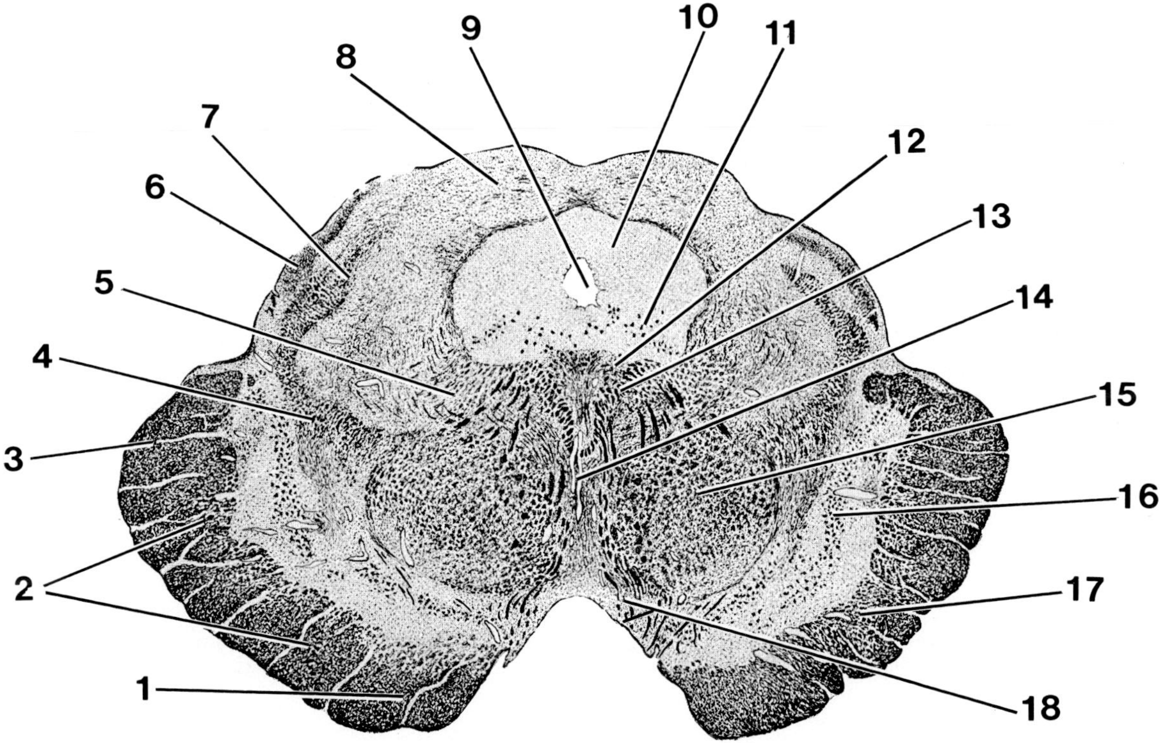

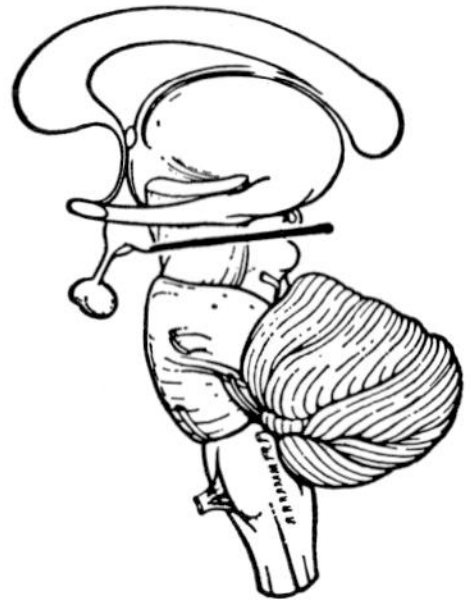

Figure 44 Modified photograph of a drawing of a transverse section through the midbrain at the level of the superior colliculus to show some nuclear areas, ascending and descending fiber tracts, and the course of the root fibers of C.N. III. ×4.5 (Modified from M. B. Carpenter: *Human Neuroanatomy*, 7th ed. Courtesy of Williams & Wilkins.)

The Cranial Nerves (Figs. 45 to 49)

1. **Spinal Accessory (C.N. XI)**—its cranial root fibers emerge with the vagus (**2**) and glossopharyngeal (**3**) between the olive (no. **2,** Fig. 46) and tuberculum cinereum. It is a motor nerve (see also no. **3,** Fig. 46).
2. **Vagus Nerve (C.N. X)**—mixed nerve with sensory and motor components. Its fibers enter or emerge from the brain stem with IXth (**3**) and XIth (**1**) fibers in dorsolateral sulcus of the medulla (see also no. **13,** Fig. 46).
3. **Glossopharyngeal Nerve (C.N. IX)**—mixed nerve with sensory and motor components and emerges with vagus (**2**) and spinal accessory (**1**) in dorsolateral sulcus (see also nos. **3**, **4**, and **13** Fig. 46).
4. **Vestibulocochlear Nerve (C.N. VIII)**—special sensory nerve fibers from internal ear enter the brain stem with fibers from the C.N. VII at the caudal border of the pons. **The cochlear division** functions in hearing. **The vestibular division** functions in equilibrium (balance) (see also no. **12,** Fig. 46).
5. **Abducens Nerve (C.N. VI)**—a motor nerve the fibers of which emerge from caudal border of pons near the midline. It supplies the lateral rectus muscle (see also no. **5,** Fig. 46).
6. **Trochlear Nerve (C.N. IV)**—this motor nerve supplies the superior oblique muscle and is the only cranial nerve to emerge from the dorsal surface of the brain. It curves around the lateral surface of the midbrain and accompanies the IIIrd and VIth cranial nerves through cavernous sinus to the orbit (see also no. **4,** Fig. 47).
7. **Oculomotor Nerve (C.N. III)**—this motor nerve, supplying all of the extraocular muscles except superior oblique and lateral rectus, emerges from the interpeduncular fossa of the midbrain rostral to the upper border of the pons (see also no. **9,** Fig. 46).
8. **Optic Nerve (C.N. II)**—located between eyeball and optic chiasma. Ganglionic fibers from the retina conduct visual impulses to the brain (lateral geniculate body). Ganglionic fibers from the medial side of each optic nerve cross to the opposite side in the **optic chiasma** to join those from the lateral side of each optic nerve to form the left and right optic tracts (located distal to the optic chiasma). The **optic tract** (composed of crossed and uncrossed ganglionic retinal fibers) conducts impulses in the visual, pupillary, and accommodation reflex pathways.
9. **Posterior Cerebral Artery**—a terminal branch of the basilar artery curves around the cerebral peduncle to reach and supply the inferior and medial surfaces of the temporal and occipital lobes. Clinically it is an important landmark as C.N. III (**7**) and C.N. IV (**6**) course between this artery and the superior cerebellar (**10**). Ruptured aneurysms of this vessel cause extraocular involvements due to damage of these two nerves which lie so close to this vessel (see also no. **5,** Fig. 65).
10. **Superior Cerebellar Artery**—branches from the basilar artery before it terminates as the left and right posterior cerebral artery. It supplies the superior aspect of the cerebellum, including the cerebellar nuclei. At its beginning this vessel courses parallel to the posterior cerebral, and C.N. III and C.N. IV emerge between these two vessels (see also no. **11,** Fig. 65).
11. **Trigeminal Nerve (C.N. V)—Sensory component.** Sensory fibers of this mixed nerve enter the pons at the junction of middle cerebellar peduncle and basal pons. It conducts general somesthetic data from most of the head area. **Motor component.** Motor fibers of this mixed curve nerve leave the pons adjacent to incoming sensory fibers to supply the muscles of mastication (see also no. **1,** Fig. 48).
12. **Facial Nerve (C.N. VII)**—mixed nerve with sensory and motor components. Its fibers enter and emerge from the lateral side of the brain stem in company with C.N. VIII at the caudal border of the pons (see also no. **11,** Fig. 46).
13. **Hypoglossal Nerve (C.N. XII)**—fibers emerge from medulla between pyramid (no. **14,** Fig. 46) and olive (no. **2,** Fig. 46) in ventrolateral sulcus. It is a motor nerve (see also no. **1,** Fig. 46).

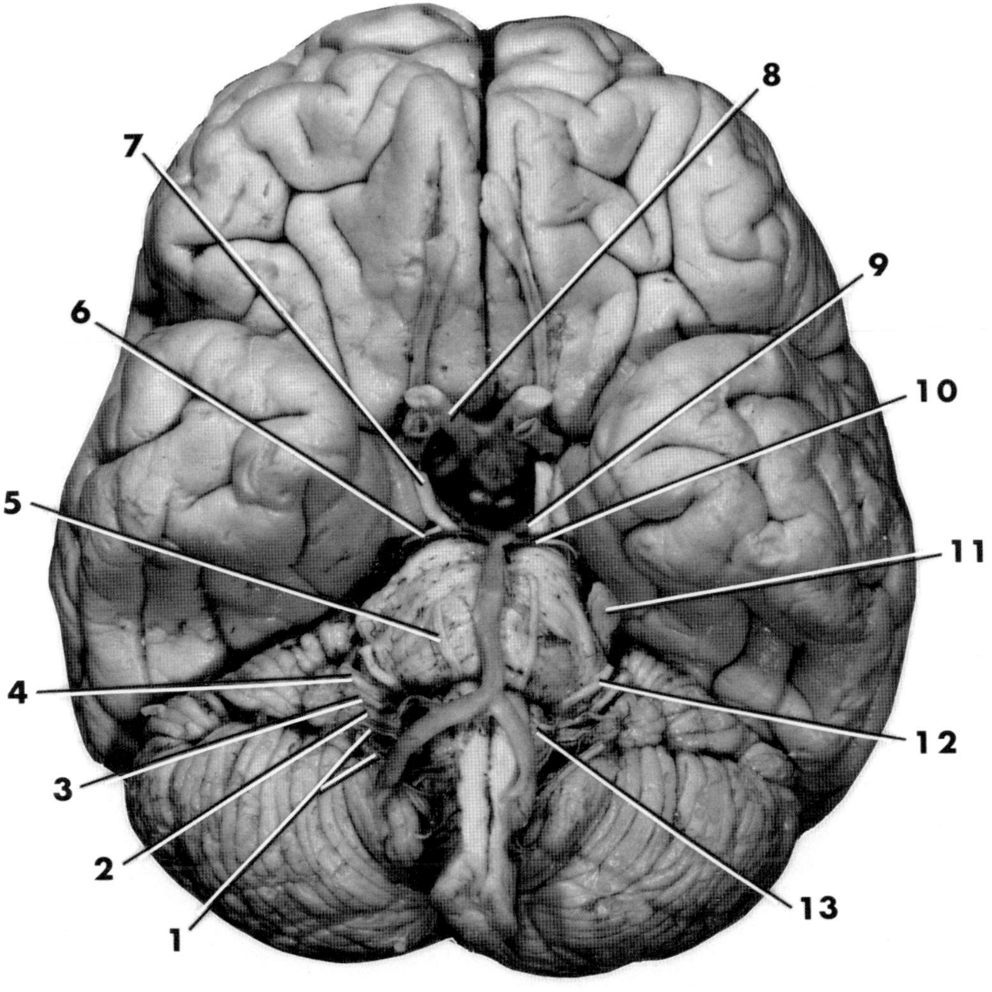

Figure 45 Ventral view of the brain showing the entering (sensory) and emerging (motor and visceromotor) fibers of the **cranial nerves** and the relationship of the third and fourth cranial nerves to the posterior cerebral and superior cerebellar arteries.

1. **Hypoglossal Nerve (C.N. XII)**—fibers emerge from medulla between pyramid (**14**) and olive (**2**) in ventrolateral sulcus. It is a motor nerve (see also no. **13,** Fig. 45).
2. **Olive**—located between pyramids (**14**) and dorsolateral sulcus. It contains the inferior olivary nucleus (see also no. **3,** Fig. 48).
3. **Spinal Accessory (C.N. XI)**—cranial root fibers of C.N. XI emerge with vagus (**13**) and glossopharyngeal (**4**) between olive (**2**) and tuberculum cinereum. It is a motor nerve (see also no. **1**, Fig. 45).
4. **Glossopharyngeal Nerve (C.N. IX)**—mixed nerve with sensory and motor components that emerge with vagus (**13**), and spinal accessory (**3**) in dorsolateral sulcus (see also no. **3**, Fig. 45).
5. **Abducens Nerve (C.N. VI)**—a motor nerve the fibers of which emerge from caudal border of pons near the midline. It supplies the lateral rectus muscle (see also no. **5,** Fig. 45).
6. **Trigeminal Nerve (C.N. V)—a. Sensory component.** Sensory fibers of this mixed nerve enter the pons at the junction of middle cerebellar peduncle and basal pons. It conducts general somesthetic data from most of the head area. **b. Motor component.** Motor fibers of this mixed nerve leave the pons adjacent to incoming sensory fibers to supply the muscles of mastication (see also no. **1**, Fig. 48).
7. **Optic Nerve (C.N. II)**—located between eyeball and optic chiasma. Ganglionic fibers from retina conduct visual impulses to brain (see also no. **9,** Fig. 49).
8. **Optic Tract**—located between optic chiasma and lateral geniculate body. Consists of ganglionic fibers from each retina. Fibers from the contralateral retina crossed in the optic chiasma. It conducts visual impulses in the visual, pupillary, and accommodation reflex pathways (see also no. **10,** Fig. 49).
9. **Oculomotor Nerve (C.N. III)**—this motor nerve, supplying all of the extraocular muscles except superior oblique and lateral rectus, emerges from the interpeduncular fossa of the midbrain rostral to the upper border of the pons (see also no. **7**, Fig. 49).
10. **Trochlear Nerve (C.N. IV)**—this motor nerve supplies the superior oblique muscle and is the only cranial nerve to emerge from the dorsal surface of the brain. It curves around the lateral surface of the midbrain and accompanies the IIIrd and VIth cranial nerves through cavernous sinus to the orbit (see also no. **4,** Fig. 47).
11. **Facial Nerve (C.N. VII)**—mixed nerve with sensory and motor components. Its fibers enter and emerge from the lateral side of the brain stem in company with C.N. VIII at the caudal border of the pons (see also no. **12,** Fig. 45).
12. **Vestibulocochlear Nerve (C.N. VIII)**—special sensory nerve fibers from internal ear enter the brain stem with fibers from the C.N. VII at the caudal border of the pons. **a. Cochlear division** functions in hearing. **b. Vestibular division** functions in equilibrium (balance) see also no. **4**, Fig. 45).
13. **Vagus Nerve (C.N. X)**—mixed nerve with sensory and motor components. Its fibers enter or emerge from the brain stem with C.N. IX and XI fibers in dorsolateral sulcus of the medulla (see also no. **2,** Fig. 45).
14. **Pyramid**—located between ventral median fissure and ventrolateral sulcus of medulla. Consists of corticospinal fibers which decussate (**15**) and descend into the spinal cord (see also no. **16,** Fig. 38).
15. **Decussation of Pyramids**—approximately 85% of pyramidal (corticospinal tract) fibers cross to contralateral side of the caudal medulla or upper cervical cord in the ventral median fissure (see also no. **17**, Fig. 38).

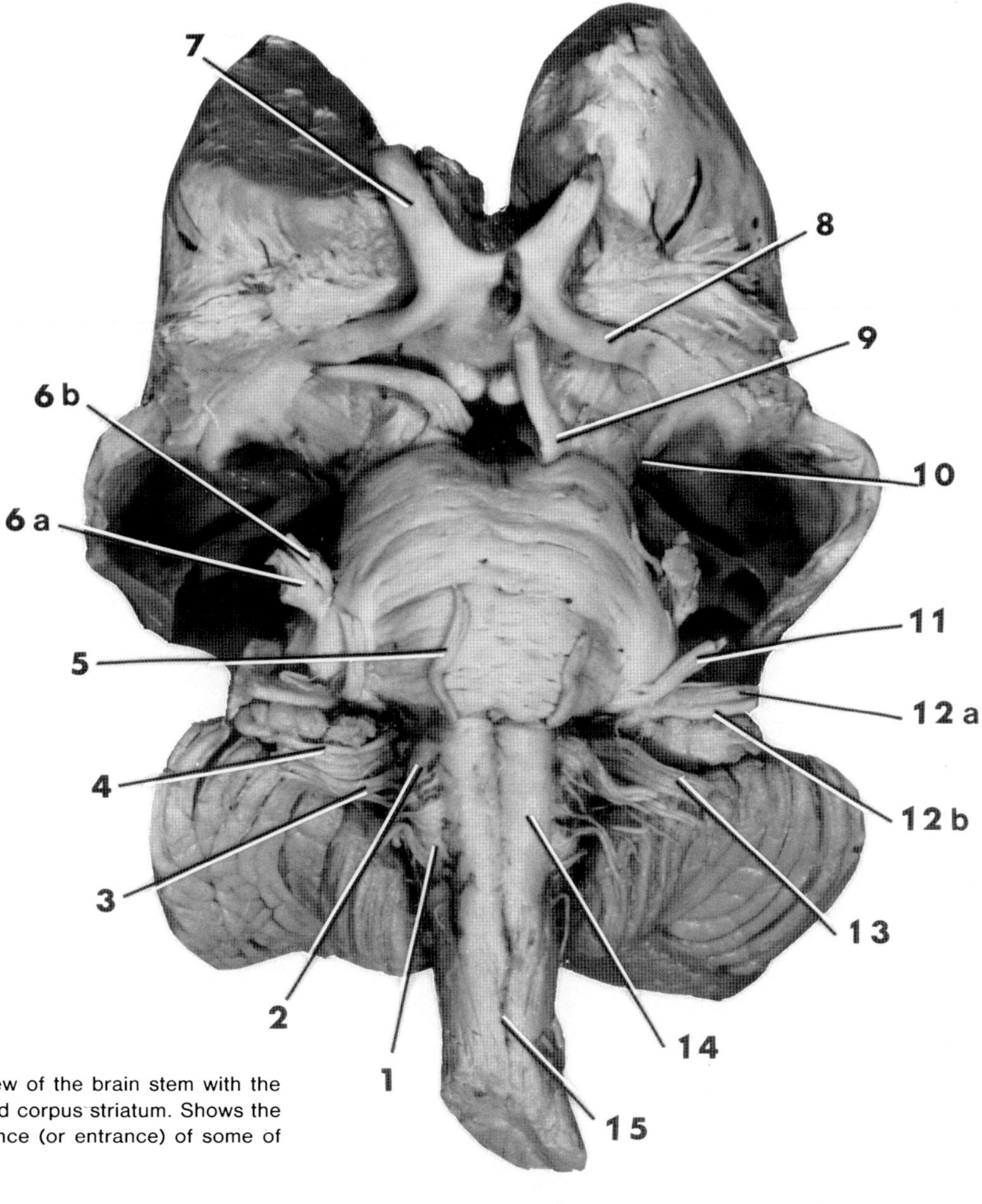

Figure 46 Ventral view of the brain stem with the attached cerebellum and corpus striatum. Shows the location of the emergence (or entrance) of some of the cranial nerves.

1. **Spinal Cord**—the first cervical segment is contained within the vertebral canal. It ends at the superior border of the atlas (1st cervical vertebra) by enlarging to form the expanded cone-shaped medulla oblongata (**2**) which passes through the foramen magnum. On the dorsal surface of the cord the dorsal median and the dorsal intermediate sulci can be seen, as well as the fasciculus gracilis and fasciculus cuneatus.
2. **Medulla Oblongata**—the expanded upward continuation of the spinal cord through the foramen magnum for approximately 3.7 cm into the posterior cranial fossa. It consists of closed (**a**) and open (**b**) portions. The caudal half of the floor of the fourth ventricle occupies the open portion of the medulla (**b**).
3. **Middle Cerebellar Peduncle (Brachium Pontis—Cut Surface)**—the longest of the three cerebellar peduncles. It consists of fibers from the contralateral pontine neurons that are located amongst the corticospinal, corticobulbar, and corticopontine fibers in the basal pons (see also no. **5**, Fig. 37*A*).
4. **Trochlear Nerve (C.N. IV)**—this motor nerve is the only cranial nerve to emerge from the dorsum of the brain stem. It emerges (**7**) caudal to the inferior colliculus of the midbrain (**5a**) and passes inferiorly around the lateral side of the midbrain. With C.N. III, it crosses the upper part of the pontine cistern to enter the lateral wall of the cavernous sinus. It then passes forward and enters the orbit via the superior orbital fissure to supply the superior oblique muscle. Damage to this nerve impairs the ability to turn the eye downward and outward (see also no. **6**, Fig. 45).
5. **Corpora Quadrigemina**—consists of four rounded elevations, the paired inferior (**a**) and superior (**b**) colliculi that form the tectum (L. roof) of the dorsal surface of the midbrain. The inferior colliculi function with the auditory pathways and the superior colliculi function with visual pathways.
6. **Point of Emergence of C.N. IV**—the trochlear nerve fibers leave the trochlear nucleus, wind around the periaqueductal gray matter with a caudal slope, to decussate in the superior medullary velum with fibers from the same nucleus of the opposite side, and emerge just behind the inferior colliculus. The nerve passes inferiorly along the lateral surface of the midbrain to terminate as described in **4.**
7. **Basis Pedunculi**—the prominent elevation on each side of the ventral surface of the midbrain. It consists mainly of corticospinal, corticobulbar, and corticopontine fibers. The basis pedunculi is the most ventral portion of the cerebral peduncle. The lateral lemniscus (**8**) and inferior brachium are located on the lateral surface of the midbrain, dorsal to the basis pedunculi.
8. **Lateral Lemniscus**—fibers of the auditory pathway from the cochlear nuclei (ipsilateral and contralateral), as well as the superior olivary nucleus, pass rostrally through the tegmentum of the pons and midbrain. This tract is situated lateral to the medial lemniscus. At this level it forms part of the lateral wall of the midbrain (see also no. **3**, Fig. 43).
9. **Superior Cerebellar Peduncle (Brachium Conjunctivum)**—consists mainly of cerebellar efferent fibers (from dentate, emboliform, and globose nuclei) that course rostrally into the tegmentum of the midbrain where they decussate. The beginning portion of these peduncles and the superior medullary velum form the rostral part of the roof of the fourth ventricle. The trochlear fibers (**4**) emerge where this velum and these peduncles approach the midbrain (see also no. **11**, Fig. 54).
10. **Floor of the IVth Ventricle (Rhomboid Fossa)**—is broad at its midportion and narrow toward the cerebral aqueduct and the obex (L. barrier). The obex is a small transverse fold overhanging the opening of the fourth ventricle into the central canal of the closed portion of the medulla. The median sulcus and the sulcus limitans divide each side of the floor into medial and lateral areas. On each side the medial area has mainly a motor function and the lateral area a sensory function.

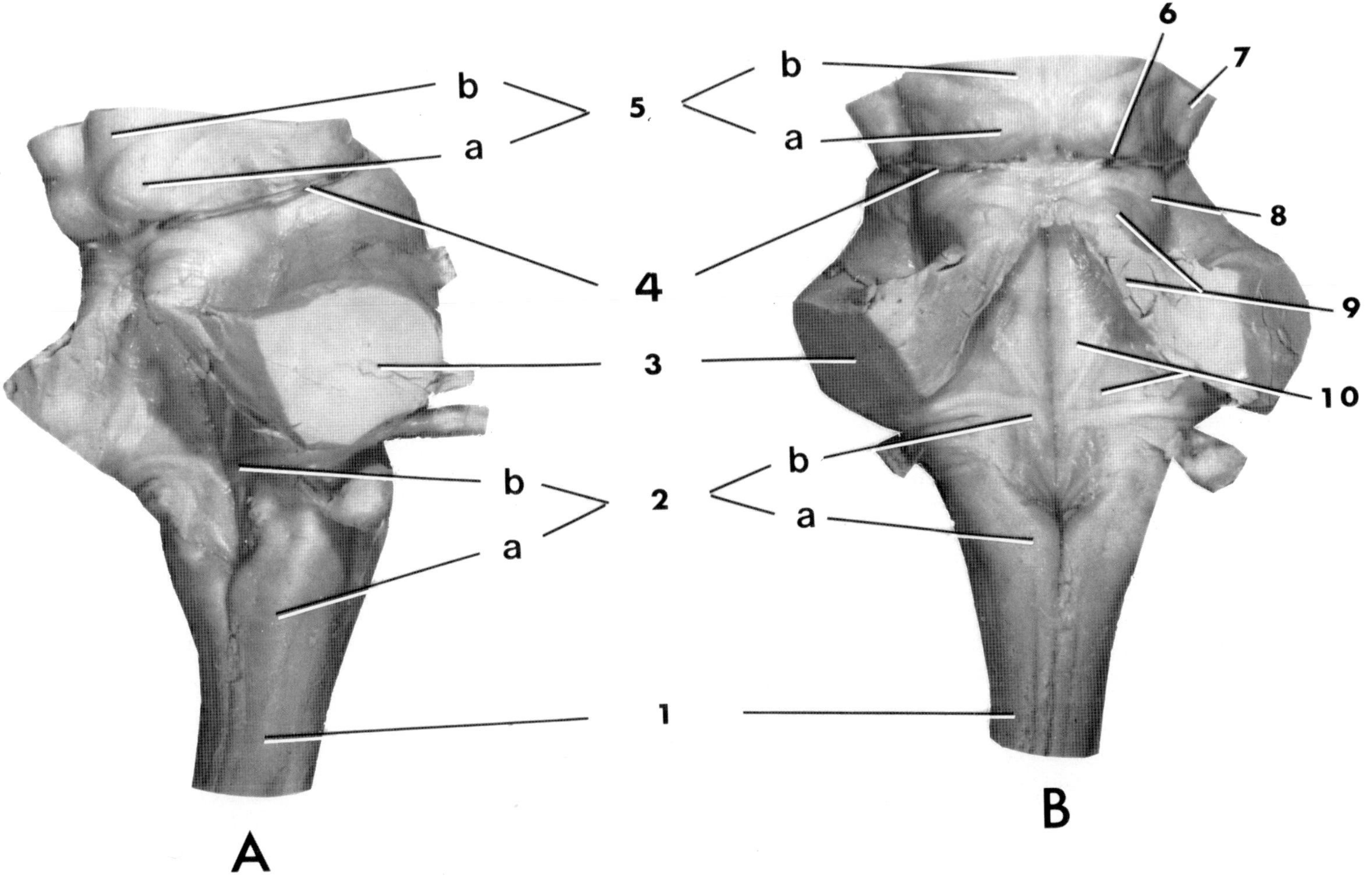

Figure 47 Lateral **(A)** and dorsal **(B)** views of the brain stem showing the trochlear (C.N. IV) nerve as it emerges from the dorsum of the brain stem.

1. **Trigeminal Nerve Fibers (C.N. V) (Sensory)**—axons from neurons in the sensory trigeminal ganglion (semilunar, Gasserian ganglion) enter the pons laterally at the junction of the basal pons and the middle cerebellar peduncle. The entering fibers form the spinal tract of the trigeminal nerve (see also no. **6a,** Fig. 46).
2. **Spinal Tract of Trigeminal Nerve**—as the sensory fibers of the trigeminal nerve enter the pons, they turn caudally and course through the dorsolateral tegmentum of the pons, the medulla, and the cephalic end of the spinal cord. As the fibers descend, they turn medially and synapse on the spinal nuclei of the trigeminal nerve that lie immediately adjacent to the fibers. These two structures form a little ridge on the lateral side of the brain stem in the dorsolateral sulcus known as the tuberculum cinereum (see also no. **5,** Fig. 41).
3. **Olive**—located betwen the pyramid and the dorsolateral sulcus in the medulla.
4. **Clava (Nucleus Gracilis)**—this club-shaped swelling is on the dorsomedial surface of the caudal (closed portion) medulla (see also no. **4,** Fig. 37*A*).
5. **Floor of Fourth Ventricle**—the dorsal surface of the tegmentum of the open medulla and pons. Some surface markings (vestibular area, facial colliculus, vagal triangle) are important landmarks.
6. **Superior Cerebellar Peduncle (Cut) (Brachium Conjunctivum)**—consists mainly of cerebellar efferent fibers passing rostrally into the caudal midbrain.
7. **Tectum of Midbrain**—consists of four rounded elevations, the corpora quadrigemina, which are also called the paired superior and inferior colliculi (see also no. **5,** Fig. 47).
8. **Corpus Callosum (Area of Splenium—Cut Fibers)**—consists of compact commissural fibers that cross in the midline from each cerebral hemisphere. The corpus callosum is formed by fibers from each cerebral hemisphere. The corpus callosum forms the roof of the lateral ventricles. Part of the corpus callosum on the right side has been removed to show the position of the crus fornix in the lateral ventricle.
9. **Lateral Ventricle**—posterior part of the body of the lateral ventricle. Fibers from the hippocampus (dissected from the inferior horn of the lateral ventricle) arch over the pulvinar of the thalamus and converge on the dorsomedial surface of the thalamus to form the body of the fornix.
10. **Internal Capsule (Exposed)**—the lentiform nucleus has been removed to show the cortical projection fibers from the corona radiata converging to form the internal capsule. The fibers of the internal capsule pass into the basis pedunculi of the midbrain (see also nos. **2** and **6,** Fig. 19).
11. **Hippocampus**—(removed from inferior horn in temporal lobe), part of the limbic system. Axons of hippocampal neurons form the crus fornix (see also no. **1,** Fig. 34).
12. **Trochlear Nerve (C.N. IV)**—emerges from the roof of the midbrain caudal to the inferior colliculus. The nerve courses inferiorly on the lateral surface of the midbrain to enter the cavernous sinus and the orbit to supply the lateral rectus muscle (see also no. **4,** Fig. 47).
13. **Right Middle Cerebellar Peduncle (Cut Fibers) (Brachium Pontis)**—consists of pontocerebellar fibers coursing from the contralateral basal pons to the cortex of the right cerebellar hemisphere.

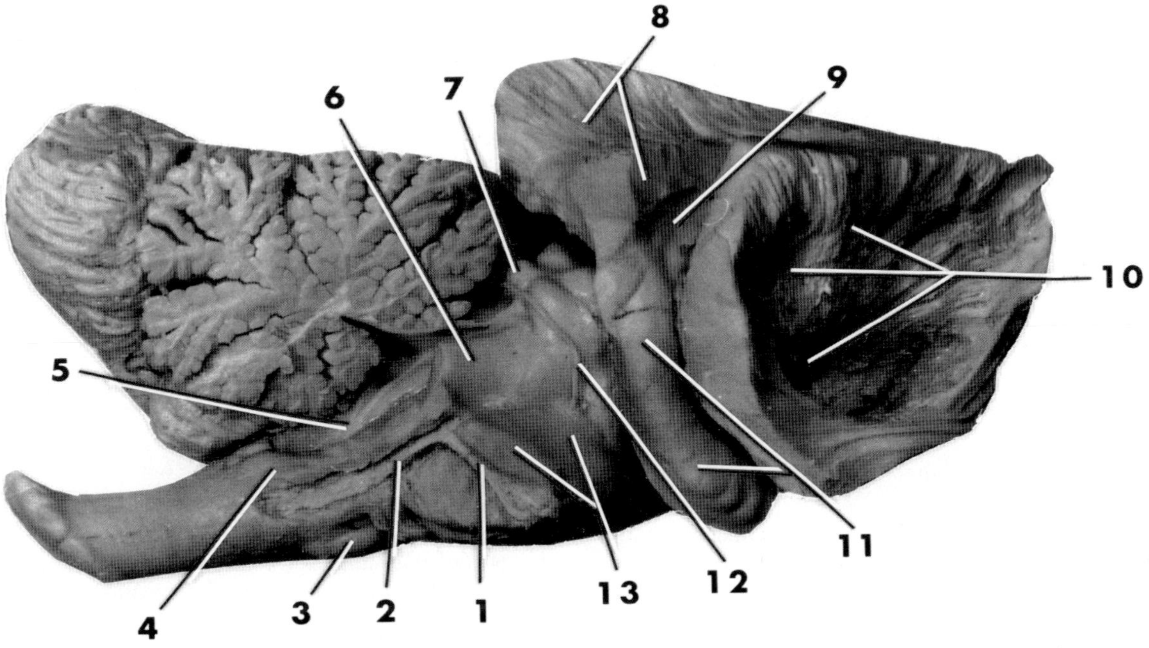

Figure 48. Lateral view of the right side of the brain stem, the hippocampus, and the internal capsule. The right cerebellar peduncles have been transected, and the right half of the cerebellum has been removed. The lateral side of the pons and the medulla has been dissected to show the course of the descending sensory fibers of the trigeminal nerve. Most of the cerebral hemisphere has been dissected away to show the hippocampus, the crus fornix, and the internal capsule.

1. **Forceps Major**—one arm of the U- or fork-shaped configuration of commissural fibers forming the posterior portion of the corpus callosum (see also no. **2,** Fig. 23).
2. **Inferior Colliculus**—nerve cell mass forming the ovoid mound (L. *colliculus*) or eminence on the caudal half of the dorsal surface of the midbrain; a relay station in the central auditory pathway.
3. **Cerebral Aqueduct (of Sylvius)**—small canal which drains cerebrospinal fluid from the lateral and third ventricles into the fourth ventricle (see also no. **9,** Fig. 44).
4. **Substantia Nigra** (L. black substance)—large nucleus consisting of a thick layer of cells containing black pigment. Extends the length of the midbrain and has motor functions (see also no. **16,** Fig. 44).
5. **Basis Pedunculi (of Cerebral Peduncle)**—the continuation of the internal capsule (see no. **17,** Fig. 44).
6. **Amygdaloid Nucleus**—exposed when much of the temporal pole cortex was removed. A flattened cell mass resembling an almond (L. from G. *amygdalē*) in size and shape.
7. **Oculomotor Nerve (C.N. III)**—see also no. **9,** Fig. 46.
8. **Olfactory Tract**—a bundle of nerve fibers connecting the olfactory bulb to the inferior surface of the cerebral hemisphere.
9. **Optic Nerve (C.N. II)**—see also no. **7**, Fig. 46.
10. **Optic Tract**—a bundle of optic nerve fibers from the optic chiasma passing to the lateral geniculate body (**11**) (see also no. **8,** Fig. 46).
11. **Lateral Geniculate Body (Nucleus)**—most of the optic tract fibers terminate in this nucleus.
12. **Meyer's Loop**—some fibers of the geniculocalcarine tract loop forward in the temporal lobe around the lateral ventricle forming Meyer's loop.
13. **Geniculocalcarine Tract**—composed of fibers from the lateral geniculate body which course to the visual cortex (see also no. **4,** Fig. 20).
14. **Visual Pathway**—ganglion fibers from the retina form the optic nerve (**9**), and the optic tract (**10**). They terminate on the lateral geniculate body (**11**). Fibers from this body form the geniculocalcarine tract (**12** and **13**) which terminates in the visual cortex (about the calcarine sulcus).
15. **Posterior Horn of Lateral Ventricle**—extends into occipital lobe.
16. **Splenium of Corpus Callosum**—the thickened, bandage-like posterior extremity of this commissure of the cerebral hemisphere.

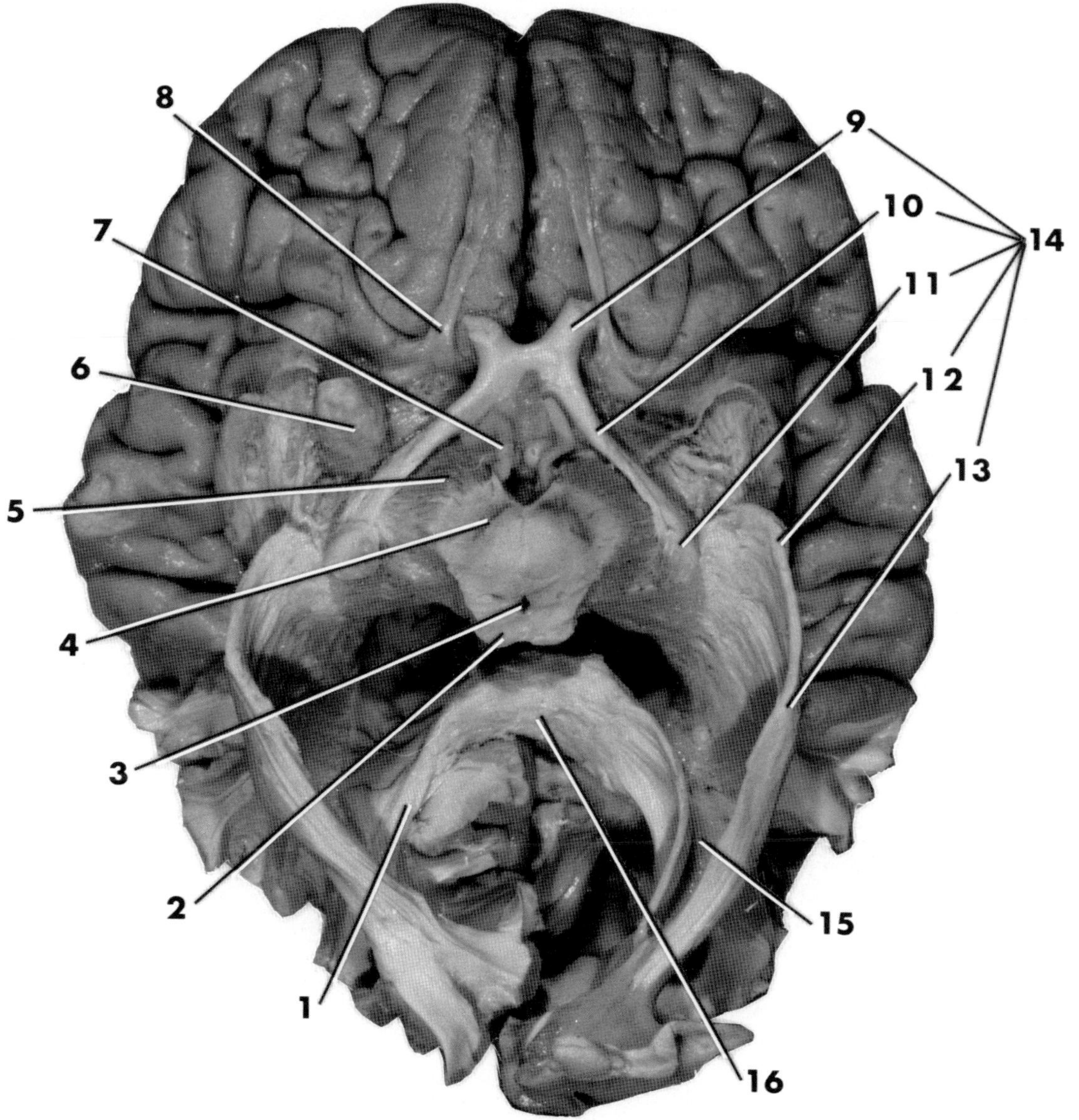

Figure 49 Dissection of the basal aspect of the cerebrum showing the visual pathways from the optic nerves to the occipital lobes.

7

The Cerebellum

1. **Posterior Incisure**—the posterior margin of the cerebellum is notched by a deep and narrow incisure which contains a fold of dura mater and the falx cerebelli. Inferiorly the posterior incisure becomes a deep medium fossa which contains the inferior vermis.
2. **Posterior Lobe of Cerebellum**—the part of the left cerebellar hemisphere posterior to the primary fissure (**4**). It also includes the inferior surface of the hemisphere. Secondary fissures divide the lobe into lobules (*i.e.*, simple, ansiform, and biventral). On the superior surface, the folia of the hemispheres are continuous with those of the vermis.
3. **Cerebellar Folia**—consists of extensive folding of the cerebellar surface into thin transverse folia (L. *folium*, leaf) on the hemispheres and vermis. On the dorsal surface of the cerebellum, the folia of hemispheres are continuous with the folia of the vermis; 85% of the cerebellar cortex is concealed between the folia.
4. **Primary Fissure**—on the dorsal surface of the cerebellum, the primary fissure separates the anterior lobe (**5**) from the posterior lobe (**2**). It is the second fissure to appear during prenatal development. The posterolateral fissure is the first fissure to appear (see no. **2**, Fig. 53).
5. **Anterior Lobe of Cerebellum**—is that part of the dorsal surface of the cerebellum that lies anterior to the primary fissure. It consists of parts of both cerebellar hemispheres, as well as the rostral portion of the superior vermis. The folia are parallel and continuous in this lobe.
6. **Cerebral Aqueduct (of Sylvius)**—the narrow cerebral aqueduct through which cerebrospinal fluid flows from the third ventricle to the fourth ventricle. It courses through the midline (central) area of the midbrain inferior to the tectum (**7**). It is surrounded by central gray matter.
7. **Tectum of Midbrain** (L. *tectum*, roof)—lies dorsal to the central gray matter and consists of the corpora quadrigemina (*i.e.*, a pair of superior and a pair of inferior colliculi). Note that the midbrain has been transected at the level of the inferior colliculi.
8. **Superior Vermis** (L. *vermis*, worm)—it is the midline part of the cerebellum which is not demarcated from the hemispheres. The folia are continuous from the cerebellar hemispheres into the vermis.
9. **Cerebellar Hemisphere** (right)—the cerebellum is composed of a midline structure called the vermis and large lateral lobes on each side known as the left and right hemispheres. The cerebellar hemispheres and the vermis are known as the corpus cerebelli. The flocculonodular lobe is a small component separate from the corpus cerebelli.
10. **Posterior Superior Fissure (Postclival Fissure)**—separates the rostral part (simple lobule) of the posterior lobe from that part of the posterior lobe (anisform lobe) that lies caudal to the posterior superior fissure.
11. **Superior Semilunar Lobule (Crus I)**—is the rostral part of the ansiform lobule that lies posterior to the posterior superior fissure. On the inferior surface the superior semilunar lobule (crus I) is separated from the inferior semilunar lobule (crus II) by the transverse fissure.

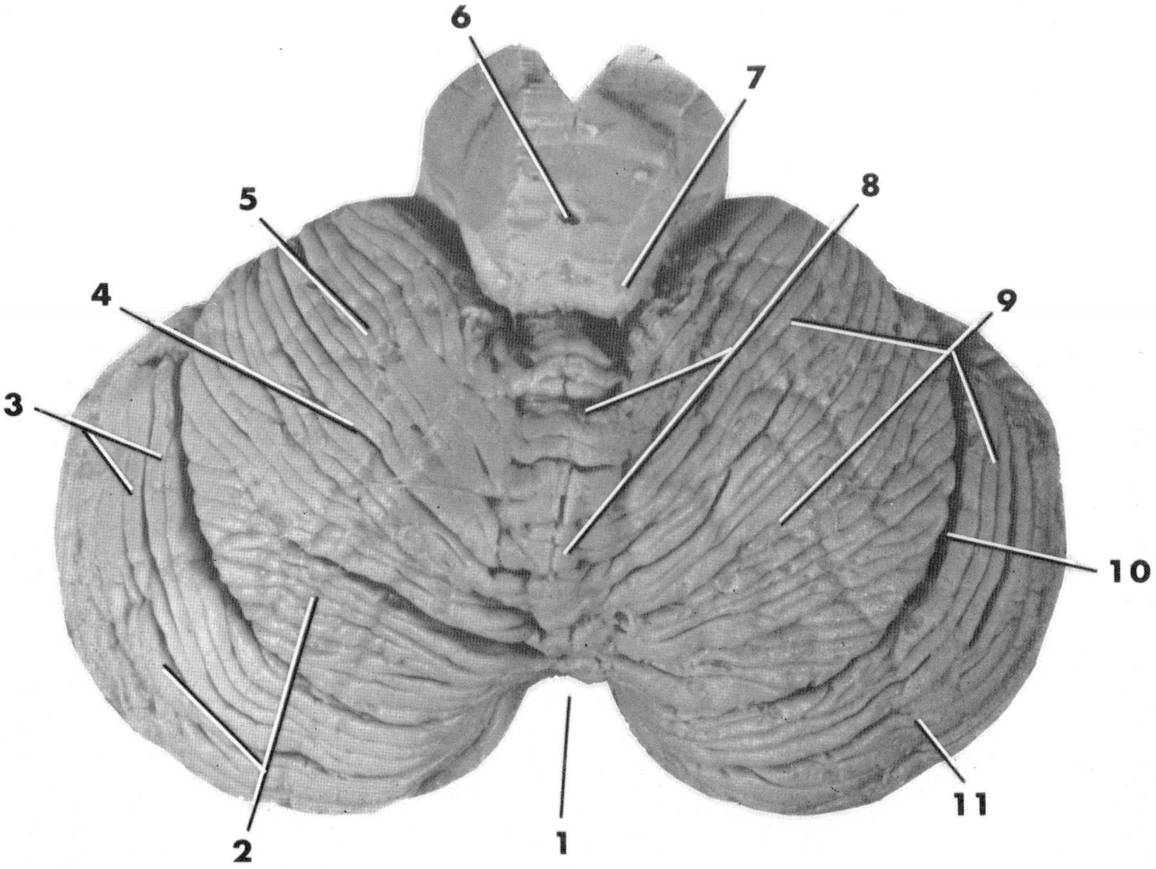

Figure 50 Superior surface of the **cerebellum** showing some of its neuroanatomical features. A cross-section of the **midbrain** at the level of the inferior colliculi is also shown.

1. **Pons (Basal)**—ventral portion of the pons consists of pontine neurons whose axons course transversely into the contralateral cerebellar hemisphere, as well as cerebral fiber pathways (corticopontine and corticospinal) that end in or pass through the basal pons.
2. **Area of Lateral Aperture (Foramen of Luschka)**—connects the lateral recess of the fourth ventricle with the pontine cistern (the large subarachnoid space between the side of the pons and the medulla, and the ventral surface of the cerebellum). Note that the arachnoid mater has been removed, thereby eliminating the cistern in this figure.
3. **Vestibulocochlear Nerve (C.N. VIII)**—passes medially beneath the flocculus (**10**) at the pontocerebellar angle to enter the brain stem at the medulla-pons junction. The cochlear fibers terminate on neurons of the cochlear nuclei, and the vestibular fibers terminate on vestibular nuclei or in the cortex of the flocculus (see also no. **5**, Fig. 53).
4. **Tonsil (Paramedian Lobule)**—is the most medial portion of the posterior lobe of the hemisphere that lies adjacent to the side of the medulla. When there is cerebellar edema or a tumor in the posterior cranial fossa, the tonsils herniate through the foramen magnum and squeeze the medulla, rendering it anemic by compressing the capillaries (see also no. **2**, Fig. 52).
5. **Posterior Lobe of Left Cerebellar Hemisphere**—consists of the rest of the hemisphere on both surfaces (superior and inferior) that lies posterior to the primary fissure. Secondary fissures subdivide this lobe into various lobules and parts which have been assigned special names (*i.e.*, simple lobule, ansiform lobule, biventer lobule, and tonsil) (see also no. **9**, Fig. 53).
6. **Horizontal Fissure**—in the posterior lobe the horizontal fissure divides the ansiform lobule into crus I (superior semilunar lobule) and crus II (inferior semilunar lobule).
7. **Vermis** (L. worm)—the midline portion of the cerebellum. The *superior vermis* (**a**) is not demarcated from the hemispheres. The folia of the vermis are continuous with the folia of the hemispheres. The **inferior vermis** (**b**) lies in a deep depression (median fossa-vallecula) and is well delineated from the cerebellar hemispheres (see also no. **8**, Fig. 55).
8. **Inferior Semilunar Lobule (Crus II)**—is part of the ansiform lobule and is separated from the superior semilunar lobule by the transverse fissure.
9. **Biventer (Biventer Lobule)**—is that part of the posterior lobe that lies between the inferior semilunar lobule, part of the ansiform lobule (**8**), and the tonsil (**4**).
10. **Flocculus (Part of Archicerebellum)**—an irregularly shaped mass on each side, located at the rostral edge of the inferior surface. It is separated from the cerebellar hemisphere by the posterolateral fissure. The flocculus is attached to the nodule, the most rostral portion of the inferior vermis, by a peduncle. These are components of the flocculonodular lobe which function in the maintenance of equilibrium (see also no. **3**, Fig. 53).
11. **Medulla Oblongata**—the medulla is conical in shape. It is the caudal end of the brain stem that connects the pons superiorly and the spinal cord inferiorly. The cerebellum rests on the rostral end (open portion) of the medulla. The pons, medulla, and cerebellum are contained in the posterior cranial fossa.

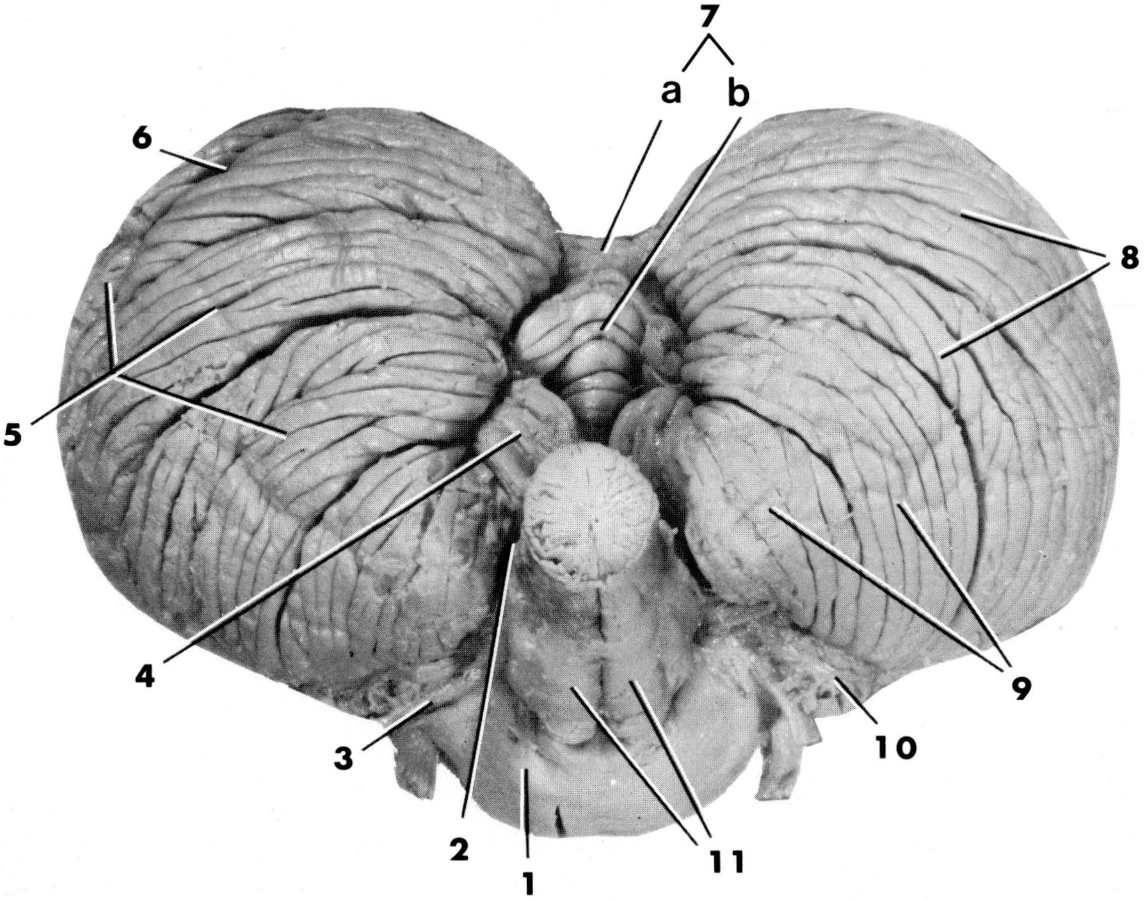

Figure 51 Posterior and inferior views of the **cerebellum** showing some of its neuroanatomical features. The medulla and the pons are also visible.

1. **Uvula of Inferior Vermis**—the part of the inferior vermis located between the nodule (nodulus), the most rostral portion of the vermis, and the pyramid. The uvula is well demarcated from the hemispheres and lies in the median fissure (vallecula cerebelli).
2. **Tonsil (Paramedian Lobule)**—located on the inferior surface, it is the most medial portion of the posterior lobe of the cerebellum. It lies adjacent to the lateral surface of the medulla. In certain pathological conditions the tonsil may enlarge, press against the medulla, and herniate through the foramen magnum.
3. **Posterior Lobe of Cerebellum**—lies between the primary and posterolateral fissures. It has superior and inferior surfaces. Secondary sulci or fissures divide it into various lobules. It forms the parts of the left and right hemispheres and the vermis that lie posterior to the primary fissure (see also no. **5**, Fig. 51).
4. **Flocculonodular Lobe**—consists of the small irregular shaped flocculus (**a**) which is separated from the hemisphere by the posterolateral fissure and the nodule (**b**) the most rostral portion of the inferior vermis. A peduncle of nerve fibers connects these two areas.
5. **Anterior Lobe of Cerebellum**—on the superior surface, the anterior lobe is that part of the corpus cerebelli (vermis and hemispheres) that lies anterior to the primary fissure. It consists of the rostral portion of the cerebellar hemispheres and the superior vermis. The folia of the hemispheres are continuous with the folia of the vermis (see also no. **5**, Fig. 50).
6. **Superior Medullary Velum and Lingula of Cerebellum**—the thin v-shaped sheet of pia mater and ependymal cells is situated between the superior cerebellar peduncles (**8**). The superior medullary velum along with the superior peduncles forms the forepart of the roof of the fourth ventricle. The lingula, the most rostral part of the superior vermis, rests on the superior surface of the superior medullary velum (see also no. **15**, Fig. 56).
7. **Superior Vermis** (L. *vermis*, worm)—on the superior surface of the cerebellum the midline area is not demarcated from the hemispheres. The parallel folia of the vermis are continuous with the folia of the hemispheres.
8. **Superior Cerebellar Peduncle (Brachium Conjunctivum)**—composed of efferent fibers from the dentate (mainly), emboliform, and globose cerebellar nuclei which extend to the contralateral ventral lateral nucleus of the thalamus and the red nucleus of the midbrain. The superior cerebellar peduncle is medial to the rostral portion of the middle cerebellar peduncle (see also no. **4**, Fig. 55).
9. **Inferior Cerebellar Peduncle (Restiform and Juxtarestiform Bodies)**—the restiform body is composed of afferent fibers from the spinal cord and the brain stem which course to the cortex of the vermal and paravermal areas. The juxtarestiform body is composed of afferents from the vestibular nuclei and ganglion cells of semicircular ducts to the vestibular nuclei. The juxtarestiform body lies medial to the restiform body, and the inferior cerebellar peduncle lies medial to the caudal area of the middle cerebellar peduncle (see also no. **1**, Fig. 55).
10. **Middle Cerebellar Peduncle (Branchium Pontis)**—the largest of the three cerebellar peduncles. It carries fibers from the nuclei pontis, located in the basal pons, to the contralateral cortex in the cerebellar hemispheres (see also no. **12**, Fig. 54).
11. **Posterolateral Fissure**—is the first fissure to develop in the cerebellum. It is located on the inferior surface of the cerebellum and separates the corpus cerebelli (vermis and hemispheres) from the flocculonodular lobe (see also no. **2**, Fig. 53).
12. **Area of Fourth Ventricle**—the tent-shaped roof of the fourth ventricle protrudes into the cerebellum. The forepart of the roof is formed by the superior medullary velum (**6**), and the lateral walls are bound by the superior (**8**) and inferior (**9**) cerebellar peduncles. The floor of the fourth ventricle is formed by parts of the medulla and the pons.

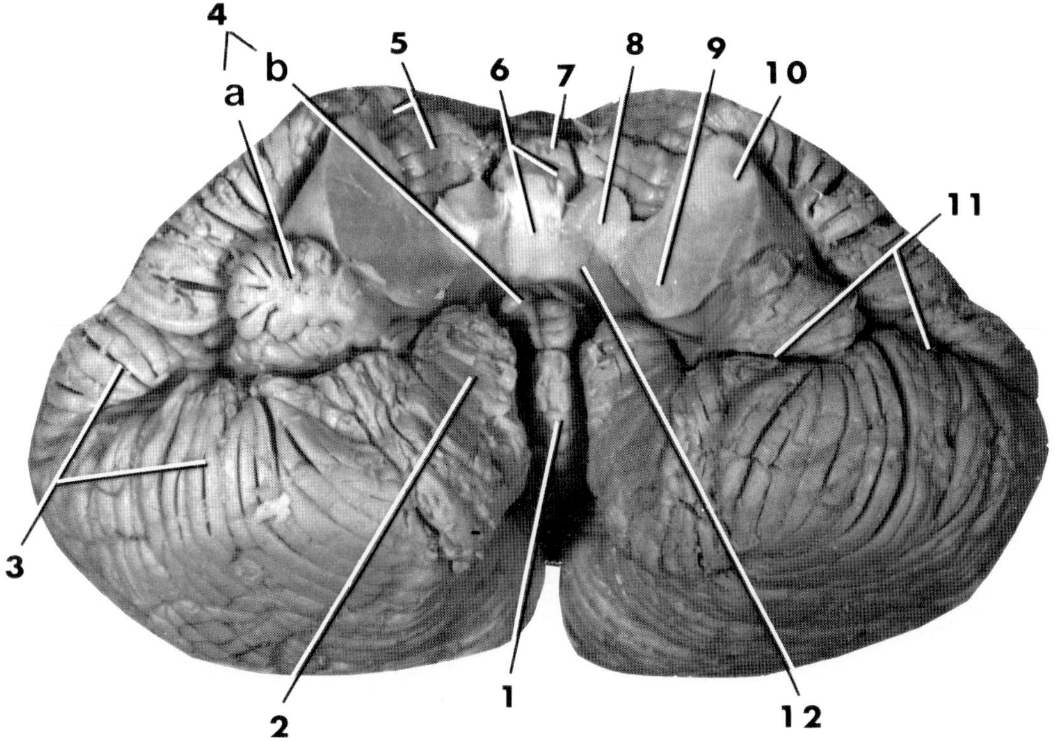

Figure 52 Inferior view of the detached **cerebellum** showing some of its neuroanatomical features and the cut surfaces of the **cerebellar peduncles**.

1. **Medulla Oblongata**—this conical shaped part of the brain stem connects the pons and the spinal cord. The rostral portion of the cerebellum rests on the pons, and its caudal portion rests on the open portion of the medulla. The IVth ventricle intervenes between the cerebellum and the pons and medulla. The pons, medulla, and cerebellum are contained in the posterior cranial fossa.
2. **Posterolateral Fissure**—this is the first fissure to develop in the cerebellum. It is located on its inferior surface and separates the corpus cerebelli (hemispheres and vermis) from the flocculonodular lobe (see also no. **11**, Fig. 51).
3. **Flocculus (Archicerebellum)**—this small irregularly shaped mass is located at the rostral edge of the inferior surface of the cerebellum. It is separated from the cerebellar hemispheres by the posterolateral fissure (**2**). A peduncle attaches the flocculus to the nodule of the inferior vermis; the whole structure is known as the flocculonodular lobe. It functions in the maintenance of equilibrium (see also no. **4a**, Fig. 52).
4. **Anterior Lobe of Cerebellum**—on the superior surface of the cerebellum, the anterior lobe is that part of the cerebellum lying anterior or rostral to the primary fissure. The cerebellar tissue posterior to this fissure comprises the posterior lobe. The anterior lobe consists of part of the left and right hemispheres and the rostral part of the superior vermis.
5. **Vestibulocochlear Nerve (C.N. VII)**—passes medially beneath the flocculus to enter the brain stem at the pontine cerebellar angle and medulla-pons junction. The cochlear fibers end on the cochlear nuclei and the vestibular fibers on the vestibular nuclei and cortex of the flocculus.
6. **Pons**—the ventral or basal portion of the pons consists of: (1) pontine neurons whose axons course transversely to enter the contralateral middle cerebellar peduncle; (2) bundles of descending corticospinal tract fibers which pass through the pons uninterrupted, as well as corticobulbar fibers which may end in the tegmental pons, and (3) descending corticopontine fibers which terminate on pontine neurons.
7. **Trigeminal Nerve (C.N. V)** (L. *trigeminus*—threefold)—the sensory and motor fibers of this large cranial nerve enter and emerge on the ventrolateral side of the pons at the junction of the basal pons and the middle cerebellar peduncle (see also no. **6**, Fig. 46).
8. **Middle Cerebellar Peduncle (Brachium Pontis)**—the largest of the three cerebellar peduncles. It consists of fibers from neurons of the contralateral pontine nuclei that course to the cortex of this cerebellar hemisphere (see also no. **3**, Fig. 55).
9. **Posterior Lobe of Cerebellum**—the part of the cerebellum exclusive of the flocculus that lies posterior to the primary fissure. The posterior lobe consists of the left and right cerebellar hemispheres and a central vermal portion. On the superior surface, the vermis is continuous with the hemisphere. On the inferior surface, the inferior vermis is well demarcated (see no. **1**, Fig. 52).
10. **Area of Lateral Aperture (Foramen of Luschka)**—the lateral aperture connects the lateral recess of the fourth ventricle with the large subarachnoid space, the pontine cistern. The flocculus and the VIIIth C.N. course beside this communication. The choroid plexus from the fourth ventricle emerges into the subarachnoid space through this aperture (see also no. **2**, Fig. 51).
11. **Tonsil (Paramedian Lobule)**—on the inferior surface the tonsil is the most medial portion of the posterior lobe. It lies adjacent to the side of the medulla. If pressure in the posterior cranial fossa is increased owing to edema or a tumor, the tonsils may herniate through the foramen magnum (see also no. **4**, Fig. 51).

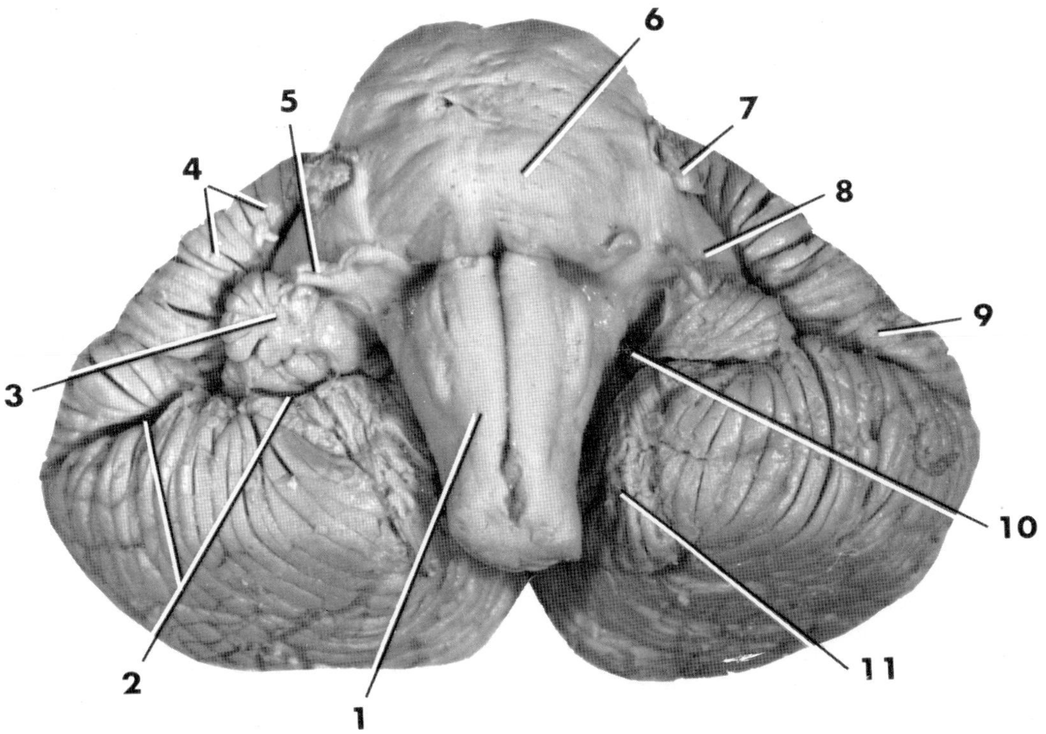

Figure 53 Anteroinferior view of the medulla, pons, and attached cerebellum showing some of their neuroanatomical features.

1. **Trochlear Nerve** (left) **(C.N. IV)**—this motor nerve is the only cranial nerve to emerge on the dorsal aspect of the brain stem. Its fibers emerge caudal to the inferior colliculus (**6**). It supplies the superior oblique muscle (see also no. **12**, Fig. 48).
2. **Basis Pedunculi**—the inferior portion of the cerebral peduncle. It is a continuation of the internal capsule and is composed of descending cortical projection fibers (see also no. **17**, Fig. 44).
3. **Inferior Brachium** (L. arm)—consists of fibers that course from the inferior colliculus (**6**) to the medial geniculate body of the thalamus. It is part of the auditory pathway (see also no. **7**, Fig. 37*A*).
4. **Cerebral Aqueduct (of Sylvius)**—located between the tectum and the tegmentum of the midbrain. It connects the third ventricle with the fourth ventricle as it passes through the midbrain.
5. **Superior Colliculus** (left)—part of the corpora quadrigemina which is the tectum (L. roof) of the midbrain. The superior colliculi are associated with the visual system.
6. **Inferior Colliculus** (left)—the left and right inferior and superior colliculi form the corpora quadrigemina. The inferior colliculi function in the auditory system.
7. **Right Cerebellar Hemisphere**—the cortex is arranged in many uniform parallel folds or folia.
8. **Vermis** (L. worm)—the midline portion of the cerebellum. The superior vermis is continuous with the cerebellar hemispheres, but the inferior vermis is well delineated from them.
9. **Fibers of Inferior Cerebellar Peduncle (Restiform Body)**—fibers from the spinal cord and the brain stem course to the cortex of the vermal (**8**) and paravermal areas. These fibers lie medial to the middle (**12**) and posterior and lateral to the superior (**11**) cerebellar peduncles (see also no. **1**, Fig. 55).
10. **Medullary Center of the Left Cerebellar Hemisphere**—consists of cortical cerebellar afferents and efferents. The left dentate nucleus is located deep within the medullary center of this hemisphere.
11. **Superior Cerebellar Peduncle (Brachium Conjunctivum)**—consists of fibers which originate from the dentate (also emboliform and globose) nucleus. The fibers pass superior and medial to the middle cerebellar peduncle, enter the tegmentum of the midbrain at the level of the inferior colliculus, decussate (cross) to the contralateral side to end on the ventrolateral thalamic and red nuclei (see also no. **14**, Fig. 56).
12. **Middle Cerebellar Peduncle** (left) **(Brachium Pontis)**—consists of pontocerebellar fibers that originate from contralateral pontine neurons in the right basal pons. The fibers course laterally, superiorly, and posteriorly to end in the cortex of the left cerebellar hemisphere (see also no. **3**, Fig. 55).

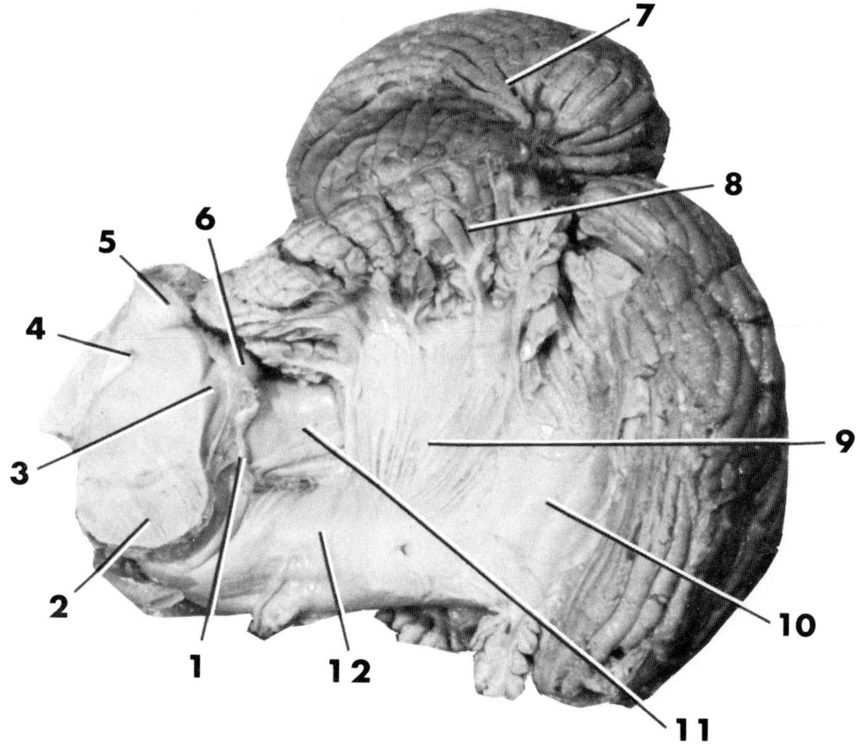

Figure 54 Lateral view of the left side of the transected midbrain, pons, and cerebellum. Much of the left cerebellar hemisphere has been removed to show the **three cerebellar peduncles** (superior, middle, and inferior).

1. **Fibers of Inferior Cerebellar Peduncle (Restiform Body)**—fibers from the spinal cord and brain stem course to the cortex of the vermal (**8**) and paravermal areas. Note that these fibers lie medial to the middle cerebellar peduncle (**3**) and posterior and lateral to the superior cerebellar peduncle (**4**) (see also no. **9**, Fig. 54).
2. **Medullary Center**—of left cerebellar hemisphere. It consists of cortical cerebellar afferent and efferent fibers.
3. **Middle Cerebellar Peduncle** (left) **(Brachium Pontis)**—it consists of pontocerebellar fibers which originate from contralateral pontine neurons in the basal pons. These fibers course laterally, superiorly, and posteriorly to end in the cortex of the left cerebellar hemisphere (see also no. **2**, Fig. 56).
4. **Superior Cerebellar Peduncle (Brachium Conjunctivum)**—consists of fibers which originate from the dentate (also emboliform and globose) nucleus. The fibers pass superior and medial to the middle cerebellar peduncle, enter the tegmentum of the midbrain at the level of the inferior colliculus, decussate to the contralateral side to end on the red nucleus or predominantly the ventrolateral thalamic nucleus (see also no. **14**, Fig. 56).
5. **Cerebral Aqueduct (of Sylvius)**—located between the tectum and tegmentum of the midbrain (connects IIIrd and IVth ventricles).
6. **Trochlear Nerve (C.N. IV)**—these motor fibers to the superior oblique muscle emerge from the dorsal surface of the midbrain posterior to the inferior colliculus (see also no. **1**, Fig. 54).
7. **Cerebellar Cortex**—covering many uniform and parallel folia of the right cerebellar hemisphere.
8. **Vermis** (L. worm)—the midline portion of the cerebellum. On the dorsal surface of the cerebellum, the vermis is continuous with the hemispheres and on the ventral surface the vermis is separate and well delineated from each hemisphere (see no. **1**, Fig. 52).

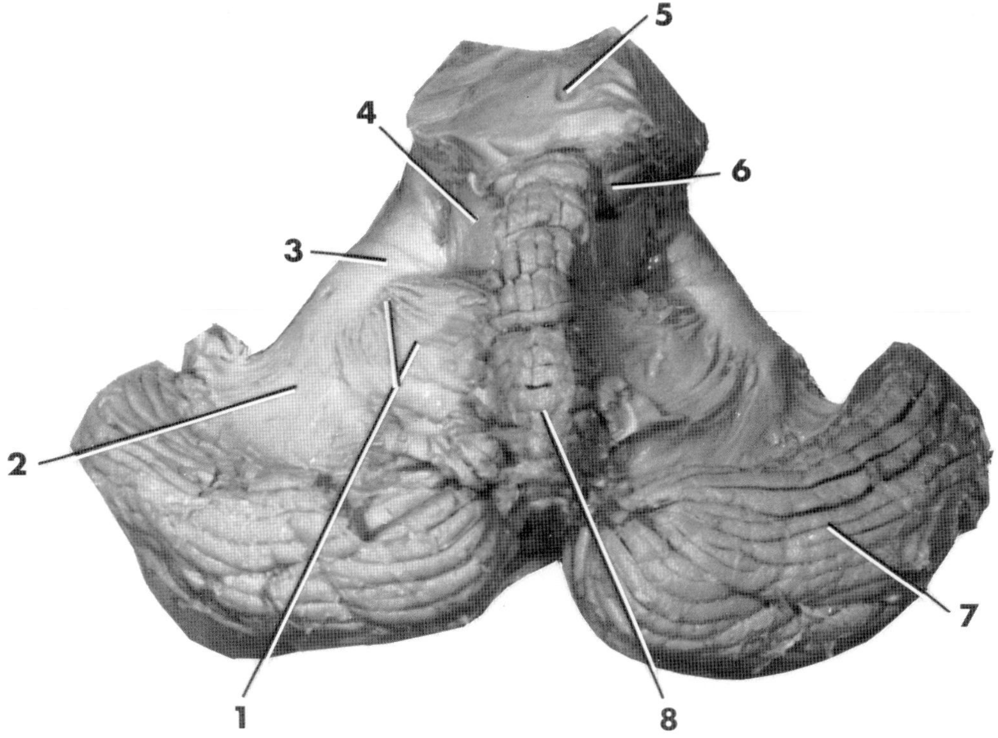

Figure 55 Superior view of the cerebellum. Much of the left cerebellar hemisphere has been removed to show the **relationship of the three cerebellar peduncles** to each other.

1. **Dentate Nucleus**—axons from neurons in this nucleus emerge to form the superior cerebellar peduncle (**14**).
2. **Middle Cerebellar Peduncle (Brachium Pontis)**, left—composed of axons from contralateral pontine neurons coursing to the cortex of the cerebellar hemisphere (see also no. **3**, Fig. 55).
3. **Trigeminal Nerve (C.N. V)**—was given its name because it has three branches (L. *trigeminus*, threefold).
4. **Hippocampus**—part of the limbic system. A gyrus which produces an elevation on the floor of the inferior horn of the lateral ventricle resembling a sea horse (G. *hippocampos*) (see also no. **1**, Fig. 34).
5. **Crus Fornix**—fibers from the hippocampus (**4**) form the fornix (**5** and **10**) which courses to the mammillary bodies. Is part of the limbic system (see also no. **11**, Fig. 36).
6. **IIIrd Ventricle**—median cleft-like cavity in the diencephalon. Part of the ventricular system of the brain. Note: The roof of IIIrd ventricle has been removed to show this.
7. **Anterior Tubercle of Thalamus**—cone-shaped mass formed by the anterior nucleus of the thalamus.
8. **Head of Caudate Nucleus**—part of the corpus striatum. It owes its name to its long tail (L. *cauda*).
9. **Internal Capsule**—projection fibers coursing between the lentiform nucleus, the head of the caudate nucleus, and the thalamus.
10. **Body of Fornix**—band of white fibers forming the main efferent tract of the hippocampus. Runs forward under the corpus callosum like an arch (L. *fornix*).
11. **Medial Geniculate Body**—nuclear relay area of the auditory system. Fibers from this nucleus course to the auditory cortex of the transverse temporal gyrus (see also no. **9**, Fig. 37*A*)
12. **Inferior Brachium**—part of the auditory pathway that connects the inferior collicular nucleus with the medial geniculate nucleus.
13. **Colliculi (Corpora Quadrigemina)**—the right superior and inferior colliculi are labelled. The latin word *colliculus* means a mound or small elevation.
14. **Superior Cerebellar Peduncle (Brachium Conjunctivum)**—composed of fibers primarily from the dentate nucleus which extend to the contralateral ventral lateral nucleus of the thalamus and to the red nucleus.
15. **Superior Medullary Velum and Lingula of Cerebellum**—this velum (L. *veil*) is a thin sheet of ependyma and pia mater stretching between the superior cerebellar peduncles (**14**). The lingula (L. dim. of *lingua*, tongue) is a tongue-shaped lobule of the cerebellum (tip of pointer) which extends forward on the velum.

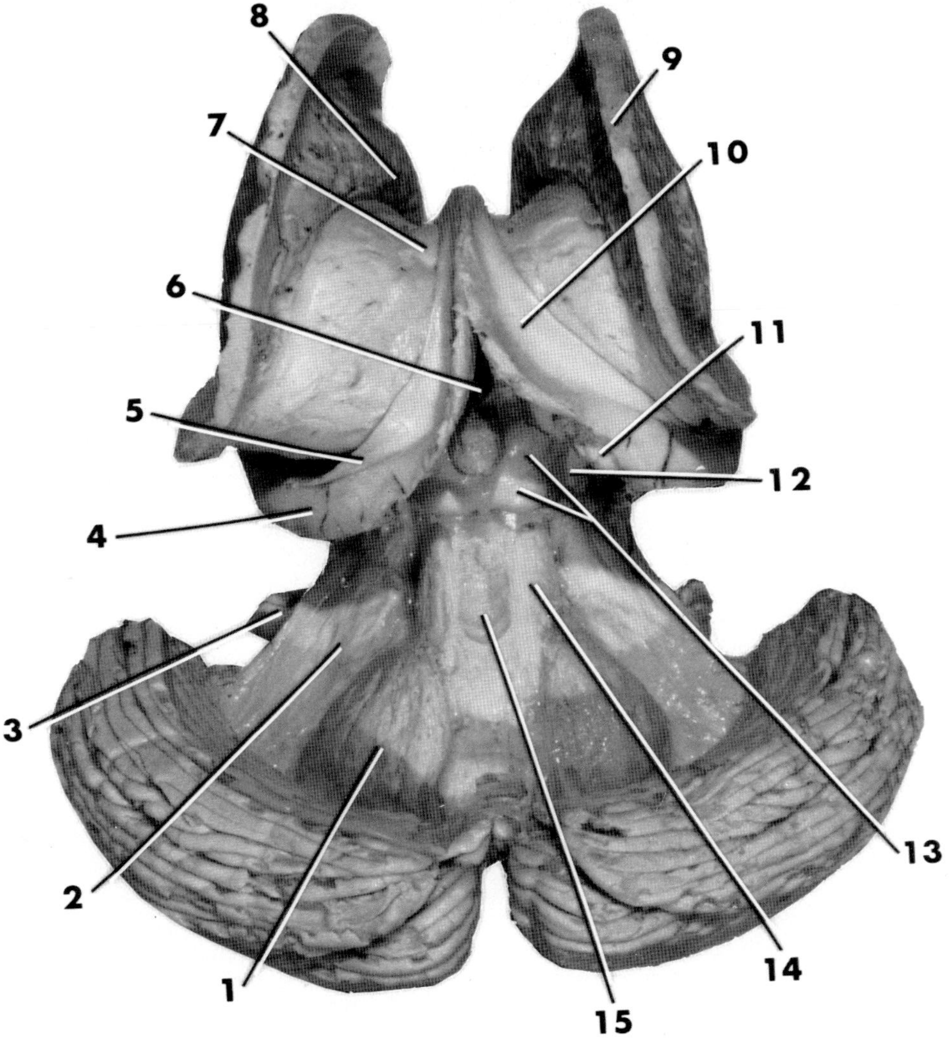

Figure 56 Dorsal view of the corpus striatum, thalamus, midbrain, and cerebellum. The superior aspect of the cerebellum has been removed to show the **cerebellar peduncles** and the **dentate nucleus**. Also shown is the relationship of some of the limbic system (hippocampus and fornix) to the thalamus.

8

The Spinal Cord

1. **Pia Mater and Dorsal Column of White Matter**—the thin investing membrane (pia mater) composed of fine reticular and elastic fibers and lined by a single layer of simple squamous epithelium covers all of the spinal cord. Many of the spinal vessels lie within this layer. The dorsal column of white matter at this level is located between the dorsal median and dorsolateral sulci, and consists of the fasciculus gracilis and fasciculus cuneatus.
2. **Dura Mater**—this dense firm membrane has been split and partly excised. Normally it takes the form of a tube which is pierced by the roots of the spinal nerves (see no. **6**, Fig. 60). It extends from the foramen magnum to the second segment of the sacrum.
3. **Left Transverse Sinus**—is located in the attached edge of the tentorium cerebelli. The left transverse sinus is usually formed when the straight sinus turns to the left.
4. **Left Cerebellar Hemisphere**—contained in the left posterior cranial fossa. The tentorium cerebelli has been removed to show the position of the cerebellum in the posterior cranial fossa.
5. **Arachnoid Mater covering the Cisterna Magna (Cerebellomedullary Cistern)**—is the large subarachnoid space beneath the arachnoid mater occupying the interval between the cerebellum and the dorsal medulla oblongata. It receives cerebrospinal fluid from the fourth ventricle through the median aperture (foramen of Magendie). **Note**—the arachnoid mater has been removed from the spinal cord inferior to the area of the foramen magnum.
6. **Occipital Squama (Cut Surface)**—much of the occipital bone has been removed to open the foramen magnum to show the spinal cord and meninges.
7. **Dorsal Rootlets of 1st Cervical Spinal Nerve**—these short horizontal dorsal rootlets can be seen entering the dorsolateral surface of the cervical region of the spinal cord, just caudal to the foramen magnum.
8. **Dorsal Rootlets of 2nd Cervical Spinal Nerve**—these rootlets are longer and more oblique than those of the 1st cervical (**7**) as they enter the dorsolateral sulcus of the cord.
9. **Right Dorsal Spinal Artery**—at this point the dorsal spinal artery can be seen descending on the dorsal surface of the spinal cord, medial to the entrance of the dorsal rootlets of the cervical nerves in the dorsolateral sulcus.
10. **Denticulate Ligament**—derived from the pia mater. It is attached along the lateral surface of the spinal cord midway between the dorsal and ventral rootlets on each side. Its lateral edge is serrated (see also no. **4**, Fig. 60).
11. **Spinal (Dorsal Root) Ganglion of Fifth Cervical Spinal Nerve**—located in the intervertebral foramen between the 4th and 5th cervical vertebrae. Note that the dorsal root fibers from this ganglion are larger and more oblique than dorsal root fibers of the upper cervical nerves.

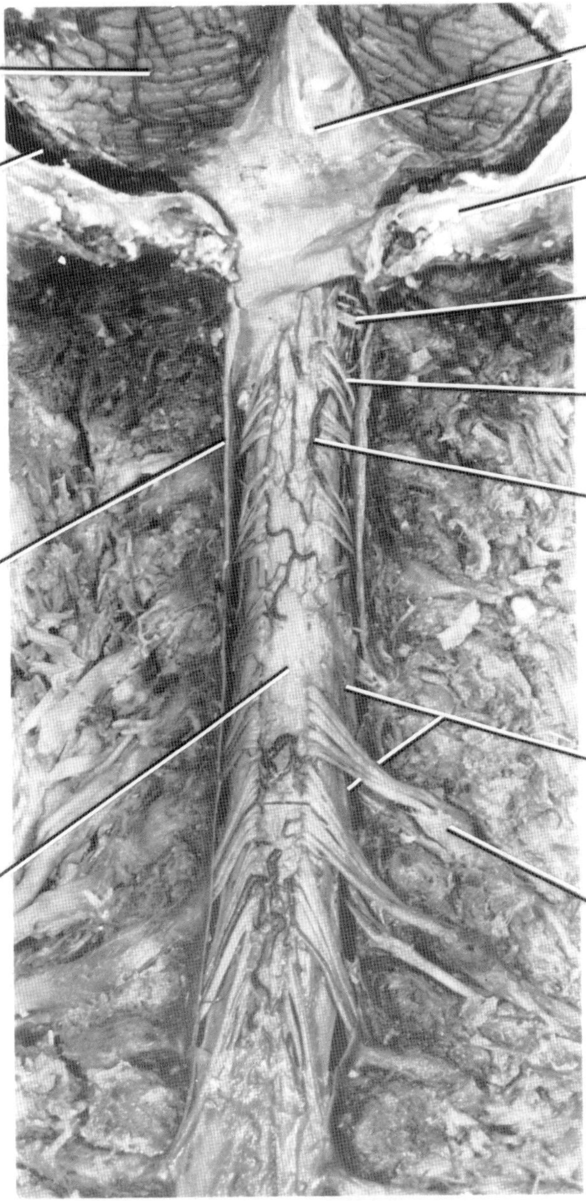

Figure 57 Dorsal view of the intact **cervical** area of the **spinal cord** showing the meningeal layers, the dorsal roots, and some spinal (dorsal root) ganglia. The spinal cord was exposed by dissecting away the muscles of the back and removing the spinous processes and arches of the cervical and thoracic vertebrae.

1. **Dorsal Root Fibers of 10th Thoracic Nerve.** These obliquely directed fibers, covered by arachnoid mater, enter the corresponding spinal cord segment via the dorsolateral sulcus.
2. **Denticulate Ligaments**—derived from the pia mater. They are attached along the lateral surface of the spinal cord midway between the dorsal and ventral rootlets on each side. Their lateral edges are serrated (see also no. **4**, Fig. 60).
3. **Spinal Ganglion of Eighth Thoracic Spinal Nerve**—located in the intervertebral foramen between the eighth and ninth thoracic vertebra. The dura mater and arachnoid mater surround the ganglion and become continuous with the epineural and perineural coverings of the spinal nerves.
4. **Dorsal Spinal Artery** (left)—descends on the dorsal surface of the spinal cord, medial to the entrance of the dorsal rootlets of the spinal nerves in the dorsolateral sulcus.
5. **Arachnoid Mater**—thin transparent membrane, located directly beneath the dura mater, completely envelopes the spinal cord and extends around the spinal rootlets as far laterally as the ganglia. The subarachnoid space is filled with cerebrospinal fluid. The pia mater lying immediately adjacent to the spinal cord and the arachnoid mater are often referred to as the pia-arachnoid membrane, or leptomeninges.
6. **Dura Mater**—this dense firm membrane forms a tube around the spinal cord which extends from the foramen magnum to the second segment of the sacrum. It is pierced by the roots of the spinal nerves. **Note** that the dorsum of the dura has been cut and removed a short distance below the pointer and that its cut edges can be seen on each side at the bottom of the figure.
7. **Dorsal Ramus (Cut End) of the Fifth Thoracic Spinal Nerve**—just distal to the spinal or dorsal root ganglion, the spinal nerve divides into dorsal and ventral rami. The dorsal ramus courses directly posteriorly and supplies the back muscles (attached to the vertebral column) and the skin of the back.
8. **Spinal (Dorsal Root) Ganglion**—sixth thoracic and its coverings.
9. **Spinal (Dorsal Root) Ganglion**—seventh thoracic. Note that the dura mater of the spinal cord extends laterally to ensheath the nerve root and becomes continuous with the epineural membranes of the spinal nerve.
10. **Ventral Ramus of the Eighth Thoracic Spinal Nerve**—after the ventral ramus leaves the intervertebral foramen between the eighth and ninth thoracic vertebra, it courses laterally in the body wall, around onto the ventral surface of the body, to supply the skin and the muscles of the comparable body segment.
11. **Dorsal Root Ganglion of the Tenth Thoracic Spinal Nerve**—note the two small white calcified plaques on the dural wall where the dorsal and ventral rootlets of the tenth thoracic nerve enter and emerge. Calcified plaques on the spinal dura are more common than on the cranial dura. Their etiology is unknown.

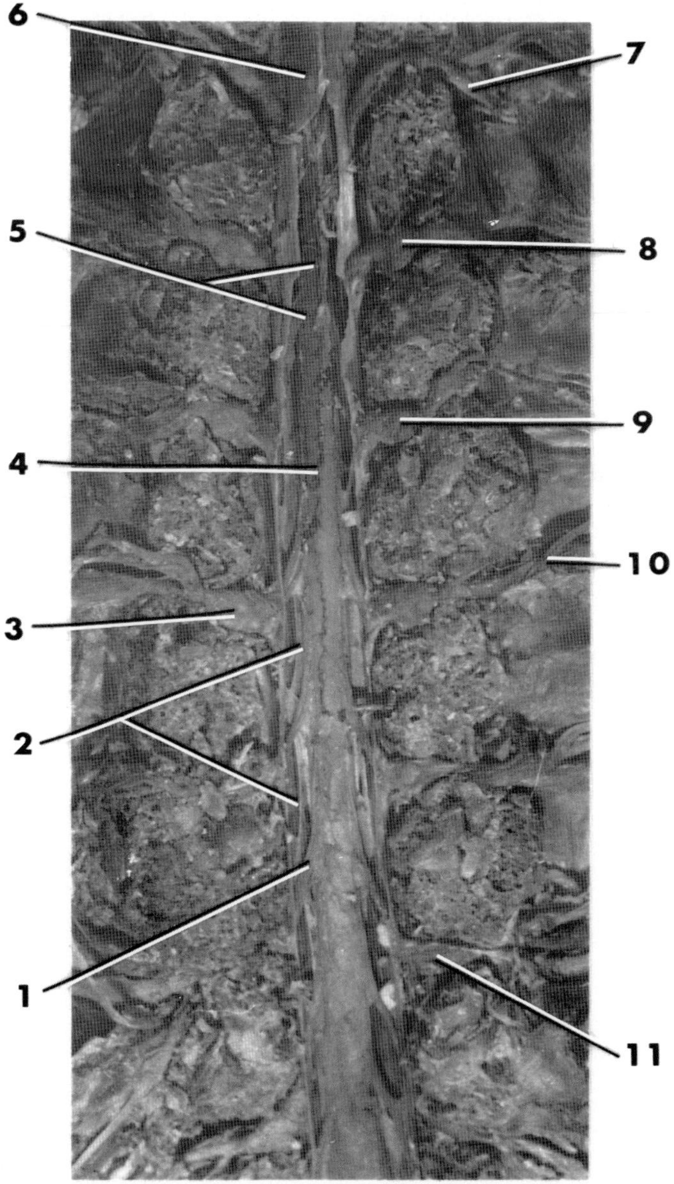

Figure 58 Dorsal view of the **thoracic area of the spinal cord** showing the meningeal layers, the dorsal roots, the spinal (dorsal root) ganglia, and the rami of the thoracic spinal nerves from T5 through to T10. The spinal cord was exposed by dissecting away the muscles of the back and removing the spinous processes, the laminae, and the articular processes of the thoracic vertebrae.

1. **Cauda Equina** (L. horse's tail)—the long lumbar and sacral spinal roots (dorsal and ventral) pass caudally in the subarachnoid space from the spinal cord segments to the intervertebral foramina of corresponding vertebral segments. The many descending roots emerging from the caudal region of the spinal cord reminds one of the long hairs of a horse's tail. The spinal roots are surrounded by cerebrospinal fluid.
2. **Conus Medullaris**—the caudal end of the spinal cord, distal to the lumbosacral enlargement, tapers rather abruptly forming the cone-shaped medullaris from which the filum terminale (**7**) arises.
3. **Spinal (Dorsal Root) Ganglion of 1st Lumbar Nerve**—located in the intervertebral foramen between the opposing left pedicles of the first and second lumbar vertebrae. The long oblique nerve roots travel in caudal (ventral root) and rostral (dorsal root) directions from the spinal cord segment to the corresponding vertebral segment.
4. **Denticulate Ligament**—one of the bilaterally symmetrical folds of pia mater which is attached along the lateral surfaces of the entire spinal cord, midway between the dorsal and ventral roots. The lateral surface is serrated where it is attached to the arachnoid and the inner surface of the dura mater at 18 to 24 points. It partially separates the subarachnoid space into dorsal and ventral compartments (see also no. **4**, Fig. 60).
5. **Lumbosacral Enlargement**—the spindle-shaped swelling of the spinal cord that innervates the lower limb. The spinal cord segments from L2 through S3 are included in it. Corresponding spinal nerves constitute most of the lumbosacral plexus responsible for the innervation of the lower limb.
6. **Dura Mater (Cut Edge)**—the tough spinal dura mater forms a cylindrical tube around the spinal cord in the vertebral canal. It is pierced by the roots of the 31 pairs of spinal nerves and blends with the connective tissue (epineurium and perineurium) of the spinal nerves. The dura extends in the vertebral column from the foramen magnum to the second segment of the sacrum. There is an epidural space between the dura and the wall of the vertebral (spinal) canal which is filled with adipose tissue and a venous plexus.
7. **Filum Terminale**—the cord tapers into a slender filament called the filum terminale which lies amongst the fibers of the cauda equina (**1**). It consists of pia mater and neuroglial elements and extends caudally to attach to the dorsum of the coccyx.
8. **Arachnoid Mater**—the thin transparent membrane located beneath the dura mater forming a cylindrical sheath that extends caudally as far as the level of the second sacral vertebra, the limit of the dural sac. The arachnoid also surrounds the spinal nerve roots as they enter and exit the intervertebral foramina. The lumbar and sacral roots (cauda equina) are located in the subarachnoid space which at this point is often referred to as the lumbar cistern. It is in this space that lumbar punctures are made for the withdrawal of cerebrospinal fluid for examination.

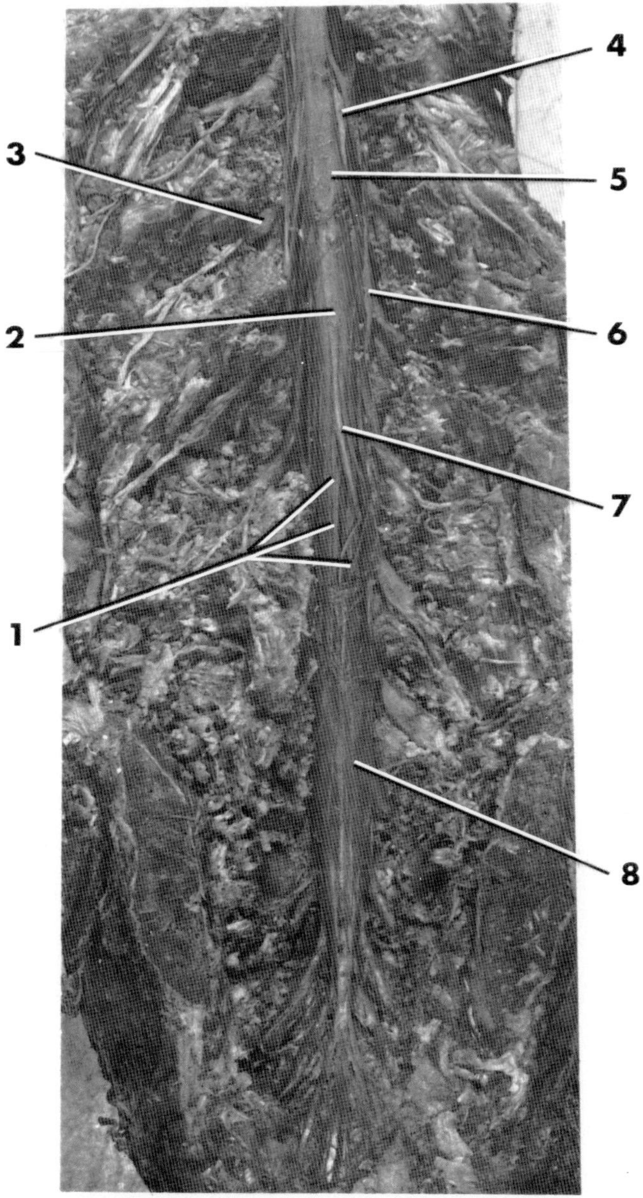

Figure 59 Dorsal view of the intact **caudal area of the spinal cord** showing the meningeal layers, the cauda equina, the filum terminale, the dorsal roots of the spinal nerves, and the spinal or dorsal root ganglia. The cord was exposed by removing the spinous processes and the vertebral arches of the lower thoracic and lumbar vertebra, the dorsal sacrum, and muscles of the back that are attached to these vertebral areas.

1. **Ventral Root Fibers**—leave the ventrolateral sulcus of the spinal cord and cross to the intervertebral foramen with the incoming dorsal root fibers. The dorsal and ventral roots are ensheathed by the arachnoid and the dura mater when they leave the vertebral canal. Note that these fibers are oblique as they leave a spinal cord segment and course to the area of a corresponding vertebral segment.
2. **Pia Mater** (L. *pius*, tender)—this microscopic and transparent layer of connective tissue adheres to the surface of the spinal cord. It covers the roots of the spinal nerves and the blood vessels for a short distance where they enter the spinal cord.
3. **Dorsal Root Fibers**—axons of neurons from the spinal ganglia enter the spinal cord at the dorsolateral sulcus. Within the vertebral canal, the fibers course in the same direction as the ventral roots and are covered by the meninges. Note the oblique direction of the sensory fibers from a vertebral segment as they course to the corresponding spinal cord segment (see also no. **1**, Fig. 58).
4. **Denticulate Ligament**—one of the bilaterally symmetrical folds of pia mater which is attached along the lateral surface of the entire spinal cord, midway between the dorsal and the ventral roots. The lateral surface is serrated where it is attached to the arachnoid and the inner surface of the dura mater at 18 to 24 points. It partially separates the subarachnoid space into dorsal and ventral compartments (see also no. **4**, Fig. 59).
5. **Arachnoid Mater**—the thin transparent membrane which forms a cylindrical sheath extending caudally as far as the level of the second sacral vertebra, the limit of the dural sac. The arachnoid also surrounds the spinal nerve roots as they enter and leave the intervertebral foramina. The lumbar and sacral roots (cauda equina) are located in the subarachnoid space. It is in this space that lumbar punctures are made for the withdrawal of cerebrospinal fluid for examination (see also no. **8**, Fig. 59).
6. **Dura Mater**—the tough spinal dura mater forms a cylindrical tube around the spinal cord in the vertebral canal. It is pierced by the roots of the 31 pairs of spinal nerves and blends with the connective tissue (epineurium and perineurium) of the spinal nerves. There is an epidural space between the dura and the wall of the vertebral canal which is filled with adipose tissue and a venous plexus (see also no. **2**, Fig. 57).
7. **Spinal (Dorsal Root) Ganglion**—located in the intervertebral foramen between the opposing left pedicles of two adjacent vertebrae (see also no. **8**, Fig. 58).
8. **Dura Mater (Reflected)**—the dura mater was split in the midline and reflected to show the underlying structures.
9. **Dorsal and Ventral Roots**—the nerve roots (dorsal and ventral) ensheathed in arachnoid mater travel in the subarachnoid space obliquely downward and lateral to their foramina of exit. Note that these roots "pierce" (are surrounded) the dural sheath as they course to or from the intervertebral foramen.

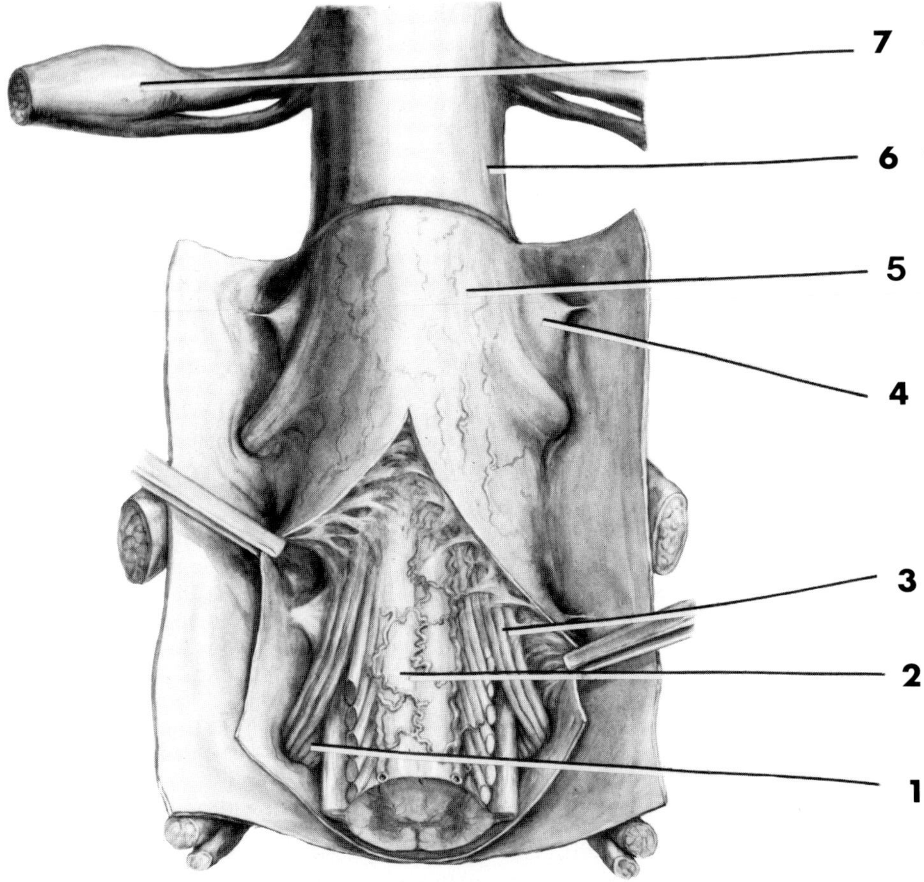

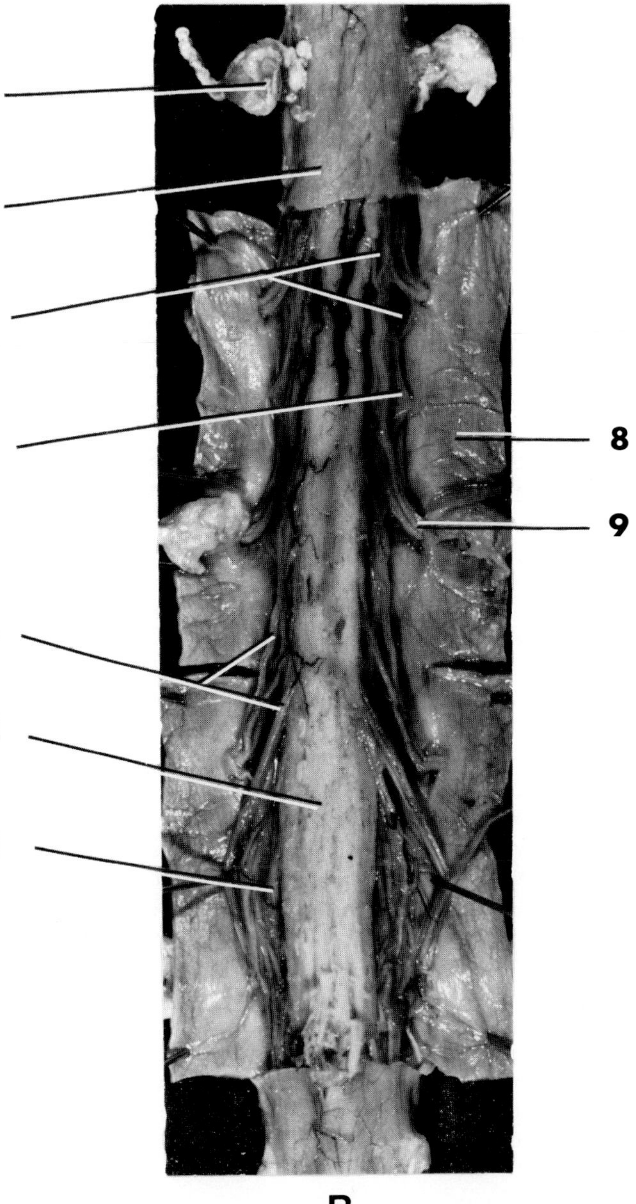

Figure 60 **A**. Drawing of a posterior view of the superior part of the thoracic spinal cord. Inferiorly, the dura mater and the arachnoid have been split in the midline to expose the spinal cord and the pial and dorsal vessels. Superiorly, the intact dura covers the spinal cord and the spinal nerve roots. (Reproduced with permission from K. L. Moore: *Clinically Oriented Anatomy*. Courtesy of Williams & Wilkins.) **B**. Photograph of a posterior view of the caudal part of the thoracic spinal cord to show the structures featured in **A**.

A

B

Sacral Segment

1. **Septomarginal Fasciculus**—located in the inferior half of the dorsal white column, immediately adjacent to the dorsal median sulcus. It consists of the descending branches of the dorsal roots that have entered the spinal cord. The fibers and their collaterals synapse with tract cells, internuncial neurons, and motor cells.
2. **Fasciculus Gracilis**—consists of heavily myelinated fibers from the spinal ganglia (T6-S5). This uncrossed tract extends the entire length of the spinal cord in the dorsal white column. The fibers terminate in the nucleus gracilis of the medulla. Inferior to the cord level of T6, it forms all the dorsal white column and superior to T8, it occupies the medial area of the dorsal white column, as the fasciculus cuneatus comes to lie lateral to it (see no. **10**, Fig. 64).
3. **Dorsal Root Fibers**—Bundles of dorsal root fibers of sacral spinal nerves enter the corresponding spinal cord segment in the area of the dorsolateral sulcus to form the dorsolateral fasciculus and the fasciculus gracilis.
4. **Nucleus Dorsomarginalis**—a thin layer of cells covering the tip (substantia gelatinosa) of the dorsal gray horn throughout the spinal cord. The axons of these cells pass into the fasciculus proprius and bifurcate into ascending and descending fibers which form intersegmental pathways. This nucleus forms Lamina I of Rexed's laminar map of the spinal gray matter.
5. **Substantia Gelatinosa (of Rolandi)**—occupies the dorsal portion of the dorsal horn (immediately under **4**) throughout the length of the spinal cord. Fibers from the dorsolateral fasciculus terminate on neurons in the substantia gelatinosa, and axons of these small Golgi type II cells terminate within the nucleus on dendrites of neurons from the subjacent nucleus proprius. Data for pain and temperature are relayed by neurons in this nucleus to some neurons in the nucleus proprius (**6**).
6. **Nucleus Proprius (Chief Sensory) of Dorsal Horn**—almost all of the dorsal horn in the entire spinal cord, except for the substantia gelatinosa and the nucleus dorsalis (confined to segments C8-L2) constitute the nucleus proprius. It consists of many internuncial neurons, together with tract cells, the axons of which contribute to ascending fasciculi (fasciculus proprius, lateral and ventral spinothalamic, etc.) in the lateral and ventral white columns.
7. **Lateral Corticospinal Tract**—a crossed tract that extends the entire length of the spinal cord in the lateral white column. At the caudal end of the medulla, about 85% of the pyramidal fibers from the motor cortex decussate to the opposite side forming the lateral corticospinal tract. The descending fibers continuously leave this tract and turn medially to synapse on ventral horn cells or intercalating neurons in the intermediate gray matter, which in turn synapse on gamma or alpha ventral horn cells. This important pathway brings the muscles of one side of the body under the voluntary control of the opposite cerebral hemisphere.
8. **Sacral Parasympathetic Nucleus**—located in the lateral area of the intermediate zone of gray matter in spinal cord segments S2 through S4. It is the source of preganglionic parasympathetic fibers for the pelvic viscera.
9. **Lateral Motor Cell Column (of Ventral Horn)**—the ventrolateral nuclear enlargement of the ventral horn extends from L2 through S3. Axons of these motor cells course in the ventral roots and lumbosacral plexus to supply the muscles in the lower limb.
10. **Lateral Spinothalamic Tract**—a crossed pathway that extends the entire length of the spinal cord in the lateral white column. It originates in the contralateral nucleus proprius, and its fibers cross in the ventral commissural gray and white matter. It transmits pain and temperature sensations from the body to the contralateral ventral posterior lateral nucleus of the thalamus.
11. **Medial Motor Cell Column (of Ventral Horn)**—occupies the medial area of the ventral horn of gray matter throughout the entire length of the spinal cord. Neurons in this area innervate the muscles attached to the axial skeleton (intercostal and abdominal muscles).
12. **Ventral Spinothalamic Tract**—a crossed pathway extending the length of the spinal cord in the ventral white column. It originates from some cells in the opposite nucleus proprius, the axons of which cross in the ventral contralateral ventral posterior lateral nucleus of the thalamus.
13. **Vestibulospinal Tract**—this uncrossed descending tract extends the entire length of the spinal cord and is located superficial (external) to the ventral spinothalamic tract in the ventral white column. It originates in the lateral vestibular nucleus of the medulla of the same side. The tract is important in the maintenance of equilibrium.

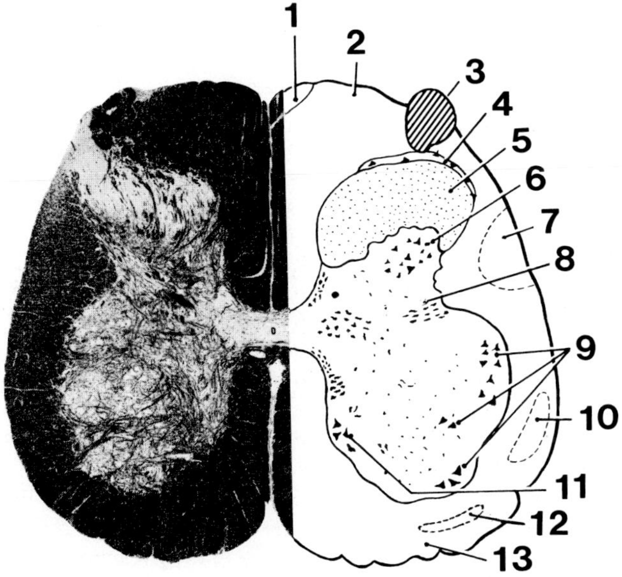

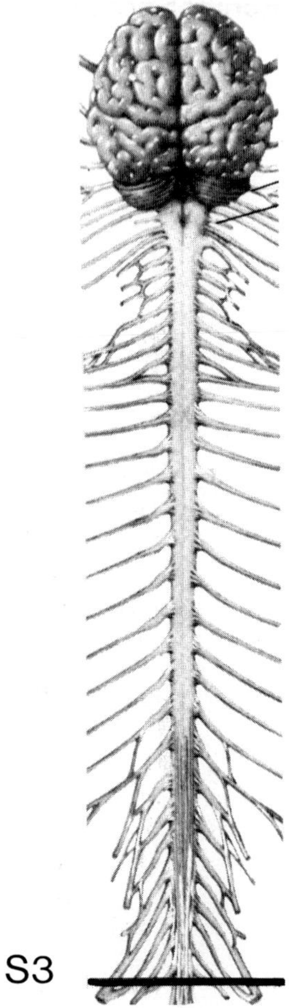

Figure 61 Modified photograph of a section through the third sacral segment of adult human spinal cord. Some of the important nuclear areas and fiber tracts are identified. (Modified from M. B. Carpenter: *Human Neuroanatomy*, 7th ed. Courtesy of Williams & Wilkins.) The inset photo of the brain and spinal cord at the right in this figure and subsequent figures 62, 63, and 64 is a modification of a photo from R. D. Collins: *Illustrated Manual of Neurologic Diagnosis*, J. B. Lippincott, Toronto, 1962.

Lumbar Segment

1. **Medial Motor Cell Column (of Ventral Horn)**—occupies the medial area of the ventral horn of gray matter throughout the entire length of the spinal cord. Neurons in this area innervate the muscles attached to the axial skeleton (intercostal and abdominal muscles).
2. **Ventral Root Fibers**—axons of ventral horn cells (alpha and gamma neurons) course through the ventral lateral column of white matter to emerge in the area of the ventrolateral sulcus to form ventral roots of respective spinal nerves.
3. **Dorsal Root Fibers (Cut Fibers)**—bundles of fibers (axons) from neurons in the spinal ganglia enter each corresponding spinal cord segment at the dorsolateral sulcus and end in the dorsolateral fasciculus, fasciculus gracilis, and fasciculus cuneatus. These fibers conduct general sensory data from the body into the spinal cord.
4. **Fasciculus Gracilis**—consists of heavily myelinated axons of neurons from the spinal ganglia (T6 through S5). This uncrossed tract extends the entire length of the spinal cord in the dorsal white column. The fibers terminate in the nucleus gracilis of the medulla. It transmits impulses for proprioception (position sense), fine or discriminative touch, and vibration sense from the inferior half of the body. In the superior half of the dorsal column (C1-T5), it occupies the medial half and in the inferior half (T6-S5) it occupies all the dorsal white column (see also no. **2**, Fig. 61).
5. **Dorsal Cornucommissurali Nucleus**—a small nuclear area located on the medial margin and the base of the dorsal horn and gray commissure that extends the length of the spinal cord. The axons of neurons in this nucleus form intersegmental tracts which comprise much of the fasciculus proprius in the dorsal white column.
6. **Substantia Gelatinosa (of Rolandi)**—occupies the dorsal portion of the dorsal horn throughout the length of the spinal cord. Fibers from the dorsolateral fasciculus terminate on neurons in the substantia gelatinosa, and axons of these small Golgi type II cells terminate within the nucleus on the dendrites of neurons from the subjacent nucleus proprius. Data for pain and temperature are relayed by neurons in this nucleus to some neurons in the nucleus proprius (see also no. **5**, Fig. 61).
7. **Nucleus Dorsomarginalis**—a thin layer of cells covering the tip (substantia gelatinosa) of the dorsal gray horn throughout the spinal cord. The axons of these cells pass into the fasciculus proprius and bifurcate into ascending and descending fibers which form intersegmental pathways. This nucleus forms Lamina I of Rexed's laminar map of the spinal gray matter.
8. **Dorsolateral Fasciculus (Zone of Lissauer)**—found throughout the entire spinal cord, it is a small uncrossed tract located between the dorsolateral sulcus and the tip of the dorsal horn of gray matter. It consists of small, fine, dorsal roots of spinal nerves that divide into short (one cord segment) ascending and descending branches after entering the cord at the dorsolateral sulcus. These fibers and their collateral branches turn medially and end on neurons in the substantia gelatinosa (of Rolandi).
9. **Lateral Corticospinal Tract**—is a crossed tract that extends the entire length of the spinal cord in the lateral white column. At the caudal end of the medulla, about 85% of the pyramidal fibers from the motor cortex decussate to the opposite side in the lateral corticospinal tract. The descending fibers continuously leave this tract and turn medially to synapse on ventral horn cells or intercalating neurons in the intermediate gray matter, which in turn synapse on gamma or alpha ventral horn cells. This important pathway brings the muscles of one side of the body under the voluntary control of the opposite cerebral hemisphere (see also no. **7**, Fig. 61).

Note: Legends for nos. **10–16** are found on page 142.

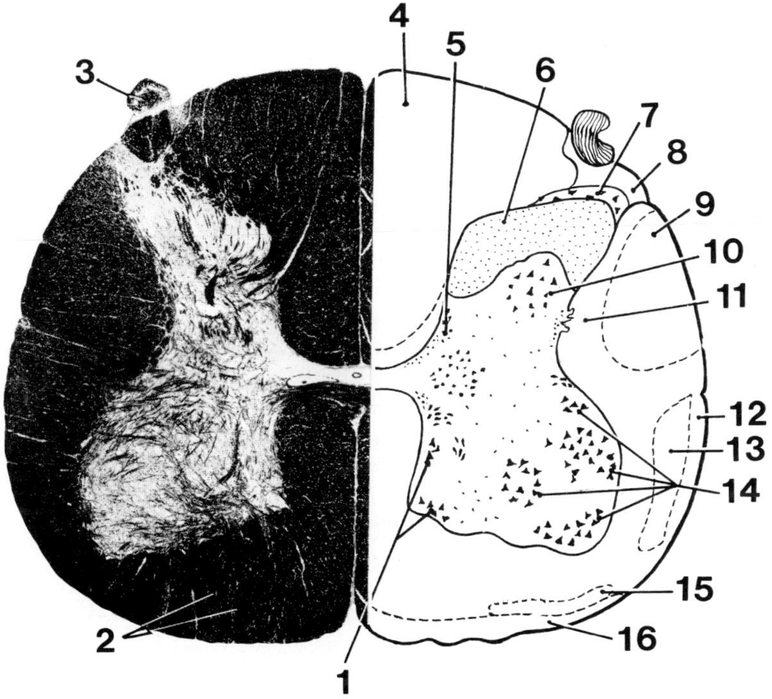

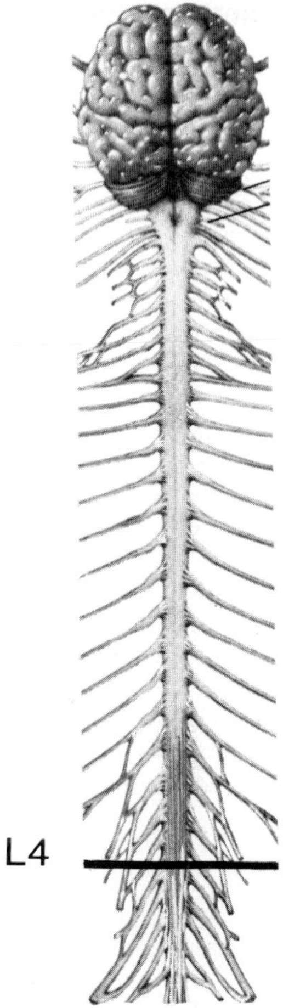

Figure 62 Modified photograph of a section through the fourth lumbar segment of the adult human spinal cord. Some of the nuclear areas and fiber tracts are identified. (Modified from M. B. Carpenter: *Human Neuroanatomy*, 7th ed. Courtesy of Williams & Wilkins.)

10. **Nucleus Proprius (Chief Sensory) of Dorsal Horn**—almost all the dorsal horn in the entire spinal cord, except for the substantia gelatinosa and the nucleus dorsalis, constitutes the nucleus proprius. It consists of many internucial neurons together with tract cells, the axons of which contribute to ascending fasciculi (fasciculus proprius, lateral and ventral spinothalamic, etc.) in the lateral and ventral white columns.
11. **Fasciculus Proprius**—surrounds the gray matter of the spinal cord. This zone of white matter consists of ascending and descending fibers connecting different spinal cord segments. The connections are important in intersegmental spinal reflexes (see also no. **6**, Fig. 61).
12. **Ventral Spinocerebellar Tract**—a crossed tract located in the ventral and marginal area of the lateral column of white matter. Fibers originating in the lumbosacral enlargement of the spinal cord and the intermediate gray matter cross in the commissure of gray and white matter in the lower lumbar region and form the ventral spinocerebellar tract. Unlike the dorsal spinocerebellar tract, this tract traverses most of the brain stem before it enters the cerebellum through the superior cerebellar peduncle. It conveys proprioception, touch, and pressure sensory data to the cerebellum.
13. **Lateral Spinothalamic Tract**—a crossed pathway that extends the entire length of the spinal cord in the lateral white column. It originates in the contralateral nucleus proprius and its fibers cross in the ventral commissural gray and white matter. It transmits pain and temperature sensations from the body to the contralateral ventral posterior lateral nucleus of the thalamus (see also no. **10**, Fig. 61).
14. **Lateral Motor Cell Column (of Ventral Horn)**—the ventrolateral nuclear enlargement of the ventral horn extends from L2 through S3. Axons of these motor cells course in the ventral roots and lumbosacral plexus to supply the muscles in the lower limb.
15. **Ventral Spinothalamic Tract**—a crossed pathway extending the length of the spinal cord in the ventral white column. It originates from some cells in the nucleus proprius, the axons of which cross in the ventral white and gray commissure. It transmits sensations for light touch and pressure from the body to the contralateral ventral posterior lateral nucleus of the thalamus (see also no. **12**, Fig. 61).
16. **Vestibulospinal Tract**—this uncrossed descending tract extends the entire length of the spinal cord and is located superficial (external) to the ventral spinothalamic tract in the ventral white column. It originates in the lateral vestibular nucleus of the medulla of the same side. The tract is important in the maintenance of equilibrium (see also no. **13**, Fig. 61).

Note: Legends for nos. **1-9** are found on page 140.

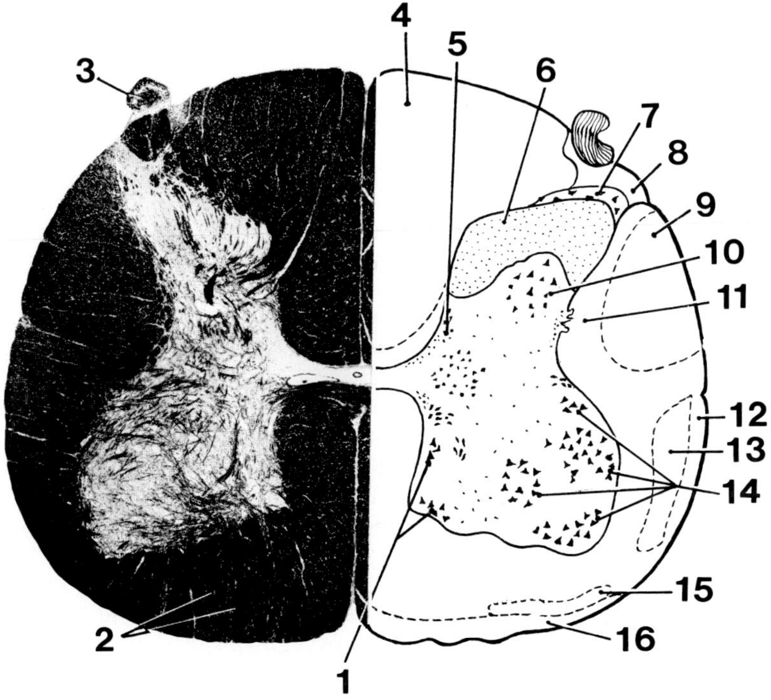

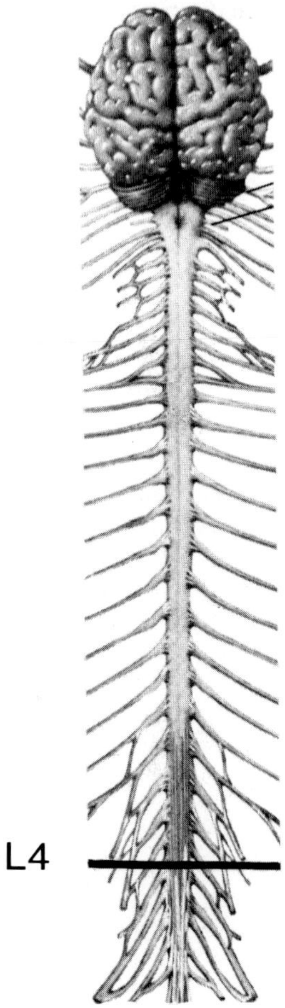

Figure 62 Modified photograph of a section through the fourth lumbar segment of the adult human spinal cord. Some of the nuclear areas and fiber tracts are identified. (Modified from M. B. Carpenter: *Human Neuroanatomy*, 7th ed. Courtesy of Williams & Wilkins.)

Thoracic Segment

1. **Vestibulospinal Tract**—this uncrossed descending tract extends the entire length of the spinal cord and is located superficial (external) to the ventral spinothalamic tract in the ventral white column. It originates in the lateral vestibular nucleus of the medulla of the same side. The tract is important in the maintenance of equilibrium (see also no. **16**, Fig. 62).
2. **Sulcomarginal Fasciculus (of Marie)**—also called descending portion of *medial longitudinal fasciculus*—consists of crossed and uncrossed fibers from neurons in the medial and inferior vestibular nuclei. It is located between the ventral corticospinal and tectospinal tracts in the cervical portion of the ventral column of white matter. The fibers terminate on neurons in the cervical ventral gray horn. It influences neck muscles in supporting the head in various positions.
3. **Fasciculus Gracilis**—consists of heavily myelinated axons of neurons from the spinal ganglia (T6 through S5). The uncrossed tract extends the entire length of the spinal cord in the dorsal white column. The fibers terminate in the nucleus gracilis of the medulla. It transmits impulses for proprioception (position sense), fine or discriminative touch, and vibration sense from the inferior half of the body. In the superior half of the dorsal column (C1-T5), it occupies the medial half, and in the inferior (T6-S5) it occupies all the dorsal white column (see also no. **4**, Fig. 62).
4. **Nucleus Dorsalis (Clarke's Column)**—a well defined nucleus extending from C8 through L2 or L3 in the ventromedial part of the dorsal horn. The cells in this nucleus are easily distinguished from other cells because they resemble cells undergoing the axon reaction. The nucleus gives origin to the ipsilateral dorsal spinocerebellar tract and conducts proprioceptive touch and pressure data to the cerebellum.
5. **Nucleus Proprius (Chief Sensory) of Dorsal Horn**—almost all the dorsal horn in the entire spinal cord, except for the substantia gelatinosa and the nucleus dorsalis, constitutes the nucleus proprius. It consists of many internuncial neurons together with tract cells, the axons of which contribute to ascending fasciculi (fasciculus proprius, lateral and ventral spinothalamic, etc.) in the lateral and ventral white columns (see also no. **6**, Fig. 61).
6. **Substantia Gelatinosa (of Rolandi)**—occupies the dorsal portion of the dorsal horn throughout the length of the spinal cord. Fibers from the dorsolateral fasciculus terminate on neurons in the substantia gelatinosa, and axons of these small Golgi type II cells terminate within the nucleus on dendrites of neurons from the subjacent nucleus proprius. Data for pain and temperature are relayed by neurons in this nucleus to some neurons in the nucleus proprius. This nucleus is comparable to Lamina II and III of Rexed (see also no. **6**, Fig. 62).
7. **Nucleus Dorsomarginalis**—a thin layer of cells covering the tip (substantia gelatinosa) of the dorsal gray horn throughout the spinal cord. The axons of these cells pass into the fasciculus proprius and bifurcate into ascending and descending fibers which form intersegmental pathways. This nucleus forms Lamina I of Rexed's laminar map of the spinal gray matter.

Note: Legends for nos. **8–15** are found on page 146.

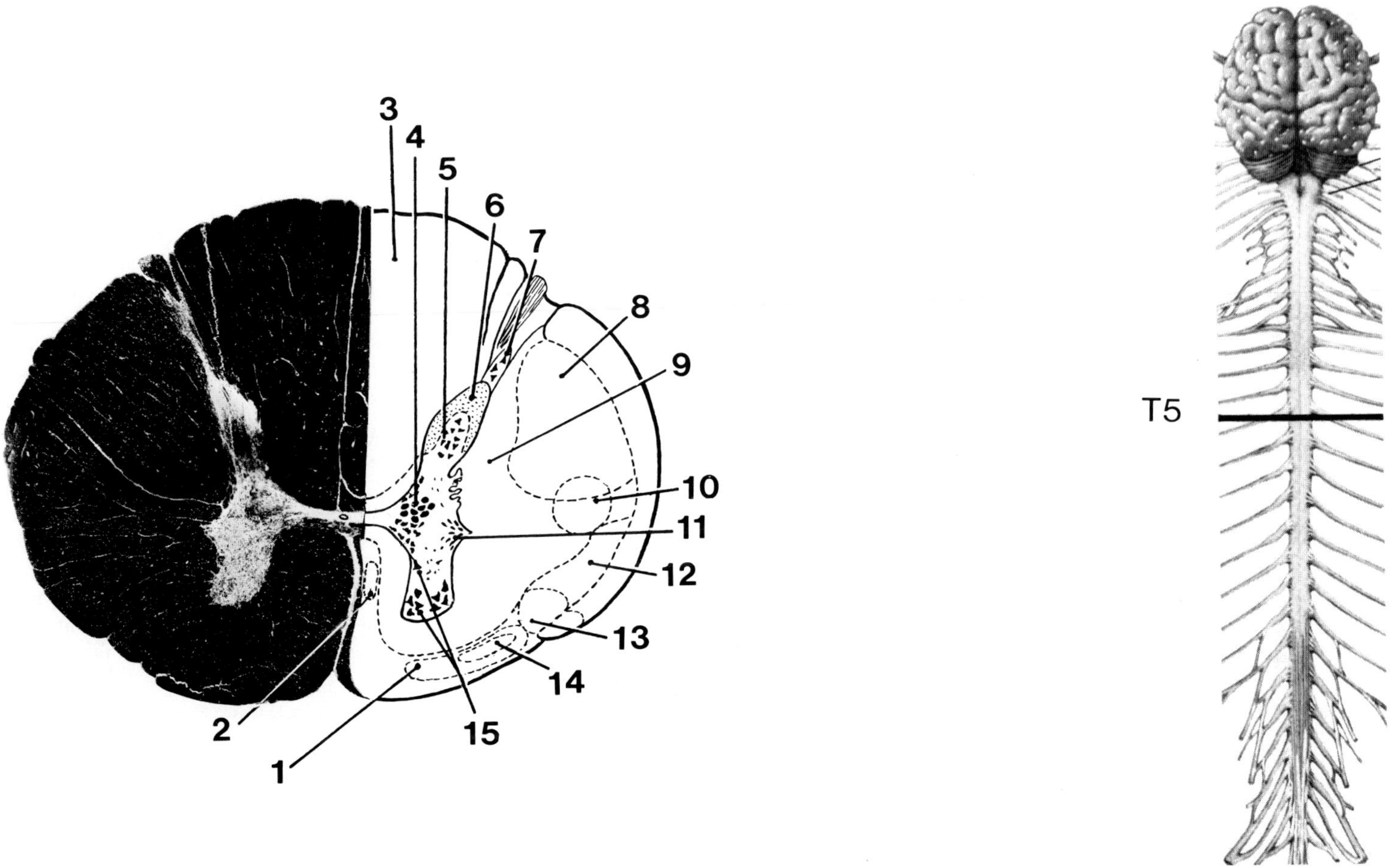

Figure 63 Modified photograph of a section through the fifth thoracic segment of adult human spinal cord. Some of the important nuclear areas and fiber tracts are identified. (Modified from M. B. Carpenter: *Human Neuroanatomy*, 7th ed. Courtesy of Williams & Wilkins.)

Thoracic Segment (*continued*)

8. **Lateral Corticospinal Tract**—a crossed tract that extends the entire length of the cord in the lateral white column. At the inferior end of the medulla, about 85% of the pyramidal fibers from the motor cortex decussate to the opposite side to form the lateral corticospinal tract. The descending fibers continuously leave this tract and turn medially to synapse on ventral horn cells or intercalating neurons in the intermediate gray matter, which in turn synapse on gamma or alpha ventral horn cells. This important pathway brings the muscles of one side of the body under voluntary control from the opposite cerebral hemisphere (see also no. **9**, Fig. 62)
9. **Fasciculus Proprius**—surrounds the gray matter of the spinal cord. This zone of white matter consists of ascending and descending fibers connecting different cord segments. The connections are important in intersegmental spinal reflexes (see also no. **11**, Fig. 62).
10. **Rubrospinal Tract**—a crossed descending tract extending the length of the spinal cord in the lateral white column. It is located ventral to the lateral corticospinal tract. It originates in the contralateral red nucleus of the midbrain, and its fibers terminate on neurons in all segments of the ventral horn of gray matter. It constitutes one of the pathways of the extrapyramidal motor system.
11. **Intermediolateral Cell Column (Nucleus Intermediolateralis or Lateral Horn)**—the small lateral horn of gray matter extends from spinal cord segment T1 through L2 or L3. The axons of its neurons are the source of preganglionic sympathetic fibers which emerge from the cord with the ventral root fibers of alpha gamma motor neurons.
12. **Lateral Spinothalamic Tract**—a crossed pathway that extends the entire length of the spinal cord in the lateral white column. It originates in the contralateral nucleus proprius, and its fibers cross in the ventral commissural gray and white matter. It transmits pain and temperature sensations from the body to the contralateral ventral posterior lateral nucleus of the thalamus (see also no. **13**, Fig. 62).
13. **Spinotectal Tract**—a crossed tract in the cord that ascends in the ventrolateral white column to end on collicular neurons in the tectum. It conducts general sensory data to the midbrain for reflex motor responses.
14. **Ventral Spinothalamic Tract**—a crossed pathway extending the length of the spinal cord in the ventral white column. It originates from some cells in the nucleus proprius, the axons of which cross in the ventral white and gray commissure. It transmits sensations from light touch and pressure from the body to the contralateral ventral posterior lateral nucleus of the thalamus (see also no. **15**, Fig. 62).
15. **Medial Motor Cell Column (of Ventral Horn)**—forms the medial area of the ventral horn of gray matter through the length of the spinal cord. In the thoracic segments this cell column is the ventral horn. Ventral horn cells from this motor cell column innervate the muscles attached to the axial skeleton (intercostal and abdominal muscles).

Note: Legends for nos. **1–7** are found on page 144.

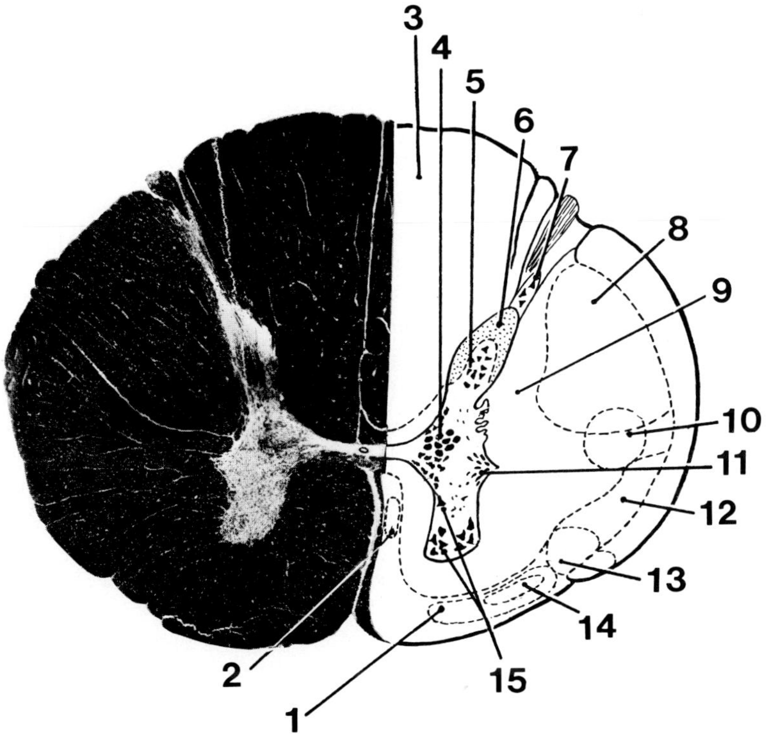

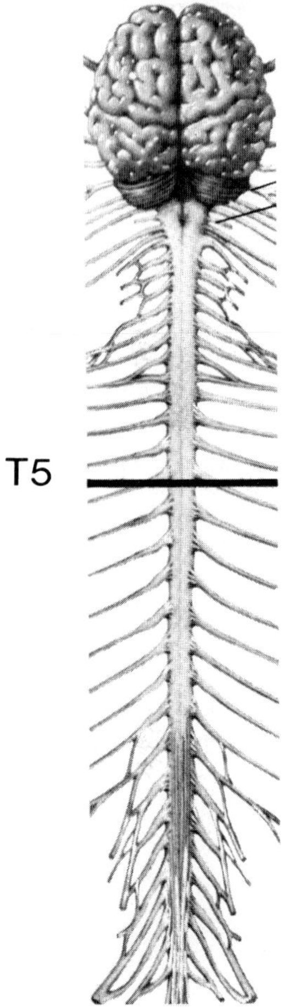

Figure 63 Modified photograph of a section through the fifth thoracic segment of adult human spinal cord. Some of the important nuclear areas and fiber tracts are identified. (Modified from M. B. Carpenter: *Human Neuroanatomy*, 7th ed. Courtesy of Williams & Wilkins.)

Cervical Segment

1. Sulcomarginal Fasciculus (of Marie).
2. Ventral Corticospinal Tract.
3. Ventral Roots (Cut Fibers).
4. Dorsolateral Fasciculus (Zone of Lissauer).
5. Dorsal Roots (Cut Fibers).
6. Dorsal Intermediate Sulcus and Septum.
7. Dorsal Median Septum.
8. Fasciculus Gracilis.
9. Fasciculus Interfascicularis.
10. Fasciculus Cuneatus.
11. Nucleus Dorsomarginalis.
12. Dorsal Spinocerebellar Tract.
13. Nucleus Proprius (Chief Sensory Nucleus) of Dorsal Horn.
14. Lateral Corticospinal Tract.
15. Fasciculus Proprius.
16. Nucleus Dorsalis (Clarke's Column).
17. Rubrospinal Tract.
18. Ventral Spinocerebellar Tract.
19. Lateral Spinothalamic Tract.
20. Lateral Motor Cell Column (of Ventral Horn).
21. Spinotectal Tract.
22. Spinoolivary Tract.
23. Vestibulospinal Tract.
24. Ventral Spinothalamic Tract.
25. Medial Motor Cell Column (of Ventral Horn).

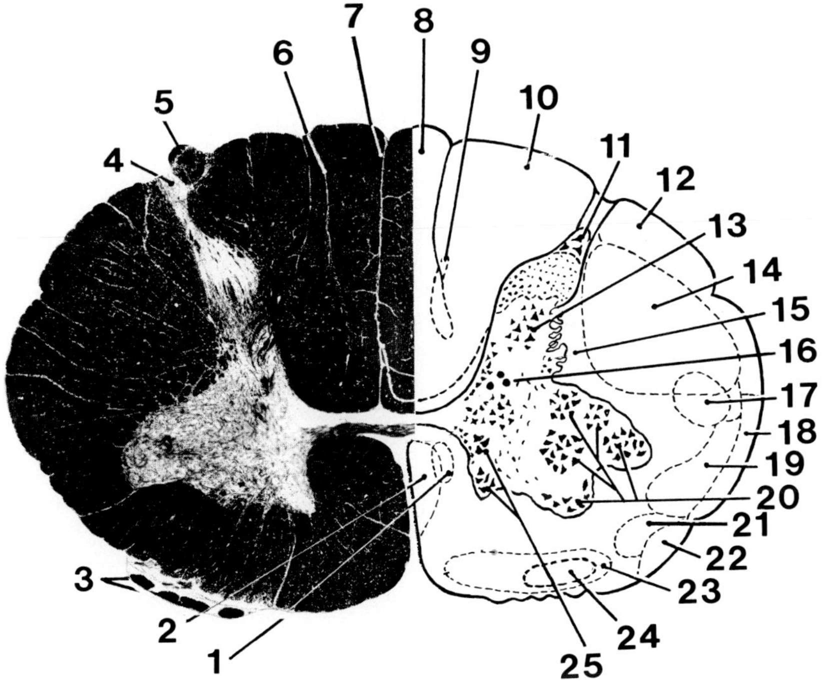

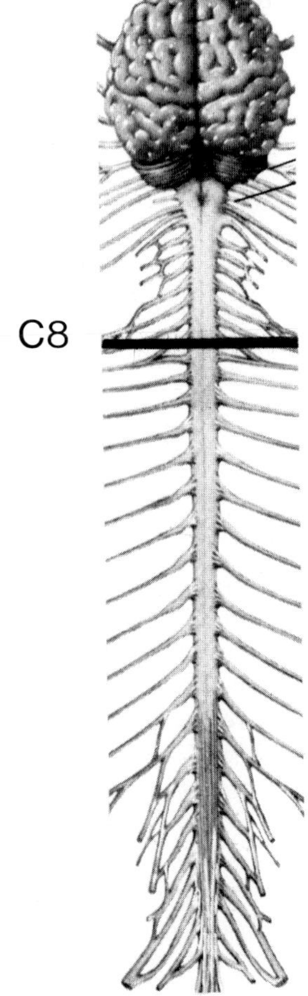

Figure 64*A* Modified photograph of a section through the eighth cervical segment of the adult human spinal cord. Some of the important nuclear areas and fiber tracts are identified. (Modified from M. B. Carpenter: *Human Neuroanatomy*, 7th ed. Courtesy of Williams & Wilkins.)

Motor Nuclei and Tracts

1. **Sulcomarginal Fasciculus (of Marie)**—also called the descending portion of the *medial longitudinal* fasciculus. It is located between the ventral corticospinal and the tectospinal tracts in the cervical portion of the ventral column of white matter in the spinal cord (see also no. **2**, Fig. 63).
2. **Ventral Corticospinal Tract**—a small uncrossed tract that descends in the ventral column of white matter, immediately adjacent to the ventral fissure as far as the midthoracic cord level.
3. **Ventral Roots (Cut Fibers)**—bundles of fibers from neurons in the ventral horn of gray matter leave the spinal cord throughout each segment and converge in a caudal and lateral direction to form the ventral root of each spinal nerve.
6. **Dorsal Intermediate Sulcus and Septum**—extends inferiorly as far as the midthoracic level. It is located between the dorsal median sulcus and the dorsolateral sulcus and separates the fasciculis gracilis (medial) from the fasciculis cuneatus (lateral).
7. **Dorsal Median Sulcus**—a shallow midline furrow on the dorsal surface of the spinal cord that extends its entire length. It separates the left column of white matter distinctly from the right column of white matter.
9. **Fasciculus Interfascicularis**—located between the fasciculus gracilis (**8**) and the fasciculus cuneatus (**10**) in the superior half of the dorsal column of the cord. It consists of the descending branches (may be several segments long) of the dorsal roots that entered the cord medial to the dorsolateral fasciculus.
14. **Lateral Corticospinal Tract**—is a crossed tract that extends the entire length of the cord in the lateral white column. At the caudal end of the medulla, about 85% of the pyramidal fibers from the motor cortex decussate to the opposite side to form the lateral corticospinal tract (see also no. **8**, Fig. 63).
15. **Fasciculus Proprius**—surrounds the gray matter of the spinal cord. This zone of white matter consists of ascending and descending fibers connecting different cord segments. The connections are important in intersegmental spinal reflexes.
17. **Rubrospinal Tract**—a crossed descending tract extending the length of the spinal cord in the lateral white column. It is located ventral to the lateral corticospinal tract.
20. **Lateral Motor Cell Column (of Ventral Horn)**—the ventrolateral nuclear enlargement of the ventral horn extends from C4 through T1. Axons of these horn cells course through the branchial plexus of nerves to supply the muscles in the upper limb.
23. **Vestibulospinal Tract**—this uncrossed descending tract extends the entire length of the spinal cord and is located superficial (external) to the ventral spinothalamic tract in the ventral white column (see also no. **16**, Fig. 62).
25. **Medial Motor Cell Column (of Ventral Horn)**—occupies the medial area of the ventral horn of gray matter throughout the entire length of the spinal cord.

Note: Leader lines with no numbers represent the sensory nuclear areas and tracts which are identified in Figure **64***C*.

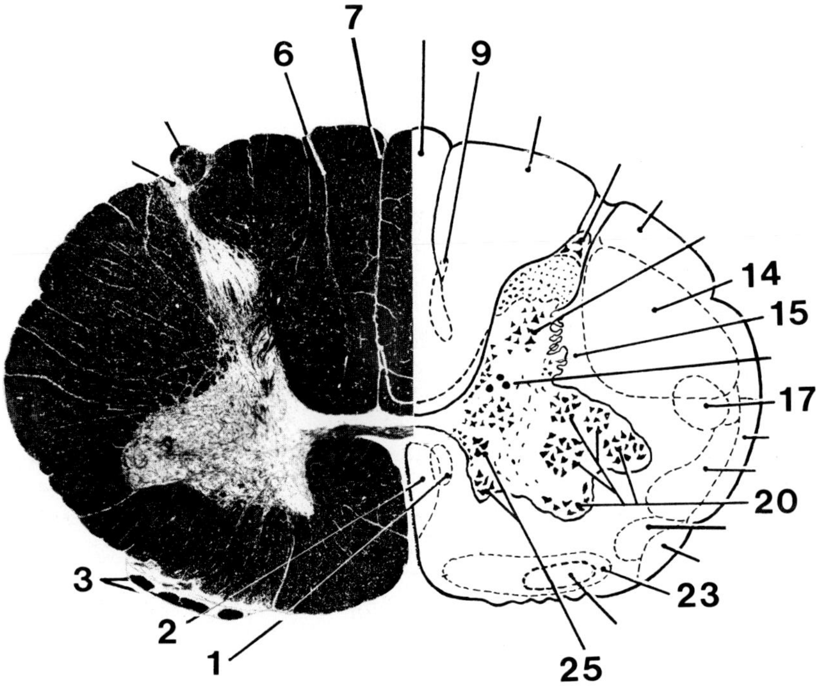

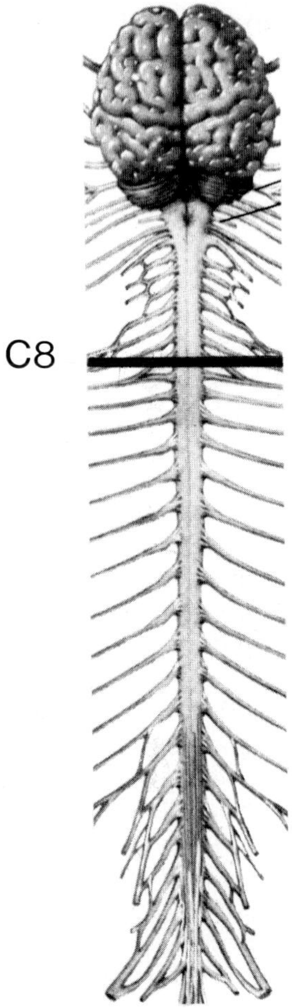

Figure 64*B* Modified photograph of a section through the eighth cervical segment of the adult human spinal cord. Some of the important **nuclear areas (motor)** of the ventral gray horn and **descending (motor) fiber tracts** are identified. (Modified from M. B. Carpenter: *Human Neuroanatomy*, 7th ed. Courtesy of Williams & Wilkins.)

Sensory Nuclei and Tracts

4. **Dorsolateral Fasciculus (Zone of Lissauer)**—found throughout the entire spinal cord, it is a small uncrossed tract located between the dorsolateral sulcus and the tip of the dorsal horn of gray matter.

5. **Dorsal Roots (Cut Fibers)**—bundles of fibers (axons) from neurons in the spinal ganglia enter each corresponding cord segment at the dorsolateral sulcus and end in the dorsolateral fasciculus, fasciculus gracilis, and fasciculus cuneatus.

8. **Fasciculus Gracilis**—consists of heavily myelinated axons of neurons from the spinal ganglia (T6 through S5). This uncrossed tract extends the entire length of the spinal cord in the dorsal white column (see also no. **3**, Fig. 63).

10. **Fasciculus Cuneatus**—consists of heavily myelinated axons of neurons from the spinal ganglia (C1 to T5). The uncrossed tract is located in the superior half (C1-T5) of the dorsal white column.

11. **Nucleus Dorsomarginalis**—a thin layer of cells covering the tip (substantia gelatinosa) of the dorsal gray horn throughout the spinal cord. The axons of these cells pass into the fasciculus proprius and bifurcate into ascending and descending fibers.

12. **Dorsal Spinocerebellar Tract**—is an uncrossed tract located in the dorsal and marginal area of the lateral column of white matter. Its fibers originate from the nucleus dorsalis (Clarke's column, **16**) extending from T1 through L2.

13. **Nucleus Proprius (Chief Sensory Nucleus) of Dorsal Horn**—almost all the dorsal horn in the entire spinal cord except for the substantia gelatinosa and the nucleus dorsalis constitutes the nucleus proprius (see also no. **5**, Fig. 63).

Note: Leader lines with no numbers represent the motor nuclear areas and tracts which are identified in Figure **64***B*.

16. **Nucleus Dorsalis (Clarke's Column)**—a well defined nucleus extending from C8 through L2 or L3 in the ventromedial part of the dorsal horn (see also no. **4**, Fig. 63).

18. **Ventral Spinocerebellar Tract**—is a crossed tract located in the ventral and marginal area of the lateral column of white matter. Fibers originating in the lumbosacral enlargement and intermediate gray matter cross in the commissure of gray and white matter in the lower lumbar region and form the ventral spinocerebellar tract.

19. **Lateral Spinothalamic Tract**—a crossed pathway that extends the entire length of the spinal cord in the lateral white column. It originates in the contralateral nucleus proprius, and the fibers cross in the ventral commissural gray and white matter (see also no. **12**, Fig. 63).

21. **Spinotectal Tract**—a crossed tract in the cord that ascends in the ventrolateral white column to end on collicular neurons in the tectum. It conducts general sensory data to the midbrain for reflex motor responses.

22. **Spinoolivary Tract**—located in the ventral white column at all levels of the spinal cord. The fibers originate from the contralateral gray matter and end in the inferior olivary complex of the medulla. Sensory data are relayed to the olivary complex which in turn are relayed to the cerebellum.

24. **Ventral Spinothalamic Tract**—a crossed pathway extending the length of the spinal cord in the ventral white column. It originates from some cells in the nucleus proprius, the axons of which cross in the ventral white and gray commissure (see also no. **14**, Fig. 63).

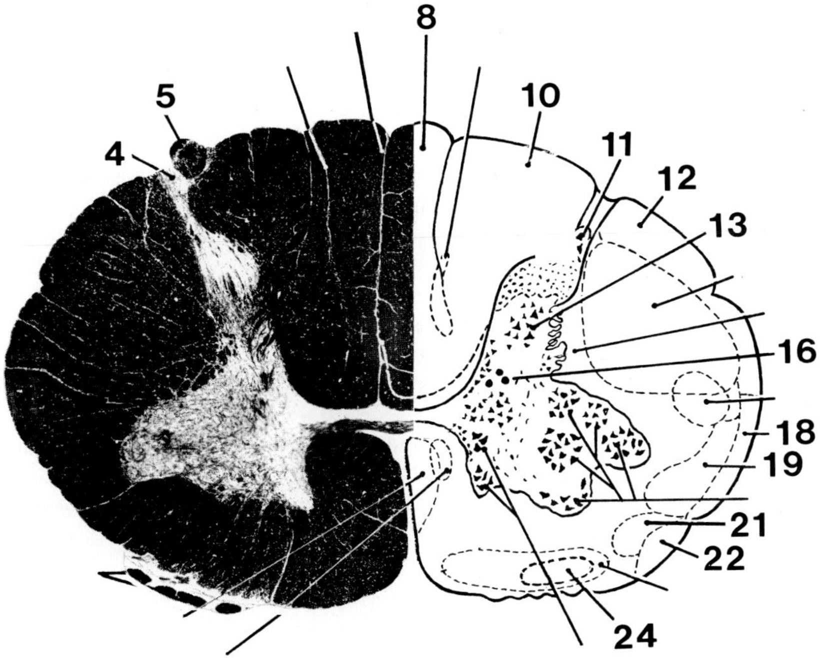

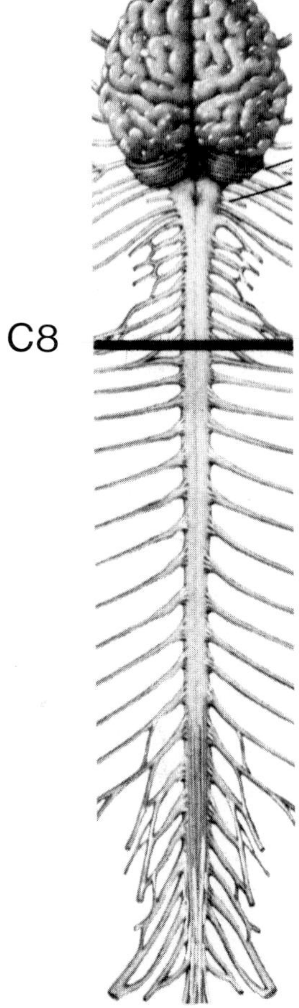

Figure 64*C* Modified photograph of a section through the eighth cervical segment of the adult human spinal cord. Some of the important **nuclear areas (sensory)** of the dorsal gray horn, and **ascending (sensory) fiber tracts** are identified. (Modified from M. B. Carpenter: *Human Neuroanatomy*, 7th ed. Courtesy of Williams & Wilkins.)

9

The Arteries of the Brain

1. **Anterior Spinal**—this small artery is formed by a branch from each vertebral artery.
2. **Vertebral**—a branch of the subclavian artery which enters the skull through the foramen magnum and runs forward beneath the medulla to join its fellow of the opposite side and form the basilar artery at the caudal border of the pons.
3. **Anterior Inferior Cerebellar**—arises from the caudal end of the basilar artery. It mainly supplies the cortex of the inferior surface of the cerebellum anteriorly. When large, the posterior inferior cerebellar artery (**13**) is small and vice versa.
4. **Basilar**—begins at the caudal border of the pons by the union of the vertebral arteries and ends at the rostral border of the pons by dividing into the two posterior cerebral arteries. In young people the basilar artery is usually in the midline; in this specimen from an elderly person, the vessel is tortuous and shows **arteriosclerotic plaques** (light areas).
5. **Posterior Cerebral**—a terminal branch of the basilar artery. Supplies the medial and inferior surfaces of the temporal and occipital lobes as far as the parietooccipital sulcus. Important branches of this artery supply the visual area.
6. **Anterior Choroidal**—branch of the internal carotid artery or middle cerebral artery. Supplies the choroid plexus in the inferior horn of the lateral ventricle (see also no. **5**, Fig. 66).
7. **Middle Cerebral**—larger terminal branch (direct continuation) of the internal carotid artery. Supplies the cortex of most of the lateral surface of one cerebral hemisphere.
8. **Internal Carotid**—a terminal branch of the common carotid artery. It enters the skull through the carotid canal, courses through the cavernous sinus, and terminates by forming the anterior and middle cerebral arteries.
9. **Anterior Cerebral**—smaller terminal branch of the internal carotid artery. Supplies the medial surface of the frontal and parietal lobes as far posterior as the parietooccipital sulcus (see also no. **7**, Fig. 66).
10. **Posterior Communicating**—arises from the internal carotid artery (sometimes middle cerebral) and joins the posterior cerebral, thereby forming part of the cerebral arterial circle (of Willis) (see also no. **8**, Fig. 68).
11. **Superior Cerebellar**—arises from the basilar artery close to its bifurcation. Supplies the superior aspect of the cerebellum and some of the dorsum of the pons and midbrain (see also no. **14**, Fig. 67).
12. **Pontine Vessels**—branches of the basilar artery supplying the basal pons (see also no. **2**, Fig. 66).
13. **Posterior Inferior Cerebellar**—large branch of the vertebral artery which supplies much of the posterior and inferior cerebellum and the lateral side of the medulla. Occlusion of this vessel gives rise to the lateral medullary (Wallenberg's) syndrome.

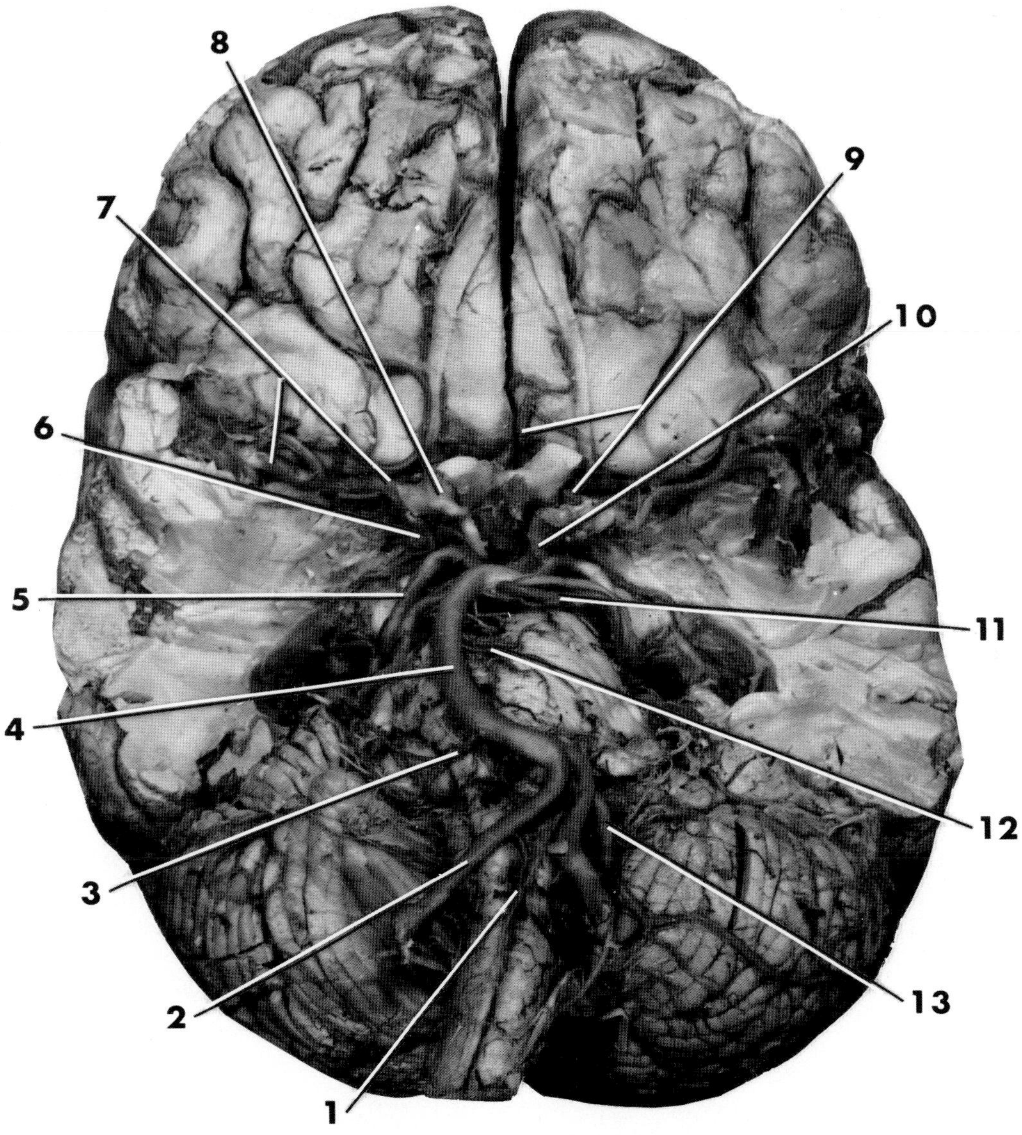

Figure 65 Basal surface of the brain showing some of the branches of the **major arteries to the brain**. Note that much of the temporal lobe on each side has been removed to show the course of some of these branches.

1. **Basilar (Rostral Portion)**—formed by the union of the two vertebral arteries at the lower border of the pons. Terminates at the upper border of the pons by forming the left and right posterior cerebral arteries (see no. **4**, Fig. 67).
2. **Pontine Vessels**—small branches of the basilar artery that supply the pons (see also no. **12,** Fig. 65).
3. **Posterior Cerebral** (right)—a terminal branch of the basilar artery. Curves over the cerebral peduncles to supply the medial and inferior surfaces of the temporal and occipital lobes, as far rostrally as the parietooccipital sulcus (see also no. **5,** Fig. 65).
4. **Oculomotor Nerve (C. N. III)**—emerges from the midbrain in the interpeduncular fossa. Supplies all the extrinsic muscles of the eye except the lateral rectus and the superior oblique.
5. **Anterior Choroidal**—branch of the internal carotid artery (sometimes middle cerebral). Supplies the choroid plexus of the inferior horn of the lateral ventricle (see also no. **3,** Fig. 68).
6. **Anterior Communicating**—joins the two anterior cerebral arteries and forms part of the cerebral arterial circle (of Willis).
7. **Anterior Cerebral**—smaller terminal branch of the internal carotid artery (middle is the larger). Supplies the medial surface of the frontal and parietal lobes, as far caudally as the parietooccipital sulcus.
8. **Internal Carotid**—a terminal branch of the common carotid artery. Gives off the anterior choroidal and posterior communicating branches before terminating in the middle and anterior cerebral arteries.
9. **Optic Tract (of C. N. II)**—cut surface of the right tract at the junction of the optic chiasma.
10. **Posterior Communicating** (left)—branching from the internal carotid artery (sometimes middle cerebral); it joins the posterior cerebral artery, forming part of the cerebral arterial circle of Willis).
11. **Superior Cerebellar**—arises from the rostral end of the basilar artery (near the posterior cerebral arteries). Supplies the cortex on the superior aspect of the cerebellum and the underlying nuclei (see also no. **9,** Fig. 68).
12. **Trigeminal Nerve (C. N. V) (Sensory Portion)**—fibers enter the lateral surface of the basal pons to terminate on the sensory spinal nucleus of the fifth cranial nerve.

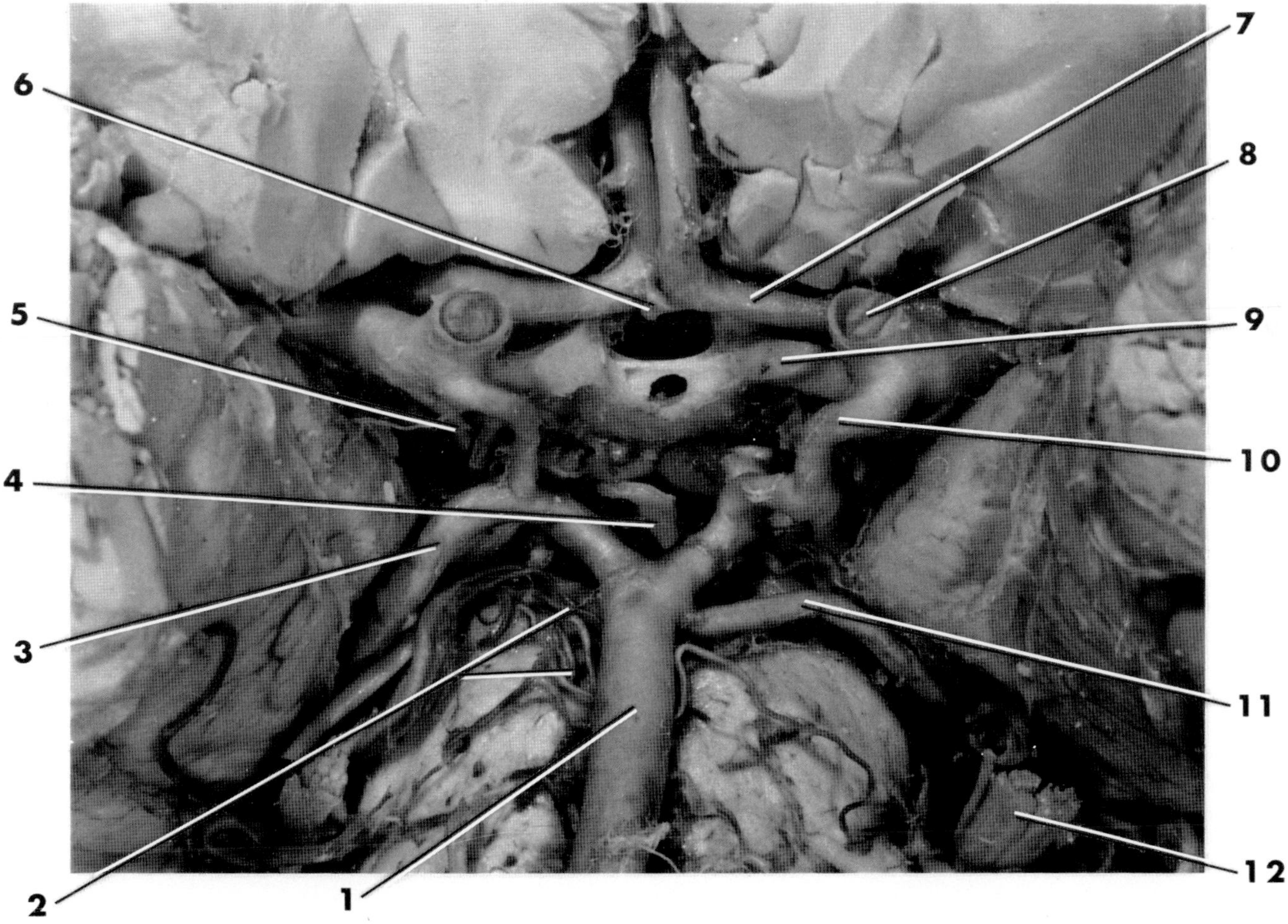

Figure 66 Enlarged area on the base of the brain showing the formation and some of the branches of the **cerebral arterial circle** (of Willis). Note—the circular opening (*black*) is the cut chiasmatic recess of the third ventricle between the optic nerves.

1. **Anterior Spinal**—formed by a branch from each vertebral artery (**2**). It descends in the ventral median fissure of the spinal cord and assists in the supply of the anterior half of the superior part of the spinal cord (see also no. **1**, Fig. 65).
2. **Vertebral Arteries** (left and right)—branches of the subclavian arteries. Within the skull they course beneath the ventrolateral medulla, where they unite at the caudal border of the pons to become the single basilar artery (**4**).
3. **Anterior Inferior Cerebellar**—arises from the caudal end of the basilar artery. It mainly supplies the cortex and medullary center of the anterior and inferior areas of the cerebellum (see also no. **3**, Fig. 65).
4. **Basilar Artery**—this single artery, formed by the union of the two vertebral arteries (**2**), courses in the basilar sulcus of the basal pons to terminate as the two posterior cerebral arteries at the upper border of the pons. In older persons it may be curved as in this specimen.
5. **Pontine Vessels**—several small arteries arising from the basilar artery to supply the tegmental pons.
6. **Posterior Communicating** (left and right)—arise from the corresponding internal carotid artery (or middle cerebral) and join the left and right posterior cerebral arteries (**13**) to form part of the cerebral arterial circle (of Willis) (see also no. **10**, Fig. 66).
7. **Optic Chiasma Vessels**—branches of the anterior median ganglionic (central) arteries. These small vessels also supply the preoptic and supraoptic hypothalamic areas.
8. **Anterior Cerebral**—the smaller terminal branch of the internal carotid artery. It supplies the medial surface of the cerebral hemisphere (frontal and parietal lobes), as far posterior as the parietooccipital sulcus (see also no. **7**, Fig. 68).
9. **Internal Carotid**—terminates at the base of the brain, lateral to the optic chiasma, by dividing into the middle cerebral (**10**) and the anterior cerebral arteries (**8**).
10. **Middle Cerebral**—the main continuing branch of the internal carotid artery. It courses in the lateral sulcus, giving off many cortical branches which ramify on most of the lateral surface of the frontal, parietal, and temporal lobes, and the insula.
11. **Central (Ganglionic or Striate)**—anterior lateral group. Arise from the middle cerebral artery and supply the corpus striatum, much of the internal capsule, the external capsule, the claustrum, and some of the hypothalamus.
12. **Anterior Choroidal**—branch of the internal carotid artery (**9**), sometimes a branch of the middle cerebral artery. It supplies the choroid plexus in the inferior horn of the lateral ventricle, as well as the optic tract, the amygdaloid nucleus, and part of the internal capsule (see also no. **3**, Fig. 68).
13. **Posterior Cerebral** (left)—curves around the cerebral peduncle to reach and supply the cortex and deeper structures of the medial and inferior surfaces of the temporal and occipital lobes. Its terminal branches also supply the lateral surface of the occipital pole (see also no. **5**, Fig. 65).
14. **Superior Cerebellar**—arises from the rostral end of the basilar artery. Note that two separate vessels arise on this side and curve around the cerebellar peduncle to reach and supply the superior area of the cerebellum (see also no. **11**, Fig. 65).

Figure 67 The terminal branches of the **basilar and internal carotid arteries** on the left side of the brain were exposed by removing much of the left temporal lobe.

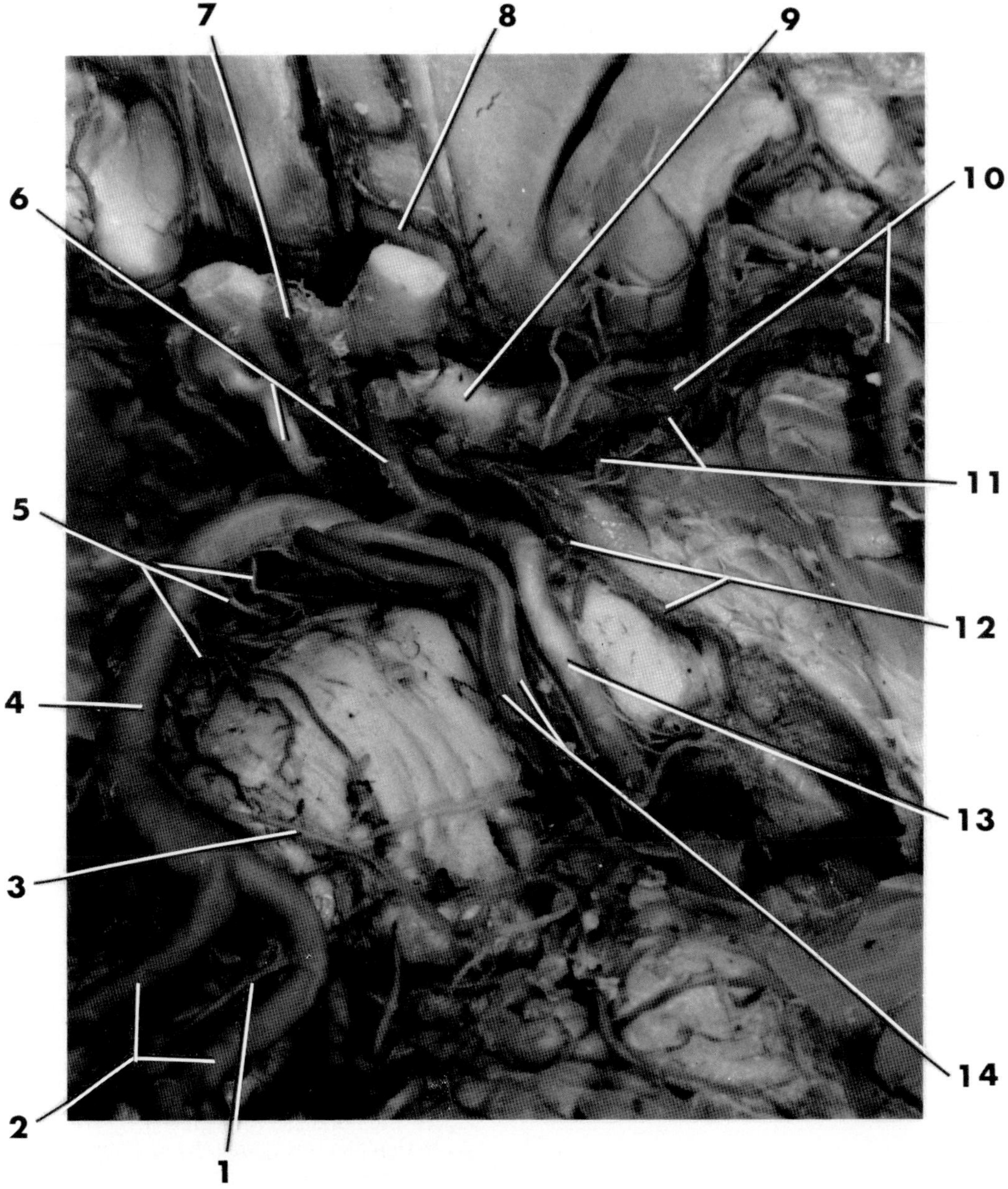

Figure 67

1. **Posterior Choroidal**—a branch of the posterior cerebral artery (**2**) which courses in the transverse fissure beneath the corpus callosum. It supplies the choroid plexus of the body of the lateral ventricle and the third ventricle, as well as the thalamus, fornix, and tectum of the midbrain.
2. **Posterior Cerebral** (right)—a terminal branch of the basilar artery which curves around the cerebral peduncle to reach and supply the inferior and medial surfaces of the temporal and occipital lobes. Some of its terminal branches also supply the inferolateral surface of the brain (see also no. **3,** Fig. 66).
3. **Anterior Choroidal**—branch of the internal carotid artery (**6**). It supplies the choroid plexus in the inferior horn of the lateral ventricle, as well as the optic tract, the amygdaloid nucleus, and part of the internal capsule (see also no. **12,** Fig. 67).
4. **Middle Cerebral**—this terminal branch, a direct continuation of the internal carotid artery, passes laterally into the lateral sulcus, where it gives off many branches that supply most of the lateral surface of the frontal, parietal, and temporal lobes (see also no. **7,** Fig. 65).
5. **Amygdaloid**—branch of the anterior choroidal artery (**3**). It passes laterally to supply the amygdaloid and the surrounding area of the temporal pole.
6. **Internal Carotid**—terminates at the base of the brain, lateral to the optic chiasma, by dividing into the middle cerebral (**4**) and the anterior cerebral arteries (**7**).
7. **Anterior Cerebral (Beginning Portion)**—the smaller terminal branch of the internal carotid artery. It supplies the medial surface of the cerebral hemisphere (frontal and parietal lobes), as far posterior as the parietooccipital sulcus (see also no. **7,** Fig. 66).
8. **Posterior Communicating** (left and right)—they arise from the internal carotid artery (sometimes middle cerebral) and join the posterior cerebrals to form part of the arterial circle (of Willis) (see also no. **10,** Fig. 66).
9. **Superior Cerebellar** (left and right)—branches of the rostral end of the basilar artery. They curve around the middle cerebellar peduncle to reach and supply the superior area of the cerebellum (see also no. **14,** Fig. 67).
10. **Pontine Vessels**—many small arteries arise from the basilar artery to supply the basal and tegmental pons.
11. **Basilar**—formed by the union of the two vertebral arteries at the caudal border of the pons. It is usually located in the midline (as shown here) on the ventral surface of pons, and terminates as the left and right posterior cerebrals at the rostral border of the pons.
12. **Internal Auditory (Labyrinthine)**—branch of the basilar artery (sometimes anterior inferior cerebellar) which supplies the internal ear.

Figure 68 Branches of the **cerebral arterial circle** on the right side at the base of the brain. Note that the temporal pole has been removed to show the course of the choroidal vessels in the lateral ventricle.

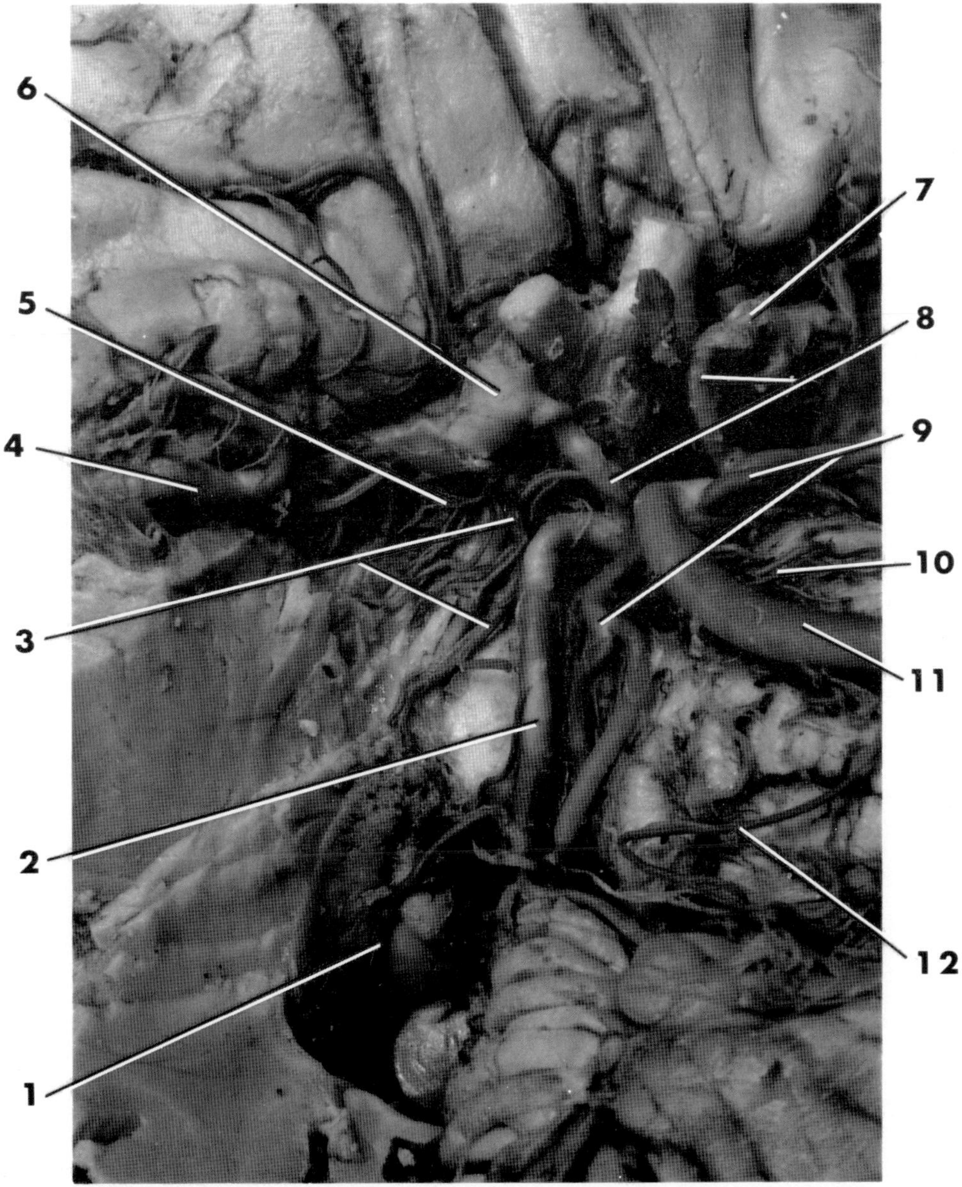

Figure 68

1. **Anterior Spinal**—this small vessel is formed by branches from the left and right vertebral arteries. It descends in the ventral median fissure on the anterior surface of the spinal cord (see also no. **1,** Fig. 65 and no. **1**, Fig. 67).
2. **Vertebral**—a branch of the subclavian artery. It enters the skull through the foramen magnum, courses beneath the ventral lateral medulla, and joins its fellow of the opposite side at the caudal border of the pons to form the single basilar artery (see also no. **2,** Fig. 67).
3. **Pontine Vessels**—many small branches from the basilar artery which supply the basal and tegmental pons.
4. **Posterior Cerebral** (right)—a terminal branch of the basilar artery. Curves around the cerebral peduncle to reach and supply the cortex of the medial and inferior surfaces of the temporal and occipital lobes. Its terminal branches supply the lateral surface of the occipital pole (see also no. **13,** Fig. 67).
5. **Superior Cerebellar**—arises from the rostral end of the basilar artery near the posterior cerebral arteries; curves onto the superior surface of the cerebellum to supply the cortex and underlying cerebellar nuclei (see also no. **9,** Fig. 68).
6. **Basilar**—formed by the union of the left and right vertebral arteries (**2**) at the caudal border of the pons. Courses along the midline of the ventral pons and terminates at the rostral border of the pons by forming the left and right posterior cerebral arteries (**4**) (see also no. **4,** Fig. 65).
7. **Anterior Inferior Cerebellar**—arises from the caudal part of the basilar artery. It mainly supplies the cortex and medullary center of the anterior and inferior areas of the cerebellum (see also no. **3,** Fig. 65).
8. **Internal Auditory (Labyrinthine)**—branch of the basilar artery (sometimes anterior inferior cerebellar). Supplies internal ear structures (see also no. **12,** Fig. 68).
9. **Posterior Inferior Cerebellar**—large branch of the vertebral artery. Supplies much of the posterior and inferior cerebellum and the lateral side of the medulla. Occlusion of this vessel gives rise to many cerebellar and brain stem disorders, *e.g.*, Wallenberg's syndrome (see also no. **13,** Fig. 65).
10. **Dorsal Spinal**—arises from the vertebral artery (sometimes posterior inferior cerebellar). Each vessel descends the length of the cord in the dorsolateral sulcus on its dorsal surface.

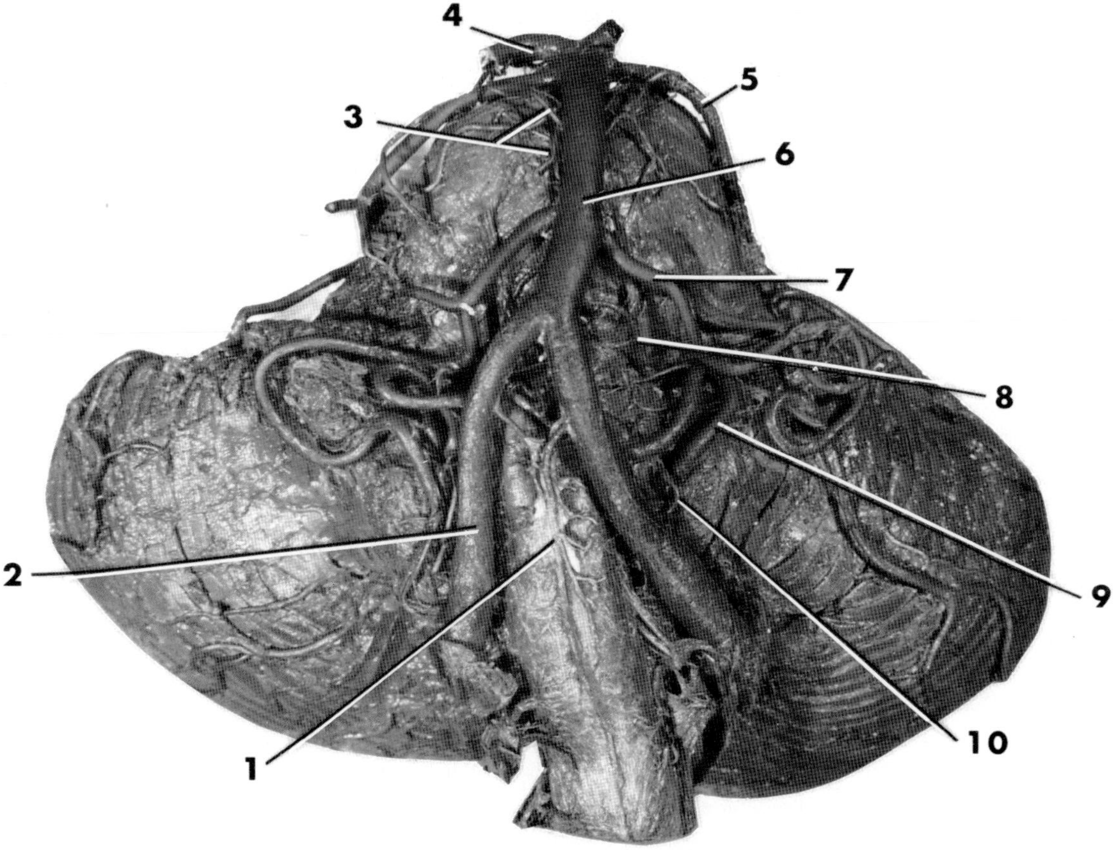

Figure 69 Basal (ventral) surface of the brain stem and the cerebellum showing the branches of the **vertebral and basilar arteries**.

10

Horizontal Serial Sections and Representative CT Scans of the Brain

Horizontal serial sections were cut through a whole brain, approximately 12 mm in thickness. The sections were then surface-stained by the modified Mulligan technique (blue, gray matter; white, white matter), photographed, mounted, and the important structures in each section numbered. In sections where there were more than 15 important structures illustrated, a duplicate photograph was used to identify the additional structures.

Throughout the series, a small drawing of the brain appears in the upper right-hand corner of each figure with a line drawn through the brain to indicate the level through which the section was taken.

The computed tomographic (CT) scans of the head were made at approximately 20° to the horizontal plane, and were of living, apparently normal persons. Because of this, and because heads vary in shape (bradycephalic, normocephalic, dolichocephalic), they do not correspond exactly to the stained horizontal sections of the brain; however, the following scans indicate the similarity of structures seen in the stained sections and in CT scans. On each legend page there is a small orientation diagram of a lateral view of the skull, cerebrum, brain stem, and lateral ventricle. The lines **A** and **B** indicate the planes of the CT scans.

1. **Longitudinal Cerebral Fissure**—separates the anterior, posterior, and superior parts of the cerebral hemispheres.
2. **Postcentral Gyrus**—bounded by the central sulcus and postcentral sulcus—landmark for general sensory area of cortex.
3. **Central Sulcus (Fissure or Sulcus of Rolando)**—important landmark because the general sensory area lies immediately behind the sulcus, and the motor area lies immediately in front of it.
4. **Precentral Gyrus**—landmark for motor area of cerebral cortex.
5. **Frontal Pole**—convex anterior end of frontal lobe.
6. **Superior Frontal Gyrus**—located between the superior frontal sulcus on the lateral surface and the cingulate sulcus on the medial surface.
7. **Parietal Lobe**—located between central sulcus and parietooccipital sulcus (fissure).

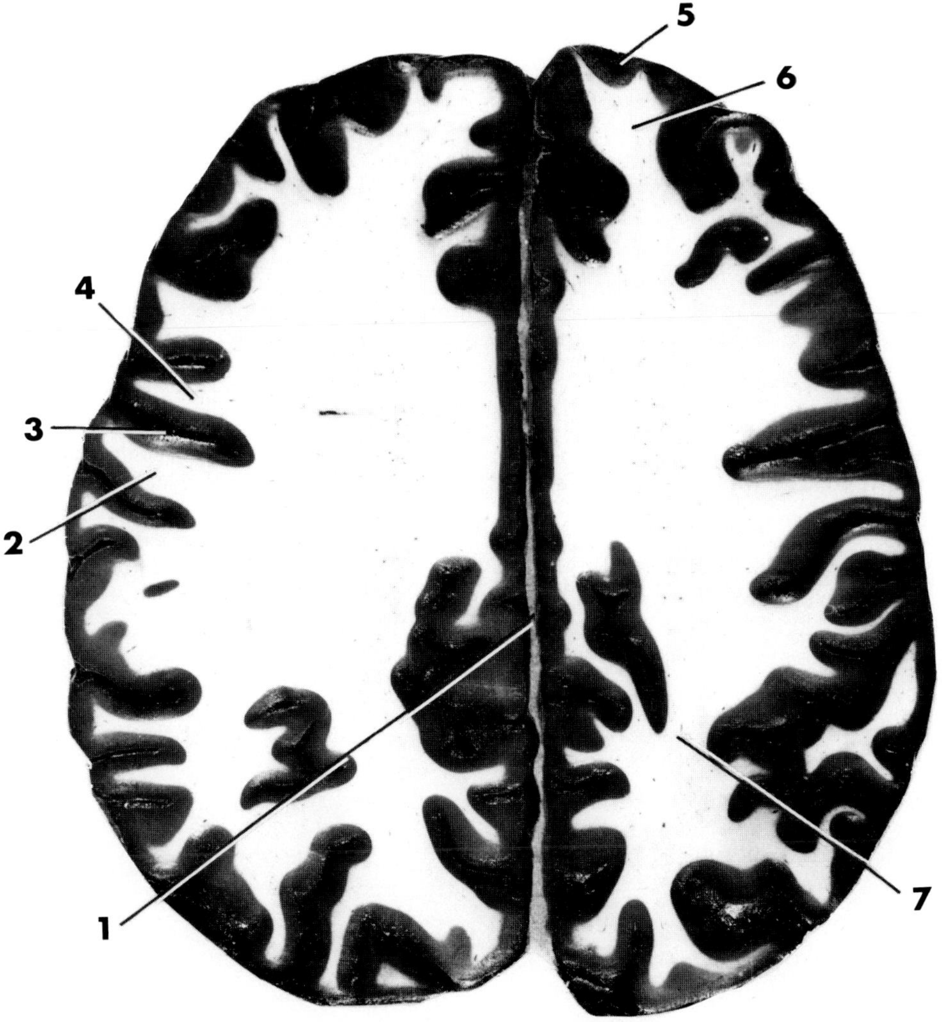

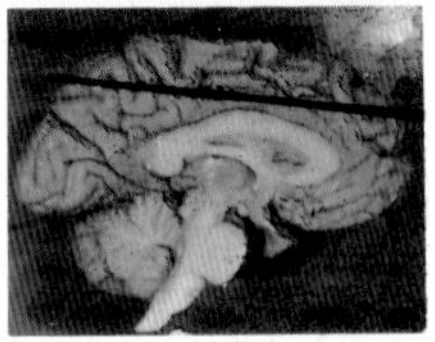

Figure 70

1. **Anterior Horn of Lateral Ventricle**—bounded by fibers of the body of the corpus callosum above and fibers of the genu of the corpus callosum in front.
2. **Body of Corpus Callosum**—composed of compact commissural fibers that cross in the midline.
3. **Head of Caudate Nucleus**—bulges into the anterior horn of the lateral ventricle.
4. **Forceps Minor**—composed of radiating commissural fibers that pass through the genu of the corpus callosum connecting the frontal lobes.
5. **Frontal Pole**—anterior convex end of frontal lobe.
6. **Precentral Gyrus**—located between the central and precentral sulci (landmark for primary motor cortex).
7. **Central Sulcus (of Rolando)**—lined by sensorimotor cortex.
8. **Postcentral Gyrus**—bounded by the central and postcentral sulci—landmark for general sensory area cortex.
9. **Occipital Pole**—posterior convex end of occipital lobe.

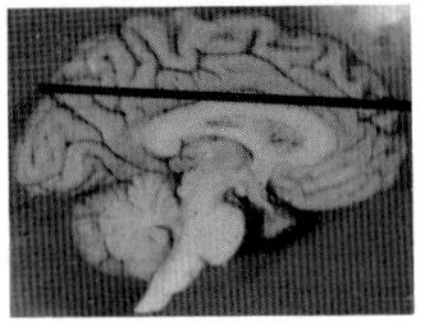

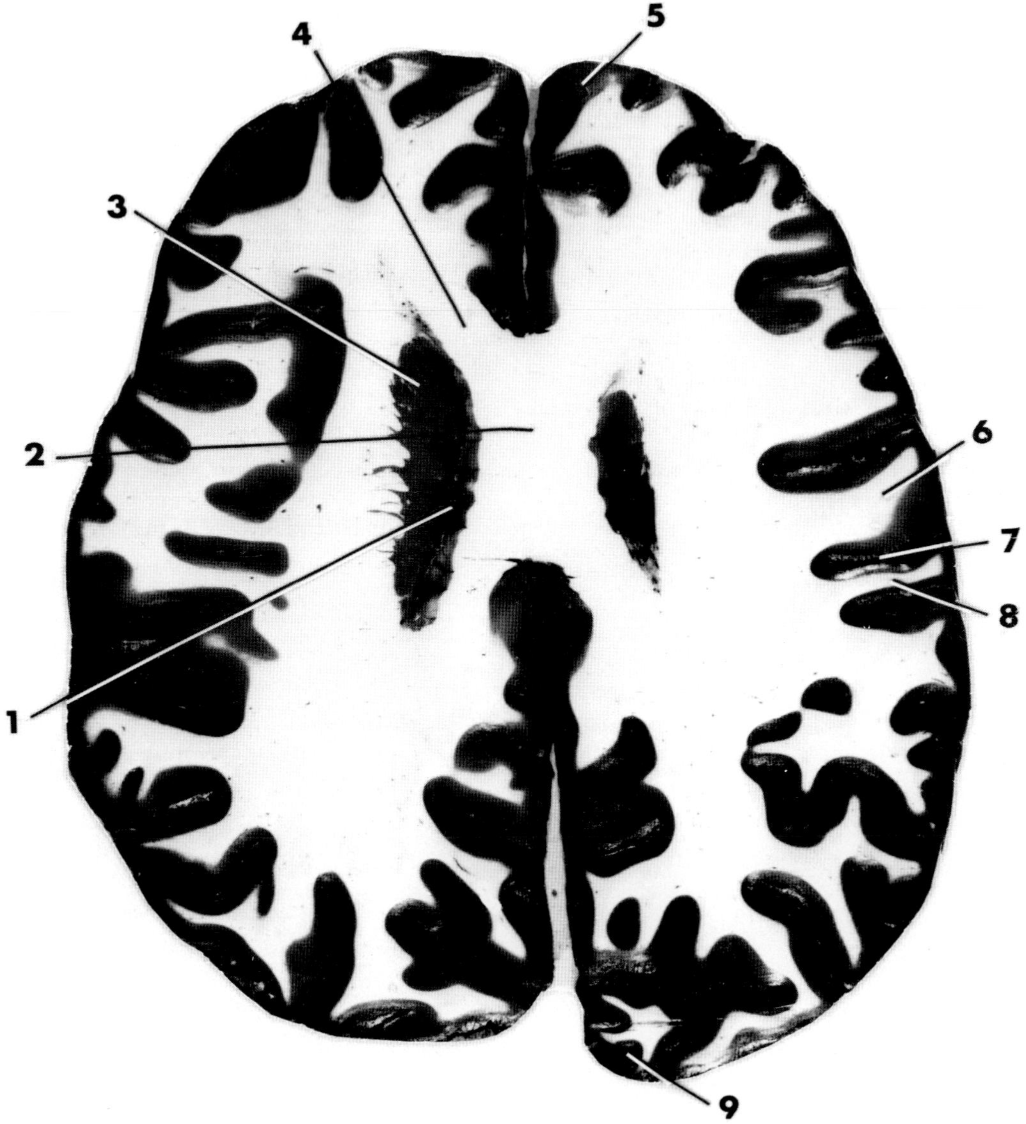

Figure 71

1. **Parietooccipital Sulcus (Fissure)**—extends from the calcarine sulcus on the medial surface to intersect the superior border approximately 4 cm from the occipital pole and continues for a short distance on the lateral surface. On the medial surface it separates occipital lobe from parietal lobe.
2. **Body of Fornix**—formed by a continuation of fibers from the crus fornix. Fibers of the fornix are part of the limbic system connecting the hippocampus with the mammillary bodies.
3. **Dorsal Thalamic Area**—part of dorsolateral nucleus of thalamus lying medial to internal capsule.
4. **Claustrum**—thin sheet of gray matter located between external and extreme capsules.
5. **External Capsule**—thin layer of white matter located between the claustrum and lenticular nucleus. It consists of association, projection, and some commissural fibers.
6. **Putamen**—lateral portion of lenticular nucleus; separated from globus pallidus (medial portion of lentiform nucleus) by a lateral medullary lamina of nerve fibers.
7. **Genu of Corpus Callosum**—anterior end of corpus callosum which thins or tapers into the rostrum (L. beak). It is composed of commissural fibers which radiate into the frontal lobes forming the forceps minor.
8. **Septum Pellucidum**—a membrane (sometimes double) located between the anterior part of corpus callosum and the fornix. It separates the anterior horns of the lateral ventricles.
9. **Head of Caudate Nucleus**—bulges into anterior horn of lateral ventricle from its lateral wall and floor.
10. **Thalamic Tubercle (Anterior Thalamic Nucleus)**—part of limbic system. The internal medullary lamina bifurcates and surrounds this nucleus as well as separating the thalamus into medial and lateral nuclear masses. Note that only a small portion of the tubercle is shown.
11. **Splenium of Corpus Callosum**—posterior portion of corpus callosum. Commissural fibers pass through this area and radiate into the occipital lobes as the forceps major (see no. **1**, Fig. 73A).

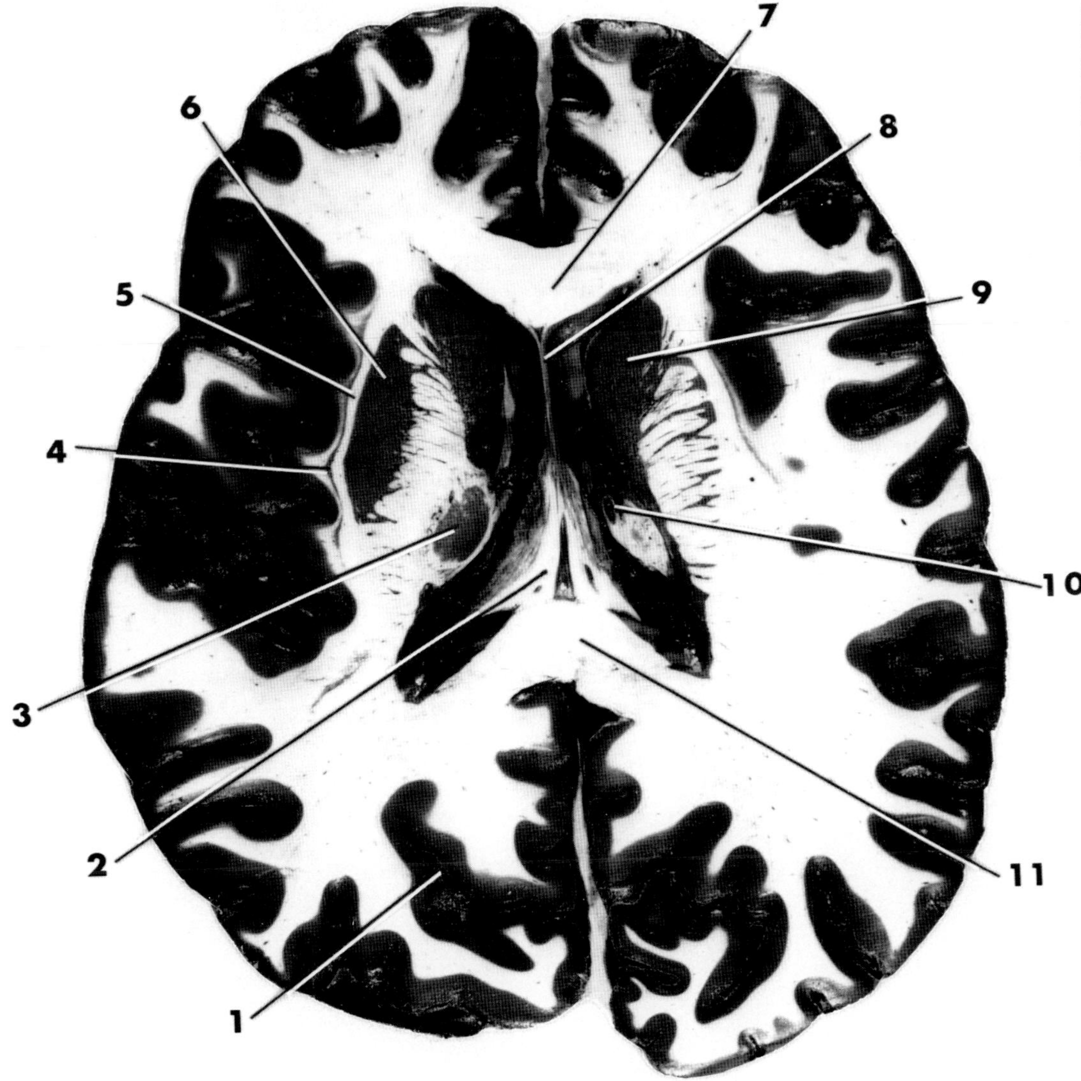

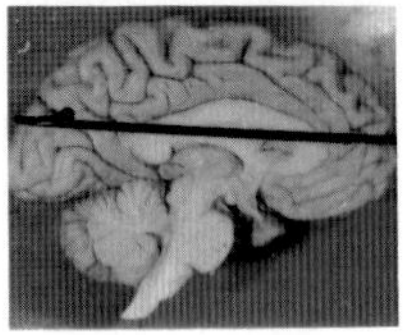

Figure 72

1. **Forceps Minor**—composed of radiating commissural fibers that pass through the splenium (**11**) from each occipital medullary center. It has the appearance of a pair of tongs. (L. *forceps*).
2. **Crus Fornix**—a continuation of the fimbria which is composed of fibers that emanate from the hippocampus. The crus (L. leg) joins its partner to form the body of the fornix.
3. **Tail of Caudate Nucleus**—the tail follows the contour of the lateral ventricle on the dorsal thalamus and continues into the roof of the inferior horn of this ventricle.
4. **Column of Fornix**—the two columns continue from the body and curve ventrally in front of the interventricular foramen (**9**) and continue through the hypothalamus to the mammillary bodies.
5. **Septum Pellucidum**—a membrane (sometimes double) separating the anterior horns of the lateral ventricles (no. **1**, Fig. 86).
6. **Genu of Corpus Callosum** (L. *genu*, the knee)—anterior end of corpus callosum where comissural fibers radiate into the frontal lobes forming forceps minor.
7. **Head of Caudate Nucleus**—bulges into anterior horn of lateral ventricle.
8. **Anterior Horn of Lateral Ventricle**—extends forward as far as genu of corpus callosum. The septum pellucidum (**5**, *see* no. 1, Fig. 86) separates the anterior horns of the two lateral ventricles.
9. **Interventricular Foramen (of Monro)**—located between lateral and third ventricles. It is bounded in front by the column of the fornix (**4**) and behind by the anterior thalamic tubercle (no. 4, Fig. 88).
10. **Posterior Horn of Lateral Ventricle**—from its beginning at the collateral trigone, it extends from the body of lateral ventricle into the medullary center of the occipital lobe.
11. **Splenium of Corpus Callosum** (G. *splēnion*, bandage)—thickened posterior extremity of corpus callosum (see no. **11**, Fig. 72).

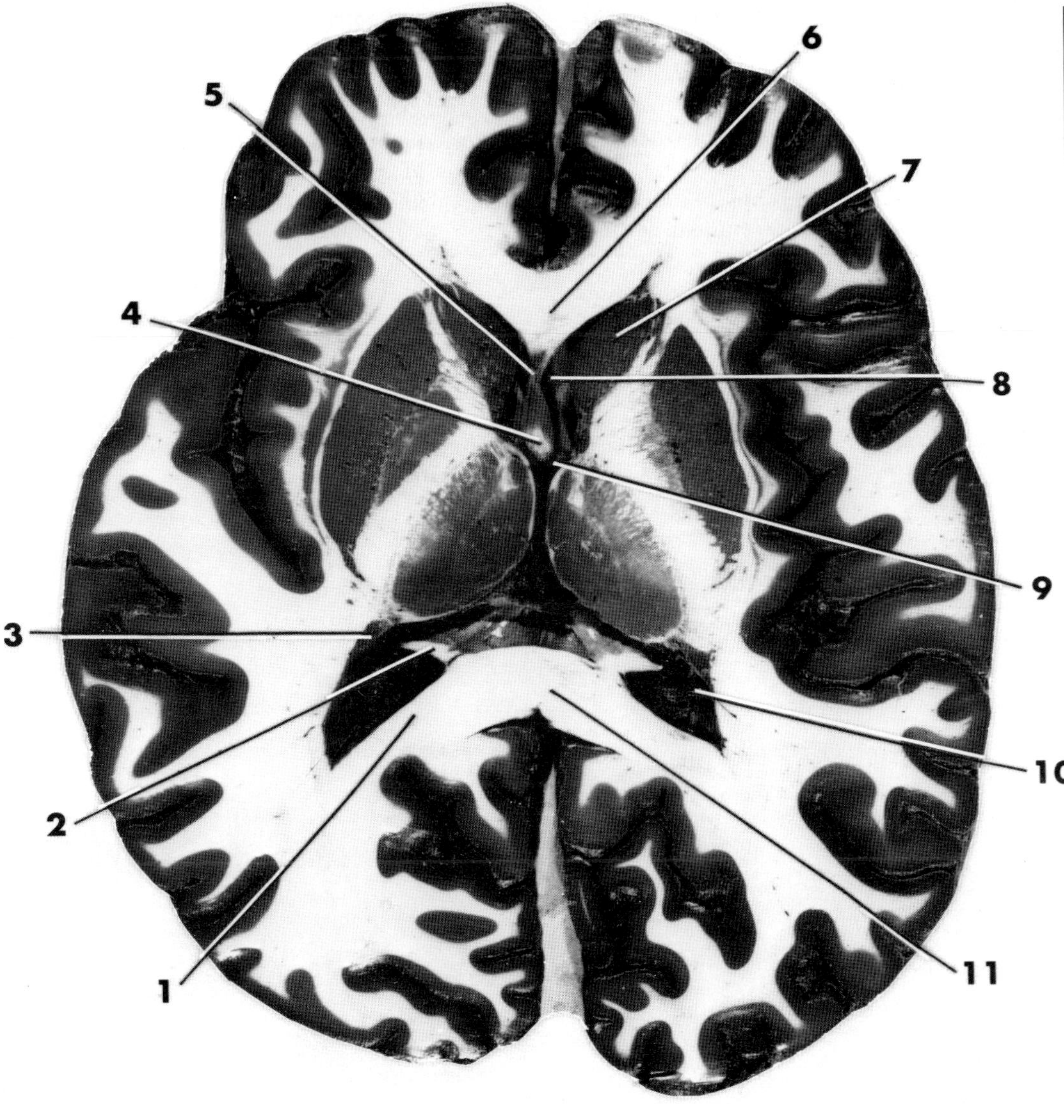

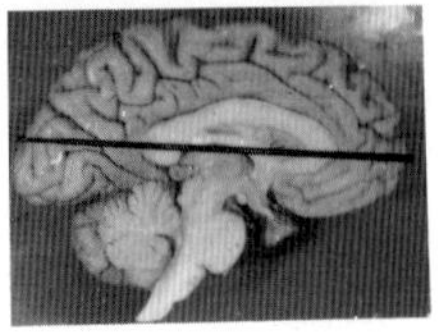

Figure 73*A*

1. **Globus Pallidus** (L. a ball + pale)—medial part of the lentiform nucleus. It is separated from the putamen (**5**, *see* no. **6**, Fig. 74*B*) by the lateral medullary lamina and from the thalamus (**10**) by the posterior limb of the internal capsule (**8**).
2. **Extreme Capsule**—separates the claustrum (**3**) from the insula (**9**).
3. **Claustrum** (L. a barrier)—a thin nuclear area (one of the cerebral ganglia) situated between the external capsule (**4**) and the extreme capsule (**2**).
4. **External Capsule**—consists mainly of projection fibers and some commissural and association fibers. It is located between the putamen (no. **12**, Fig. 87) and the claustrum (**3**).
5. **Putamen** (L. shell)—the larger and lateral part of the lentiform nucleus of the corpus striatum (see also no. **6**, Fig. 74*B*).
6. **Anterior Limb of Internal Capsule**—composed of projection fibers partially separating head of caudate nucleus and putamen (no. **4**, Fig. 86).
7. **Genu of Internal Capsule**—medial to the apex of the globus pallidus (**1**), it partially separates head of caudate nucleus from thalamus.
8. **Posterior Limb of Internal Capsule**—composed of projection fibers separating lentiform nucleus from thalamus. In addition to this lenticulothalamic portion, there are retrolenticular and sublenticular portions of the posterior limb.
9. **Insula** (L. island)—composed of hidden cortex at the bottom of the lateral sulcus (fissure). Also called the *insular lobe*.
10. **Ventrolateral Thalamic Area**—located medial to the posterior limb of internal capsule (**8**). It is composed of the ventral anterior, lateral, and posterior thalamic nuclei.
11. **Medial Thalamic Area**—forms part of the wall of the third ventricle. It is subdivided into medial and midline thalamic nuclei.

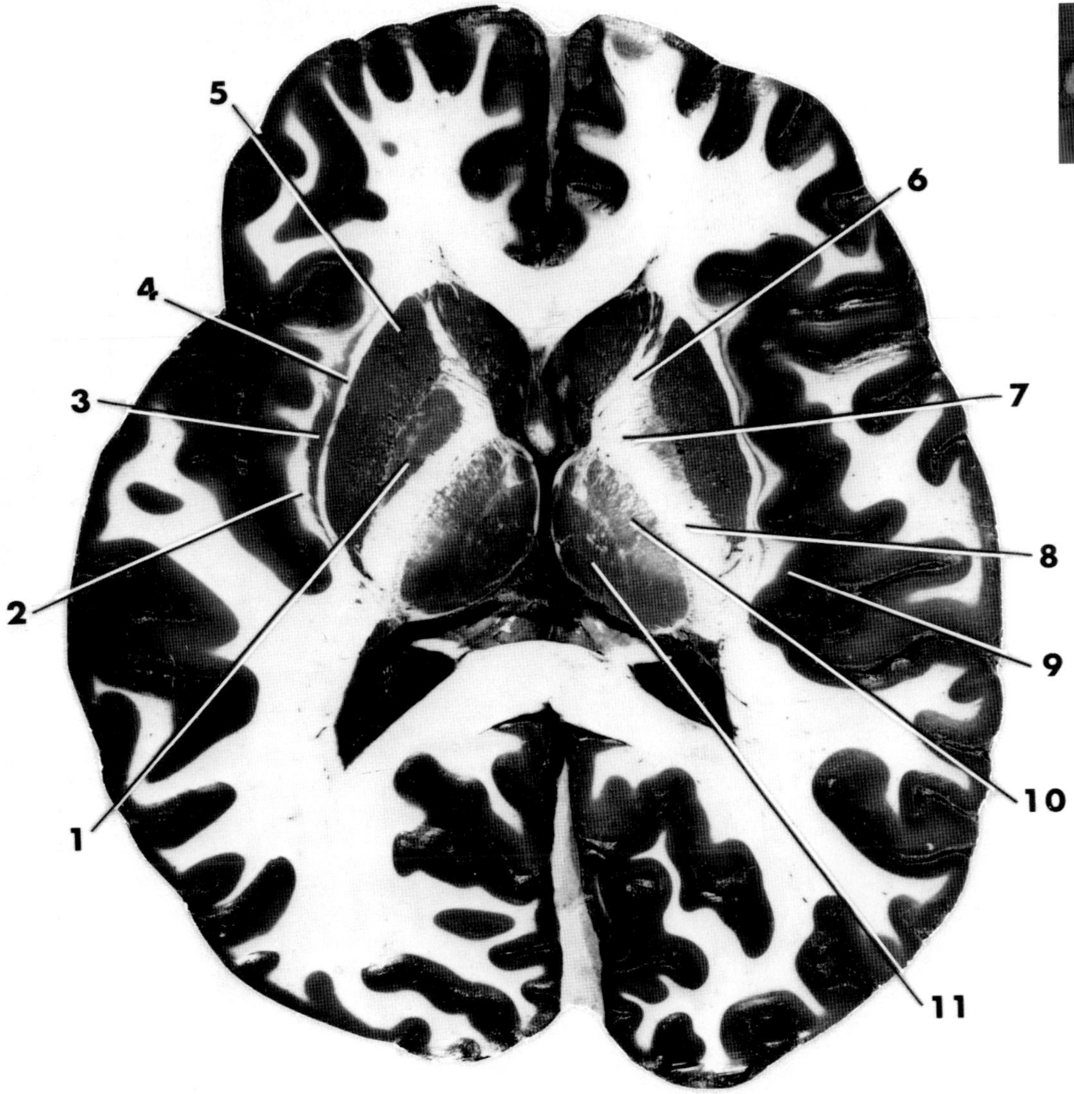

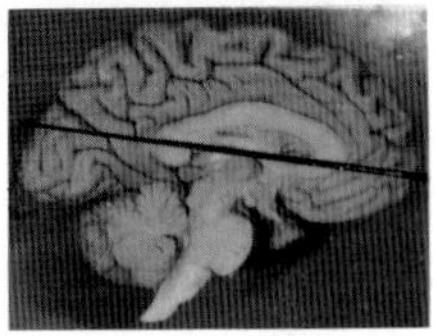

Figure 73*B*

1. **Collateral Trigone of Lateral Ventricle (Junction of Inferior and Posterior Horns)**—posteriorly the body of the lateral ventricle in the parietal lobe divides into posterior and inferior horns which extend into the occipital and temporal lobes, respectively (see also **1d**, Fig. 29).
2. **Hippocampus** (G. sea horse)—part of limbic system occupying floor of inferior horn of lateral ventricle. Its efferent fibers form the alveus, fimbria, crus, body, and columns of the fornix which terminate in the mammillary bodies.
3. **Crus Fornix**—its fibers are a continuation of the fimbria which originates in the hippocampus (**2**). This crus (L. leg) joins its partner to form the body of the fornix (see also no. **2**, Fig. 73*A*).
4. **Mammillothalamic Tract (Bundle of Vicq d'Azyr)**—part of limbic system. Composed of reciprocal fibers passing through hypothalamus, connecting mammillary body and anterior nucleus of thalamus (see no. **3**, Fig. 75*B*).
5. **Column of Fornix**—part of limbic system. The column of the fornix is a division of the body. It passes through the hypothalamus to terminate in the mammillary body. As the column curves ventrally it passes in front of the interventricular foramen (see no. **4**, Fig. 73*A*).
6. **Head of Caudate Nucleus**—lies in and on the floor of the anterior horn of lateral ventricle. Inferiorly and laterally it is continuous with the putamen (no. **5**, Fig. 73*B*) to form the corpus striatum.
7. **Anterior Commissure**—composed of reciprocal commissural fibers that cross the midline and pass through the corpus striatum on their way to the temporal lobes (see also no. **13**, Fig. 88).
8. **Globus Pallidus**—medial part of lentiform nucleus (no. **1**, Fig. 73*B*). The lateral medullary lamina separates it from the putamen (no. **5**, Fig. 73*B* and no. **5**, Fig. 89*A*).
9. **Tail of Caudate Nucleus**—continues into the roof of inferior horn of lateral ventricle (see no. **3**, Fig. 73*A*). It rests on the dorsolateral surface of the thalamus in the body of the lateral ventricle.
10. **Geniculocalcarine Tract**—part of visual pathway passing lateral to posterior horn of lateral ventricle in the medullary center. It connects the lateral geniculate body with visual cortex which forms lips of calcarine sulcus (see no. **9**, Fig. 74*B*).

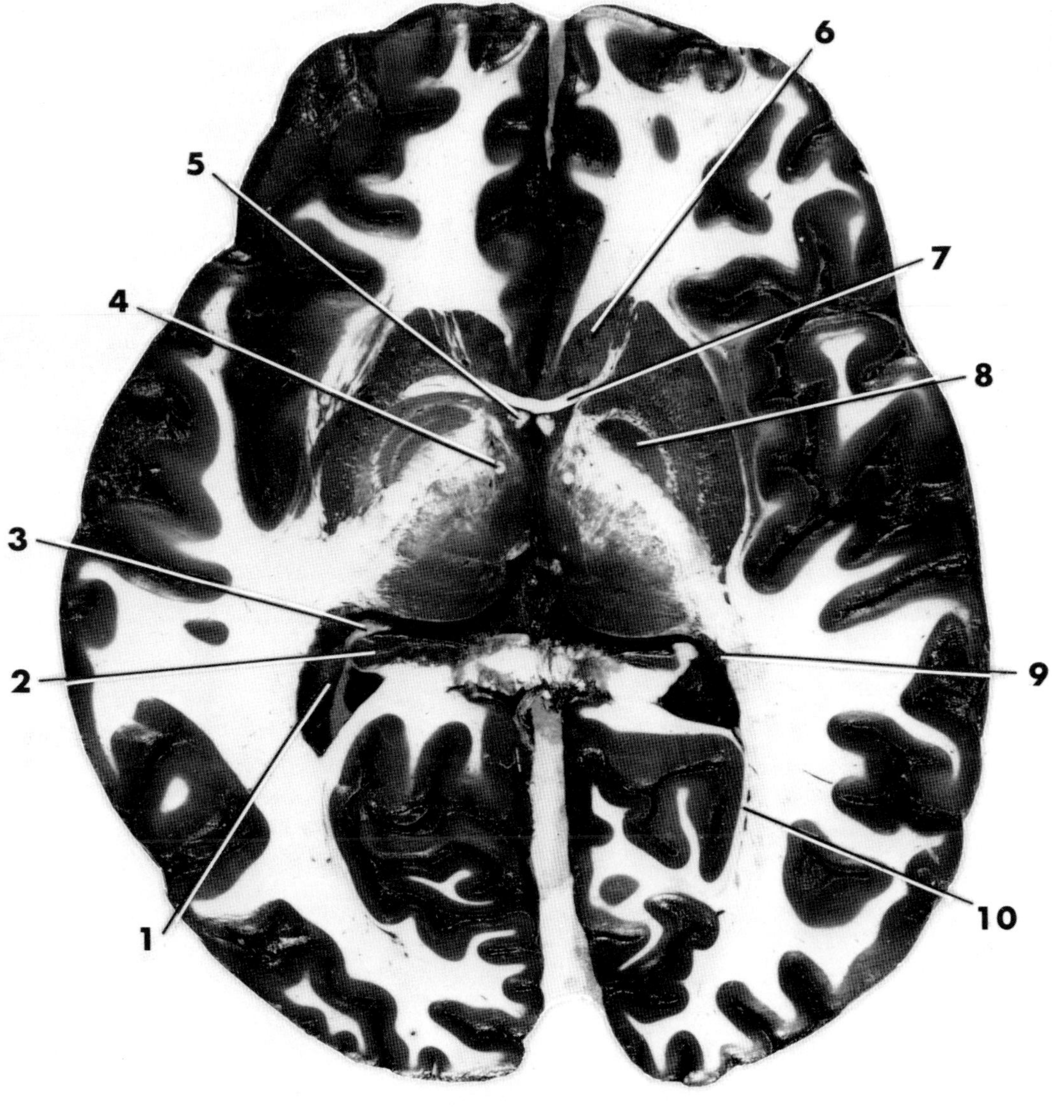

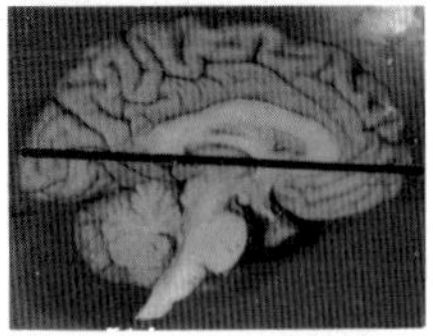

Figure 74*A*

1. **Pulvinar** (L. cushioned seat)—the posterior cushion-like projection of the thalamus that overhangs the medial and lateral geniculate bodies. Each pulvinar rests on the dorsolateral aspect of the midbrain.
2. **Posterior Limb of Internal Capsule**—composed of projection fibers that continue into the midbrain as basis pedunculi (no. **2**, Fig. 75*A*). The posterior limb separates thalamus from lentiform nucleus (globus pallidus + putamen).
3. **Lateral Medullary Lamina**—consists of nerve fibers that separate globus pallidus (no. **2**, Fig. 89*A*) and putamen (**6**) (see also no. **5**, Fig. 73*B* for lentiform nucleus).
4. **Medial Medullary Lamina**—consists of nerve fibers separating globus pallidus (no. **2**, Fig. 89*A*) into medial and lateral segments.
5. **External Capsule**—consists mostly of projection fibers lying between putamen and claustrum.
6. **Putamen**—the large lateral area of lentiform nucleus. Anteriorly and inferiorly it is continuous with the head of the caudate nucleus; they form part of the corpus striatum.
7. **Claustrum**—thin nuclear area, one of the basal nuclei (often called basal "ganglia"), located between the external (**5**) and extreme capsules (**8**).
8. **Extreme Capsule**—consists of association and commissural fibers separating claustrum (**7**) from insula (see also no. **9**, Fig. 73*B*).
9. **Visual Cortex (Brodmann's Area 17)**—surrounds the calcarine sulcus. It receives connections from lateral geniculate body via the geniculocalcarine tract.

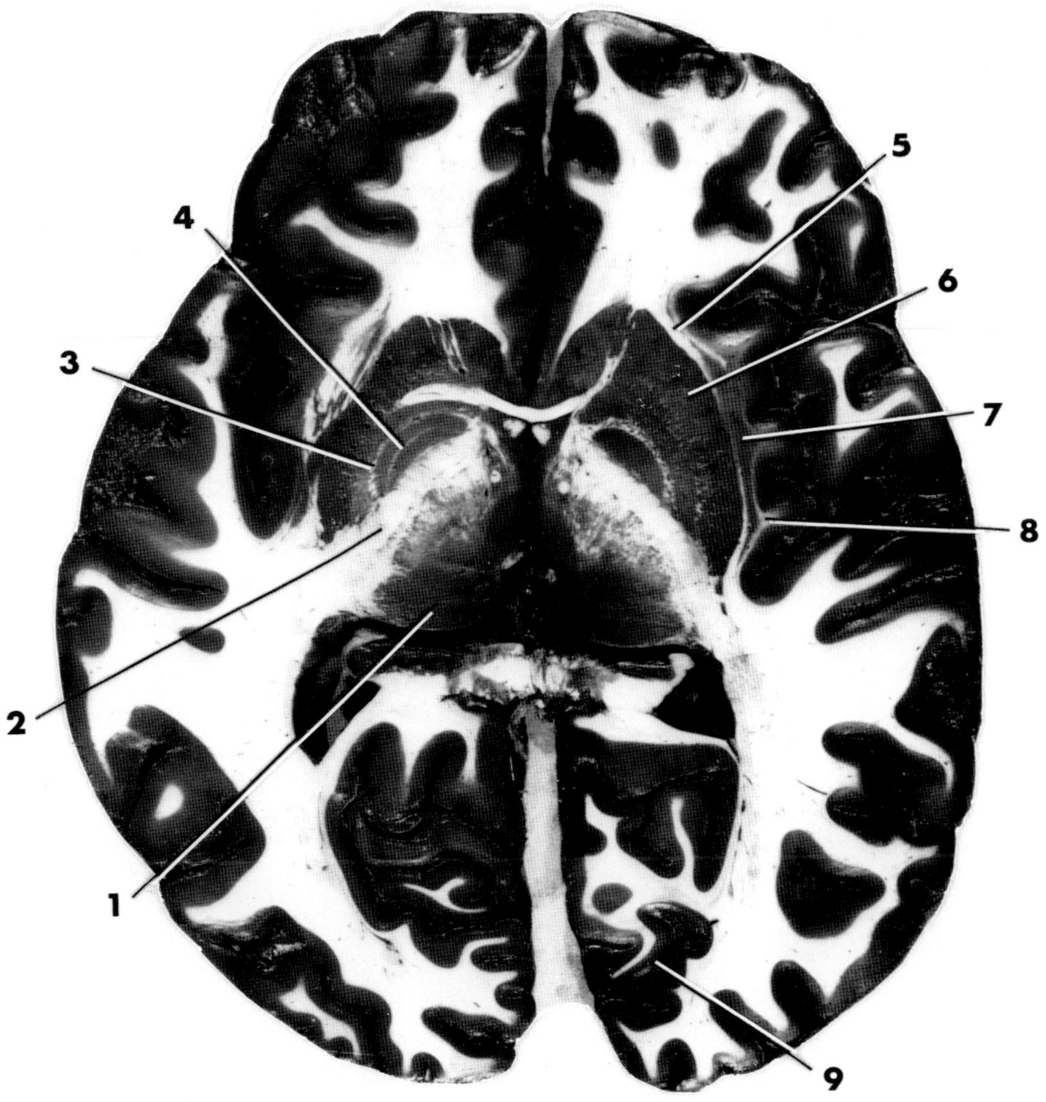

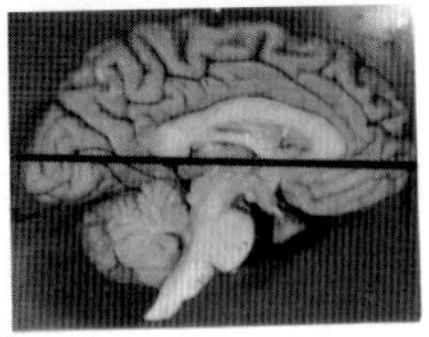

Figure 74*B*

1. **Dentatothalamic Fibers of Superior Cerebellar Peduncle (Brachium conjunctivum)**—encapsulating red nucleus. The brachium (L. arm) conjunctivum is a bundle of fibers that originates from contralateral cerebellar nuclei (dentate, emboliform, and globose) and decussates in caudal midbrain to end on ventral lateral thalamic nucleus. While coursing through midbrain, it encapsulates red nucleus (**6**), and some of its fibers end in this nucleus.
2. **Basis Pedunculi (Crus Cerebri)**—ventral part of the cerebral peduncle. It is a continuation of the internal capsule (no. **2**, Fig. 74*B*) which consists of cortical projection fibers.
3. **Ansa Lenticularis**—composed of efferent fibers from globus pallidus that curve around the medial edge of the internal capsule, then course to the ventral anterior and ventral lateral nuclei of the thalamus.
4. **Hypothalamic Area**—surrounds basal area of third ventricle. It is subdivided into medial and lateral zones of nuclei.
5. **Frontal Pole**—convex anterior end of frontal lobe lying superior to the roof of orbit (floor of anterior cranial fossa).
6. **Red Nucleus**—prominent brain stem motor nucleus located in the tegmentum of the rostral midbrain. It receives connections from cerebellar nuclei and functions in the extrapyramidal system.
7. **Optic Tract**—composed of optic nerve fibers from the optic chiasma that course around the cerebral peduncle to end in the lateral geniculate body.
8. **Substantia Nigra**—a large brain stem motor nucleus located in the midbrain between the tegmentum and the basis pedunculi (**2**). Many of its constituent cells contain dark melanin pigment, hence the term *nigra* (L. black).
9. **Superior Colliculus** (L. small elevation)—nerve cell mass on the rostral half of dorsal surface of the midbrain. It is a relay station in visual system for eye and head movements.
10. **Occipital Pole**—convex posterior end of the occipital lobe lying superior to the tentorium cerebelli and cerebellum.

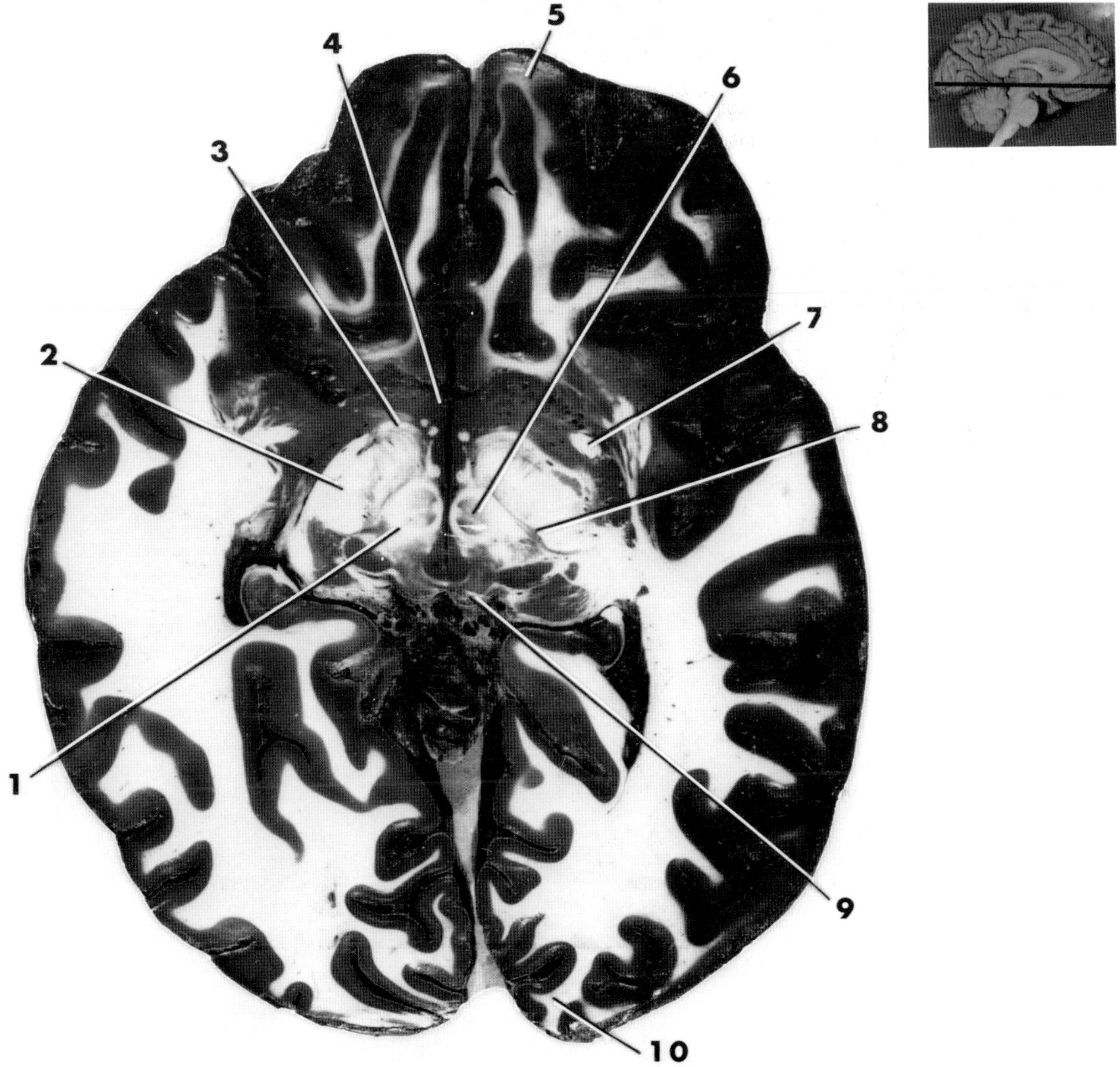

Figure 75*A*

1. **Medial Geniculate Body**—nuclear swelling formed by the medial geniculate nucleus, located beneath the pulvinar on the posterior surface of thalamus. It is on the auditory pathway.
2. **Hippocampus** (G. seahorse)—located in floor of inferior horn of lateral ventricle. It is part of limbic system and its fibers terminate in the mammillary bodies via the alveus, fimbria, and fornix (see also no. **8**, Fig. 91*B*).
3. **Mammillothalamic Tract (Fasciculus, Bundle of Vicq d'Azyr)**—component of limbic system that reciprocally connects mammillary body with anterior nucleus of thalamus. This tract courses through the hypothalamic area (see also no. **4**, Fig. 14*B*).
4. **Column of Fornix** (L. arch)—part of limbic system. Its fibers, continued from the body of the fornix, arch downwards in the midline between the anterior commissure and interventricular foramen to continue through hypothalamus to mammillary body (see also no. **5**, Fig. 74*A*).
5. **Third Ventricle (IIIrd Ventricle)**—diencephalic part of the ventricular system. The thalamus and hypothalamus form its lateral wall on each side.
6. **Pulvinar** (L. cushioned seat)—cushion-like area of the thalamus overhanging the medial and lateral geniculate bodies. This area of the thalamus bulges onto the dorsal surface of the midbrain (see also no. **1**, Fig. 74*B* and no. **3**, Fig. 91*A*).
7. **Tail of Caudate Nucleus**—located in roof of inferior horn of lateral ventricle after curving around caudal surface of pulvinar (**6**).
8. **Fimbria of Fornix**—efferent fibers leave the hippocampus and curve upwards in inferior horn of lateral ventricle to continue as the crus of the fornix (see no. **3**, Fig. 74*A*), which continues to form body of fornix.
9. **Choroid Plexus** (G. like a membrane)—of inferior horn of lateral ventricle. It is supplied by the anterior choroidal artery and produces cerebrospinal fluid.

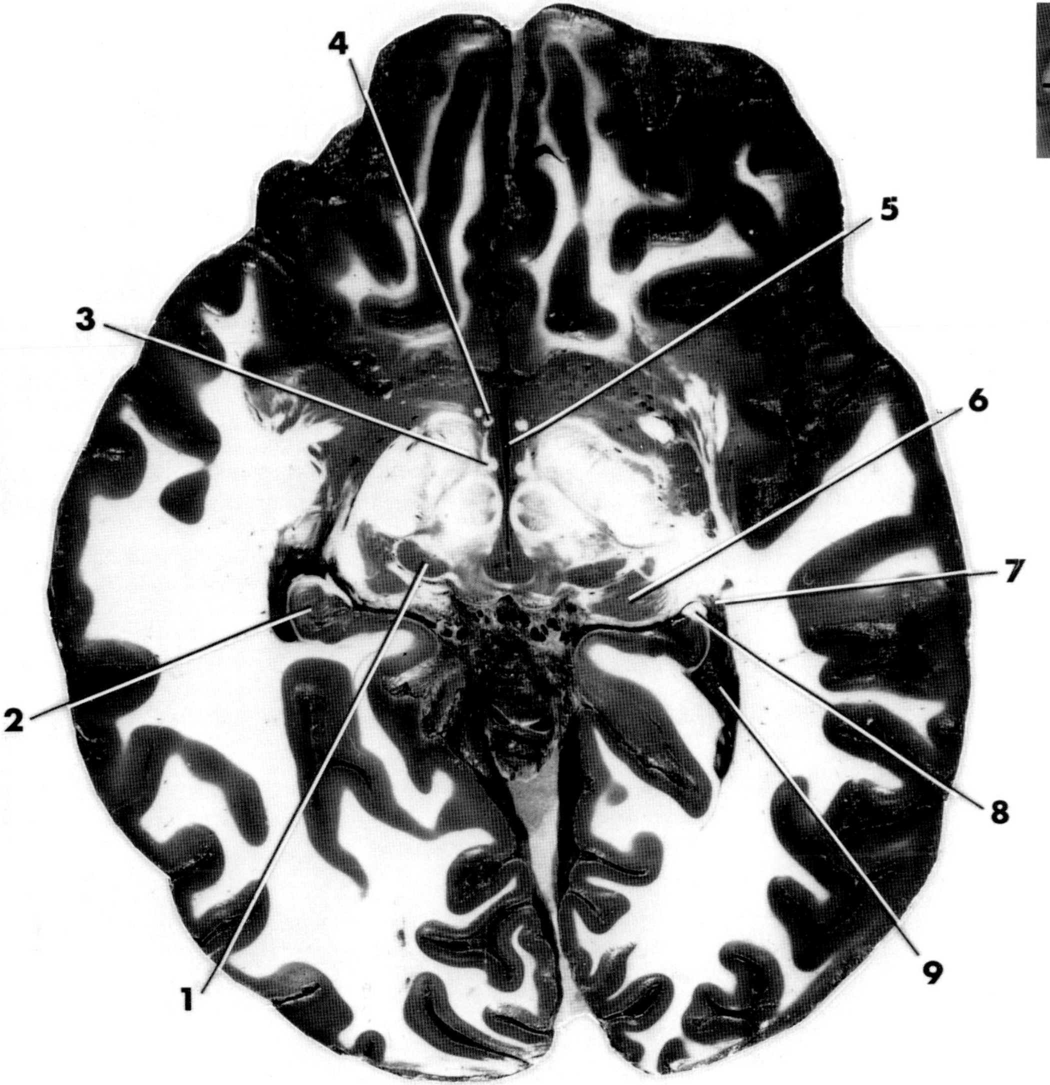

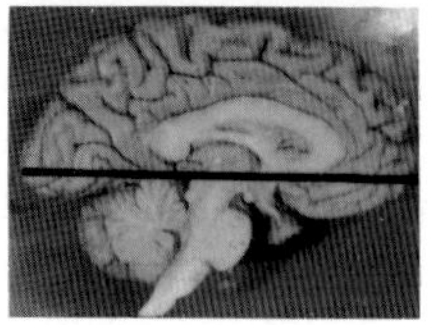

Figure 75*B*

1. **Inferior Colliculus** (L. small elevation)—nerve cell mass in the caudal half of the tectum of the midbrain. It is a relay station in the auditory system.
2. **Cerebral Aqueduct (of Sylvius)**—located ventral to the tectum (corpora quadrigemina) of midbrain. It is surrounded by central area of gray matter and connects third and fourth ventricles.
3. **Medial Lemniscus** (G. ribbon, band)—transmits impulses concerned with discriminative touch, proprioception, and vibratory sense from contralateral nucleus gracilis and nucleus cuneatus to ventral posterior nucleus of thalamus.
4. **Superior Cerebellar Peduncle (Brachium Conjunctivum)**—consists of contralateral cerebellar efferents that course to and terminate in ventrolateral and ventral anterior thalamic nuclei (see no. **10**, Fig. 73*B*).
5. **Hypothalamus (Ventral)**—basal part of hypothalamus (tuber cinereum) that extends into infundibulum (pituitary stalk).
6. **Optic Tract**—courses laterally from optic chiasma around cerebral peduncle. Most of its fibers synapse on neurons in lateral geniculate body.
7. **Mammillary Body** (L. *mamma*, breast)—basal posterior hypothalamic nucleus. Has important function in limbic system.
8. **Basis Pedunculi**—located on ventral surface of midbrain. Composed of cortical projection fibers (tracts) that course to different areas of brain stem and spinal cord, *i.e.*, corticospinal, corticobulbar, corticopontine, and corticonigral tracts.
9. **Substantia Nigra**—large nucleus in entire basal midbrain area located between basis pedunculi (**8**) and midbrain tegmentum. It functions with motor systems (see also no. **1**, Fig. 91*A*).
10. **Lateral Lemniscus** (G. band, ribbon)—part of auditory pathway, connecting cochlear nuclei with inferior colliculus (**1**).
11. **Vermis** (L. worm)—the midline worm-like portion of cerebellum. On its dorsal surface it is continuous with the cerebellar hemispheres but remains a separate structure on the ventral surface.

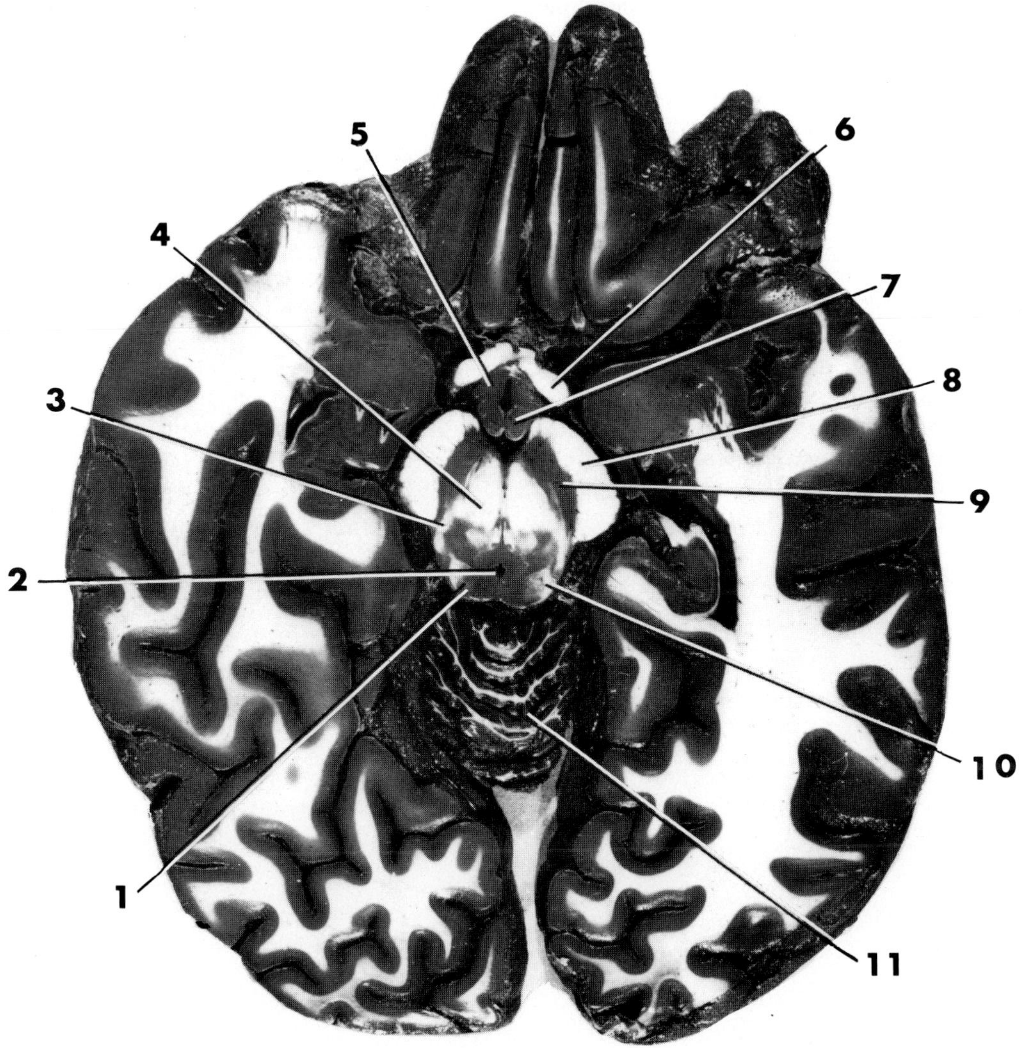

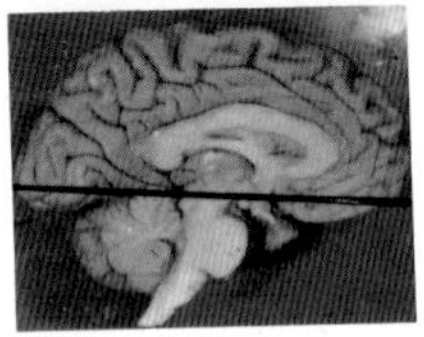

Figure 76

1. **Cerebral Aqueduct (of Sylvius)**—caudal portion enters the upper IVth ventricle and is roofed by superior medullary velum (see also no. **2**, Fig. 76, and no. **11**, Fig. 92).
2. **Central Gray Matter**—surrounds cerebral aqueduct, composed of a poorly organized nuclear area and finely myelinated fiber tracts.
3. **Medial Lemniscus**—(axons of second order neurons) a sensory pathway for proprioception, vibration sense, and discriminative touch extending through brain stem from nucleus gracilis and cuneatus to posterior ventral nucleus of thalamus.
4. **Decussation of Brachium Conjunctivum**—axons from neurons in dentate, emboliform, and globose nuclei leave the cerebellum and course into tegmentum of midbrain. They cross in the midline to the opposite side and terminate (synapse) on neurons in ventral lateral thalamus.
5. **Interpeduncular Fossa**—is the rhomboidal groove or space between the cerebral peduncles on the basal (ventral) surface of the midbrain. The fibers of the oculomotor nerve (C.N. III) emerge from this fossa.
6. **Basis Pedunculi**—composed of cortical projection fibers that continue into the brain stem from the internal capsule. The basis pedunculi forms the ventral (basal) aspect of the cerebral peduncle and is separated from its fellow of the opposite side by the interpeduncular fossa (**5**).
7. **Inferior Horn of Lateral Ventricle**—the inferior horn extends from the body of the lateral ventricle into the temporal lobe. The hippocampus is located in its floor and the tail of the caudate nucleus in its roof.
8. **Medial Longitudinal Fasciculus**—axons of neurons in vestibular nuclei form a bundle of fibers that ascend the brain stem on each side to cranial nerve nuclei (**III**, **IV**, and **VI**) that innervate extraocular muscles.
9. **Superior Cerebellar Peduncle (Brachium Conjunctivum)**—axons of neurons in the dentate, emboliform, and globose nuclei leave the cerebellum and form the superior cerebellar peduncle. These fiber bundles course into midbrain tegmentum to decussate in the midline (**4**).
10. **Vermis of Cerebellum**—the midline portion of the cerebellum. On the dorsal surface, the vermis is continuous with the hemispheres but remains a separate structure on the ventral surface.

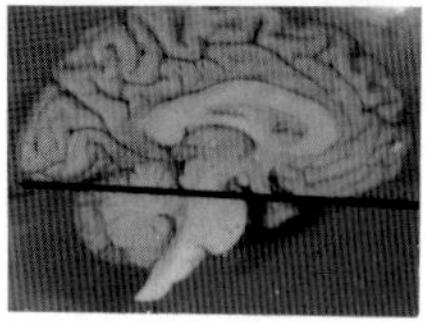

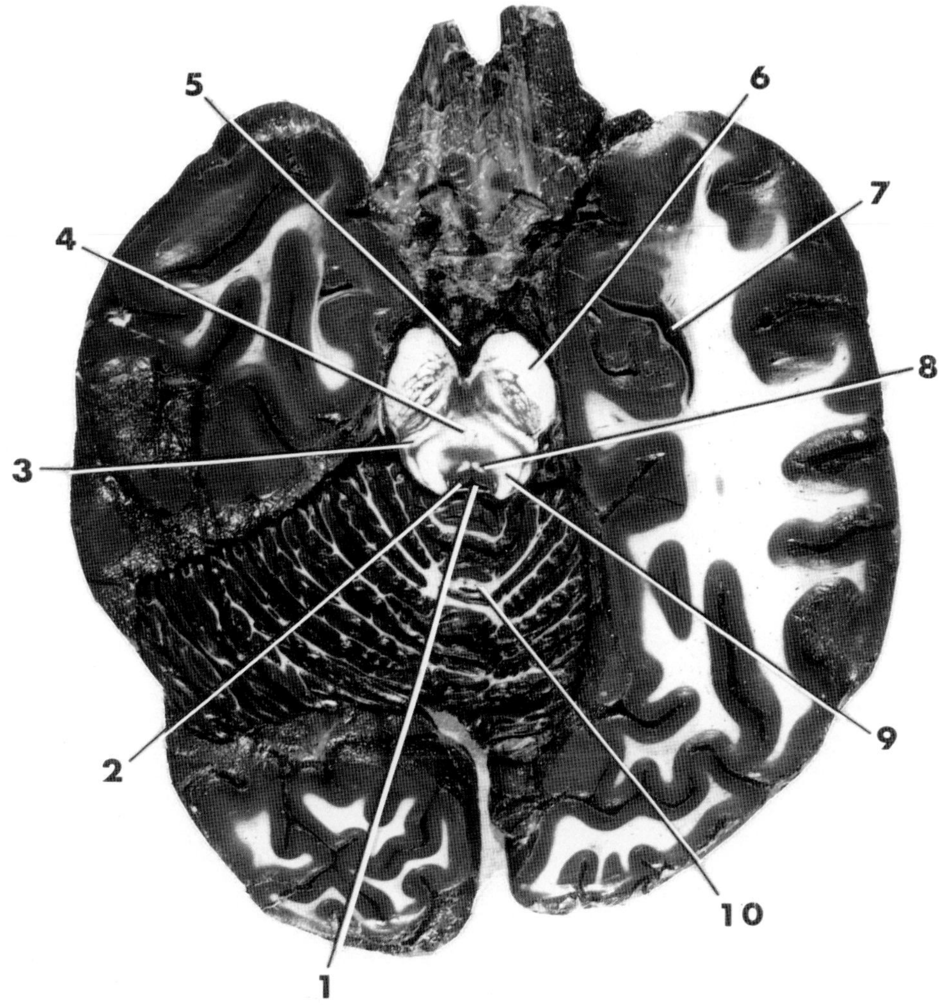

Figure 77

1. **Dentate Nucleus** (L. *dentatus*, toothed)—the largest of the four pairs of cerebellar nuclei. It is embedded deep in the medullary center of each cerebellar hemisphere.
2. **Superior Medullary Velum** (L. sail, veil)—is a thin sheet of ependyma and pia mater that bridges the space between the brachia conjunctiva (**10**) as they leave the cerebellum and course to midbrain. This velum helps to form the roof of the cranial portion of the fourth ventricle (see also no. **6**, Fig. 52).
3. **Fourth Ventricle**—is that part of the ventricular system which is located between the tegmental portion of the pons, the open medulla, and the cerebellum.
4. **Medial Longitudinal Fasciculus**—this bundle of ascending fibers originates from vestibular nuclei and courses in the midline brain stem tegmentum directly beneath motor nuclei to end on cranial nerve nuclei innervating extraocular muscles (see also no. **8**, Fig. 77).
5. **Brachium Pontis (Middle Cerebellar Peduncle)**—this is the beginning of the brachium (L. arm). It is formed when axons of contralateral pontine neurons of basal pons leave the pons and course to cerebellar hemispheres.
6. **Pontine Nuclei**—these nuclei are located in basal pons between descending corticospinal tract (**7**) and corticopontine and pontocerebellar fibers (**8**).
7. **Corticospinal Tract Fibers**—cortical projection fibers continue from internal capsule into basis pedunculi of midbrain and on through the basal pons as many separate bundles which join to form the pyramids in the medulla.
8. **Pontocerebellar Fibers**—are axons of pontine neurons that course horizontally in the basal pons and form the contralateral brachium pontis (middle cerebellar peduncle).
9. **Medial Lemniscus**—is horizontally located in the most ventral part of the pons tegmentum. It is a sensory pathway for proprioception, vibration sense, and discriminative touch which extends through brain stem from nucleus gracilis and cuneatus to ventral posterior nucleus of thalamus.
10. **Superior Cerebellar Peduncle (Brachium Conjunctivum)**—composed of axons of neurons from dentate nucleus (**1**), as well as from emboliform and globose cerebellar nuclei that course into midbrain and decussate in the midline. These fibers make up the prominent superior cerebellar peduncles that help to form the roof of the rostral part of the fourth ventricle (see also no. **9**, Fig. 77 and no. **4**, Fig. 76).

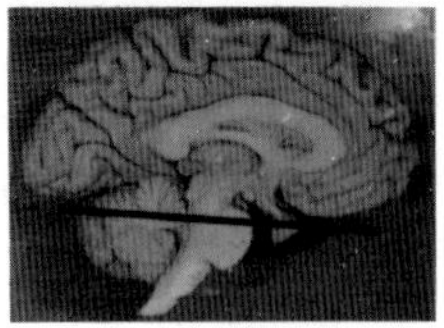

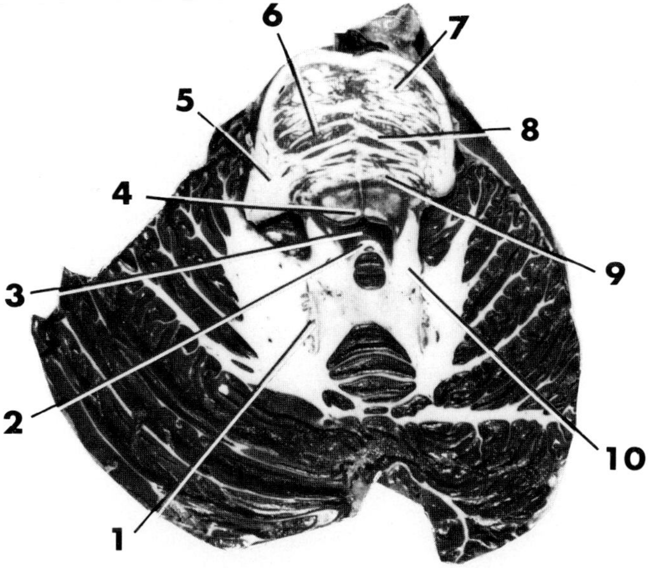

Figure 78

1. **Dentate Nucleus** (L. *dentatus*, toothed)—has the form of a toothed or notched sac. Largest of the cerebellar nuclei, it is located deep in the medullary center of the cerebellar hemispheres. Axons of its neurons converge to form the brachium conjunctivum (**2**) (see also no. **1**, Fig. 78).
2. **Superior Cerebellar Peduncle (Brachium Conjuctivum)**—composed of axons from neurons of cerebellar nuclei (except fastigial nucleus) that course into midbrain tegmentum and decussate at midline to end in contralateral ventral lateral nucleus of thalamus.
3. **Facial Colliculus**—small elevation (L. *colliculus*) at caudal end of pons. It is located in the median eminence in floor of fourth ventricle. It is formed by fibers from motor nucleus of facial nerve looping over the abducens nucleus.
4. **Middle Cerebellar Peduncle (Brachium Pontis)**—composed of pontocerebellar fibers that are axons of contralateral pontine neurons that course into the cerebellar hemisphere. These fibers make a thick peduncle or band.
5. **Basal Pons**—consists of longitudinal fiber bundles (corticospinal), transverse fibers (pontocerebellar), and collections of nerve cells (pontine nuclei) in intervals between longitudinal and transverse fasciculi (L. dim. of *facis*, bundle).
6. **Corticospinal Fibers**—bundles of projection fibers that coursed from motor cortex, through internal capsule and basis pedunculi into basal pons. In the pons the corticospinal fibers are arranged in many longitudinal bundles that pass into the pyramids of the medulla (see also no. **7**, Fig. 78).
7. **Medial Lemniscus**—its fibers are horizontally located in the ventral tegmental pons. This sensory pathway for discriminative touch, proprioception, and vibration sense originates in the nucleus gracilis and nucleus cuneatus and terminates in the ventral lateral nucleus of the thalamus. It has a vertical midline position in the medulla and a horizontal position in the pons (see also no. **9**, Fig. 78, no. **3**, Fig. 77, and no. **3**, Fig. 80).
8. **Medial Longitudinal Fasciculus**—composed of axons from ipsilateral and contralateral vestibular nuclei that ascend on each side of the midline tegmentum of rostral medulla, pons, and midbrain to end on cranial nerve nuclei innervating extraocular muscles (see also no. **4**, Fig. 78).
9. **Fourth Ventricle**—that part of the ventricular system located between tegmental portion of pons, open medulla, and cerebellum. Cerebrospinal fluid passes from the third ventricle into the fourth ventricle via the cerebral aqueduct and exits from this ventricle into the subarachnoid space via the median and two lateral apertures.
10. **Vermis of Cerebellum**—the midline portion of the cerebellum. The fastigial and emboliform nuclei are located in the medullary center of this area.

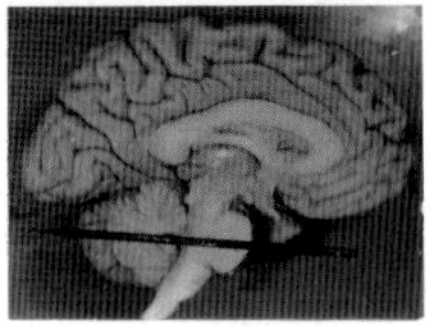

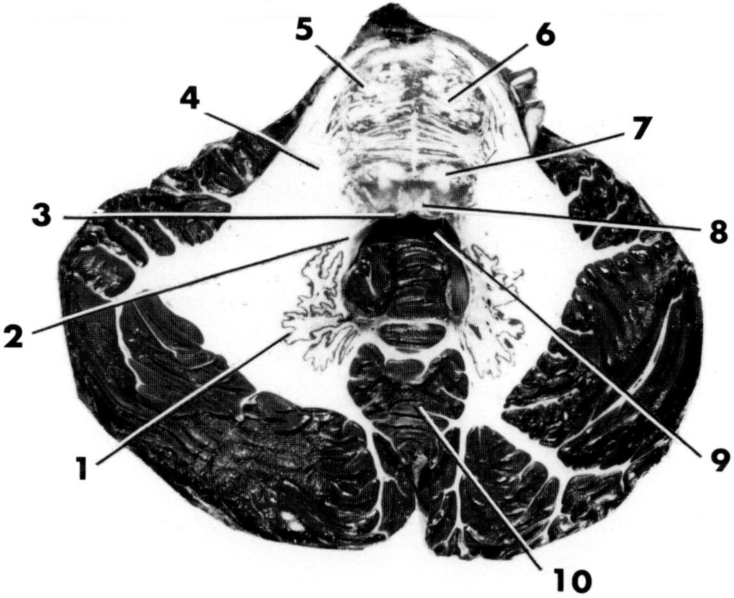

Figure 79

1. **Fourth Ventricle (Inferior or Caudal Portion)**—located between the open portion of the medulla and the cerebellum (see also no. **9**, Fig. 79, no. **3**, Fig. 78, and no. **4**, Fig. 96 for other parts of this ventricle).
2. **Restiform Body** (L. *restis*, rope + *forma*, form)—main mass of inferior cerebellar peduncle containing afferents from brain stem and spinal cord to the cerebellum.
3. **Medial Lemniscus**—composed of ascending sensory fibers (for proprioception, discriminative touch, and vibration sense) that originate from neurons in nucleus cuneatus and nucleus gracilis. In the medulla these fibers forming the medial lemniscus are arranged in two vertical columns on each side of the midline (see also no. **7**, Fig. 79).
4. **Inferior Olivary Nucleus**—located in the olive of the lateral area of medulla. Only a small portion of this nucleus is shown at this level (see no. **5**, Fig. 81 for a section through the center of the olive produced by this nucleus).
5. **Corticospinal Fibers**—longitudinal bundles of corticospinal fibers passing through basal pons into the pyramid of the medulla (see also no. **6**, Fig. 79).
6. **Vestibulocochlear Nerve (C.N. VIII)**—attached to the brain stem at the caudal border of the pons. The cochlear division ends in the dorsal and ventral cochlear nuclei, and the vestibular division penetrates the medulla deep to the inferior cerebellar peduncle to end in the vestibular nuclei.
7. **Flocculus**—irregular shaped mass of cerebellum at the rostral edge of the inferior surface. The flocculus along with the nodule comprises the flocculonodular lobe, the oldest phylogenetically of the cerebellum. It functions for balance and equilibrium (see also no. **4**, Fig. 52).
8. **Vestibular Area (Area Acoustica)**—lies beneath most of the lateral mass of the floor of the fourth ventricle. The vestibular (nuclear) area or complex is bounded medially by the sulcus limitans and is made up of the superior, medial, lateral, and inferior vestibular nuclei.

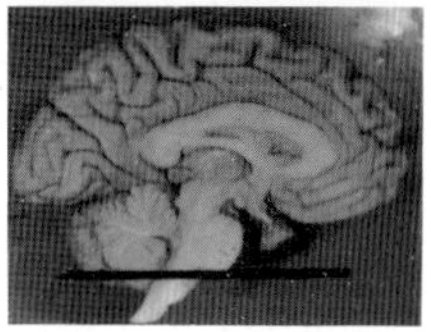

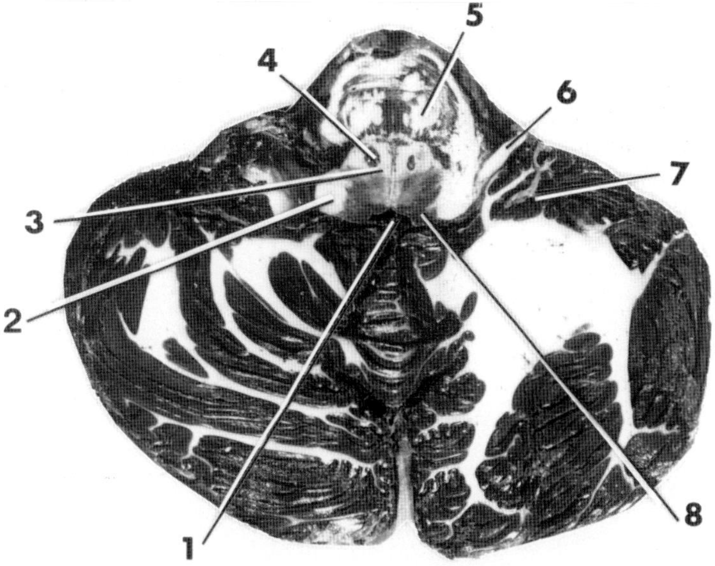

Figure 80

1. **Nucleus Gracilis** (L. slender)—contained in the clava (tubercle) on the dorsal surface of the closed portion of the medulla. The fasciculus gracilis (composed of sensory fiber tracts for proprioception, vibration sense, and discriminative touch) ascends from the spinal cord to end in this slender nucleus.
2. **Fasciculus Cuneatus**—ascending fiber tract from the dorsal column of white matter extends into the dorsal lateral area of medulla and terminates in the nucleus cuneatus located in cuneate tubercle. Fibers from the upper thoracic and cervical spinal nerves form this fasciculus. It conducts proprioceptive, discriminative touch, and vibration sensations to higher centers.
3. **Nucleus Cuneatus** (L. *cuneus*, wedge)—fibers from fasciculus cuneatus (**2**) end in the nucleus cuneatus which is located in cuneate tubercle, rostral and lateral to the nucleus gracilis.
4. **Spinal Nucleus and Tract of Fifth Cranial Nerve**—together these two structures form an area in the dorsolateral sulcus identified as the tuberculum cinereum. Fibers from the fifth cranial nerve enter the lateral pons and descend into medulla and cephalic end of spinal cord to turn in and synapse in the spinal nucleus, which lies immediately adjacent to these fibers throughout their length.
5. **Inferior Olivary Nucleus**—located in the olive which lies between the pyramid and the tuberculum cinereum. In cross-section it is shaped like a crumpled bag or purse with its opening facing medially.
6. **Pyramid**—located on the ventral surface of the medulla between the ventral median fissure and ventrolateral sulcus. It consists of corticospinal fibers that descend into the spinal cord and function with the motor systems (see also no. **1**, Fig. 96).
7. **Decussation of Pyramids**—in the caudal medulla approximately 85% of corticospinal fibers in the pyramid cross over (decussate) in the ventral median fissure to the opposite side and descend in the lateral column of white matter of the spinal cord.
8. **Cerebellum (Caudal Portion)**—the cerebellum is composed of a midline area, the vermis, and two lateral expansions, the left and right cerebellum hemispheres. It functions for muscle synergy and accuracy of nonsterotypical movements.

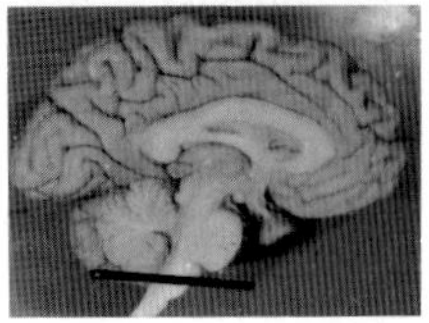

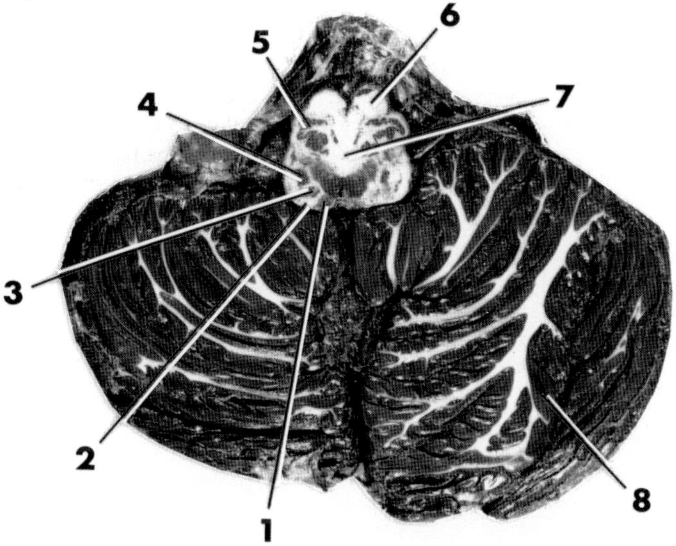

Figure 81

Scan A

1. **Frontal Bone**—articulates with the two parietal bones at the coronal suture. It lies rostrally and protects the frontal lobes of the cerebral hemispheres. It also forms the roof of the orbit on each side.
2. **Falx Cerebri (Superior Part)** (L., *falx*, a sickle)—a large, sickle-shaped vertical partition in the longitudinal fissure between the two cerebral hemispheres. Anteriorly, it is attached to the crest of the frontal bone and the crista galli of the ethmoid bone.
3. **Superior Cerebral Sulcus**—the pointer indicates the superior frontal sulcus. Cortical grooves on the superior and lateral surfaces of the cerebral hemispheres can be seen in the CT scans.
4. **Parietal Bone** (L. *paries*, a wall)—the two parietal bones form the superior part of the sides of the calvaria. These bones lie superior and lateral to and protect the parietal lobes of the cerebral hemispheres.

Scan B

1. **Calcar Avis**—an elevation on the medial aspect of the lateral ventricle at the junction of the posterior and inferior horns (see no. **2**, Fig. 25).
2. **Calcified Glomus of Choroid Plexus** (L. *glomus*, ball)—the calcified globular enlargement of the choroid plexus appears as a white dot in the lateral ventricle in this CT scan.
3. **Anterior Horn of Lateral Ventricle**—see No. **8**, Figure 73*A* in the stained horizontal series. It also shows in Figure 72 lying medial to the head of the caudate nucleus (no. **9**) but is not numbered.
4. **Body of Lateral Ventricle**—see Figure 72. The body of the lateral ventricle lies between nos. **2** and **3** in the figure, but is not numbered.
5. **Trigone of Lateral Ventricle**—compare with no. **10**, Figure 73*A*.
6. **Posterior Horn of Lateral Ventricle**—compare with no. **10**, Figure 73*A* and no. **1**, Figure 74*A*.

Figure 82 Two prints (**A** and **B**) of a CT scan taken at approximately 10° to the horizontal plane. **Scan A** was made approximately 2.0 cm inferior to the top (vertex) of the head. **Scan B** was made through the middle of the main parts of the cerebral ventricles.

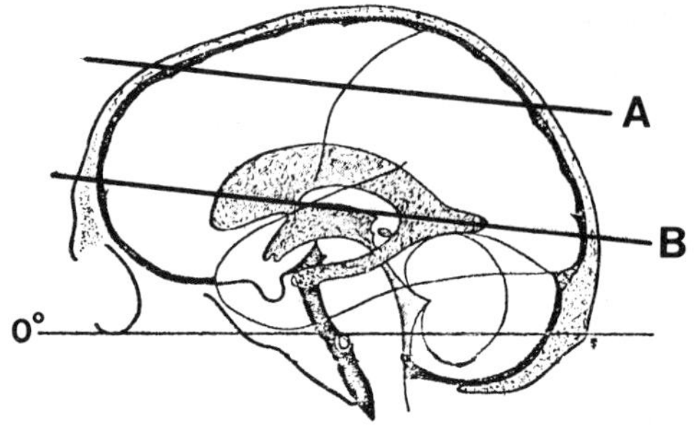

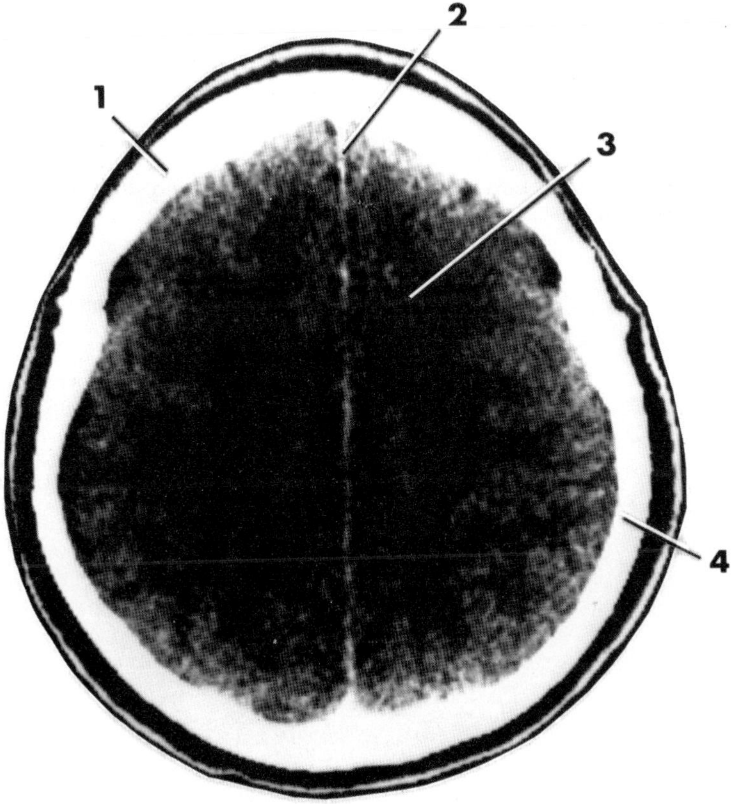

A

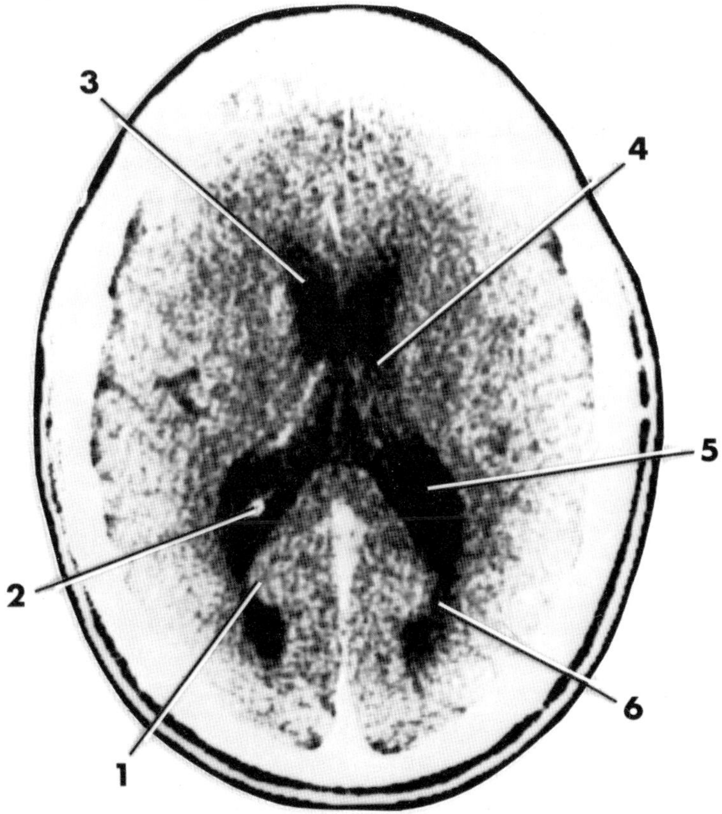

B

Scan A

1. **Posterior and Inferior Part of Falx Cerebri** (L., *falx*, sickle)—a long sickle-shaped vertical partition in the longitudinal fissure between the two cerebral hemispheres. Posteriorly, it is attached to the midline of the tentorium cerebelli at the internal occipital protuberance.
2. **Pulvinar of Thalamus (Superior Portion)**—compare with nos. **10** and **11**, Figure 73*B*. See also no. **1**, Figure 74*B*.
3. **Anterior Part of Falx Cerebri**—anteriorly the rostral portion of this sickle-shaped partition is attached to the crest of the frontal bones and to the crista galli of the ethmoid bone. Note the cerebral tissue of the frontal poles of the hemispheres on each side of the falx cerebri.
4. **Anterior Part of the Body of Lateral Ventricle**—compare with no. **8**, Figure 73*A*.
5. **Thalamus**—compare with nos. **10** and **11**, Figure 73*B*, or no. **1**, Figure 74*B*.
6. **Posterior Part of Superior Sagittal Sinus**—lies in the midline along the attached border of the falx cerebri. Posteriorly at the internal occipital protuberance, it ends by becoming the right transverse sinus.

Scan B

1. **Cistern of the Quadrigeminal Plate (Part of Superior Cistern)**—in the subarachnoid space lying dorsal to the superior and inferior colliculi (corpora quadrigemina). In Figure 75*A*, this cistern is the unnumbered space caudal to no. **10.**
2. **Third Ventricle**—compare with the unnumbered space between the left and right thalami in Figure 73*A*.
3. **Anterior End of Lateral Sulcus**—compare with the unnumbered sulcus (lateral to insular cortex) in Figure 73.
4. **Head of Caudate Nucleus**—compare with no. **9**, Figure 72 or no. **7**, Figure 73*A*.
5. **Anterior Horn of Lateral Ventricle**—compare with no. **8**, Figure 73*A* or with the unnumbered space medial to no. **8** in Figure 72.
6. **Interventricular Foramen (of Monro)**—compare with no. **9**, Figure 73*A*.
7. **Thalamus**—compare with nos. **10** and **11**, Figure 73*B* or with no. **1**, Figure 74*B*.
8. **One of the Four Colliculi**—compare with no. **9**, Figure 75*A*.
9. **Sulci of Medial Surface of Occipital Lobe**—compare with no. **9**, Figure 74*B* or with similar unnumbered sulci of the occipital lobe in Figure 75*B*.

Figure 83 Two prints (**A** and **B**) of CT scans taken at different angles to the horizontal plane. **Scan A** was made slightly inferior to the body of the lateral ventricle and **Scan B** was made through the third ventricle.

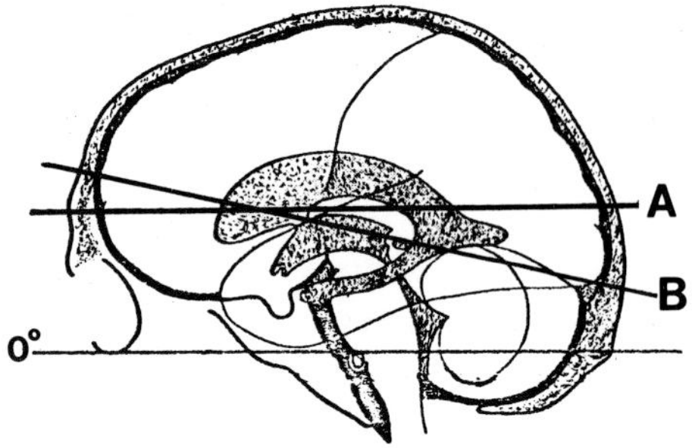

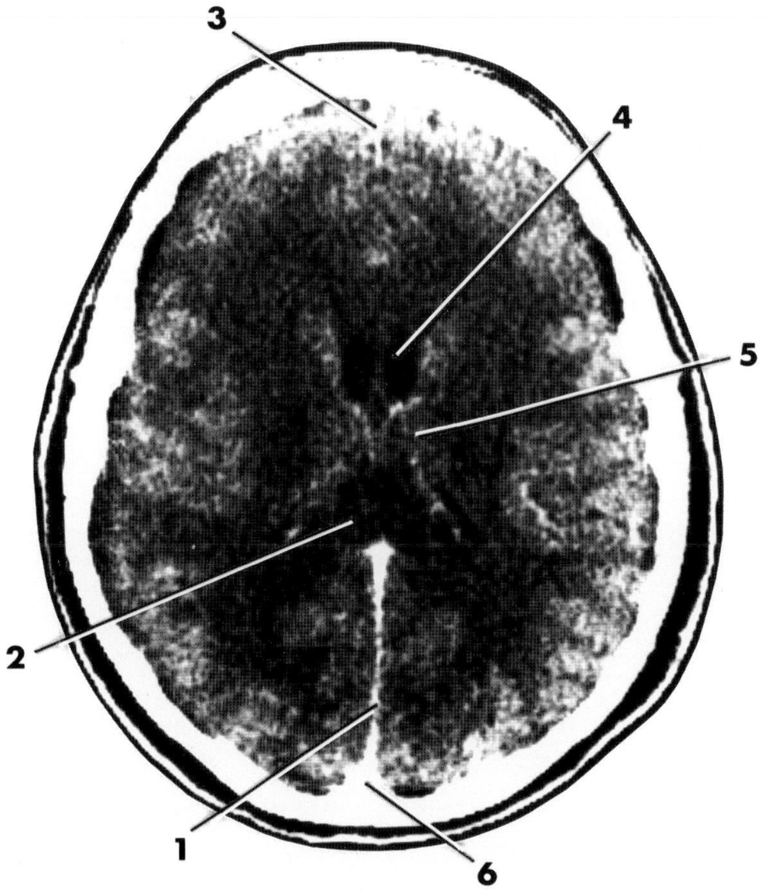

A

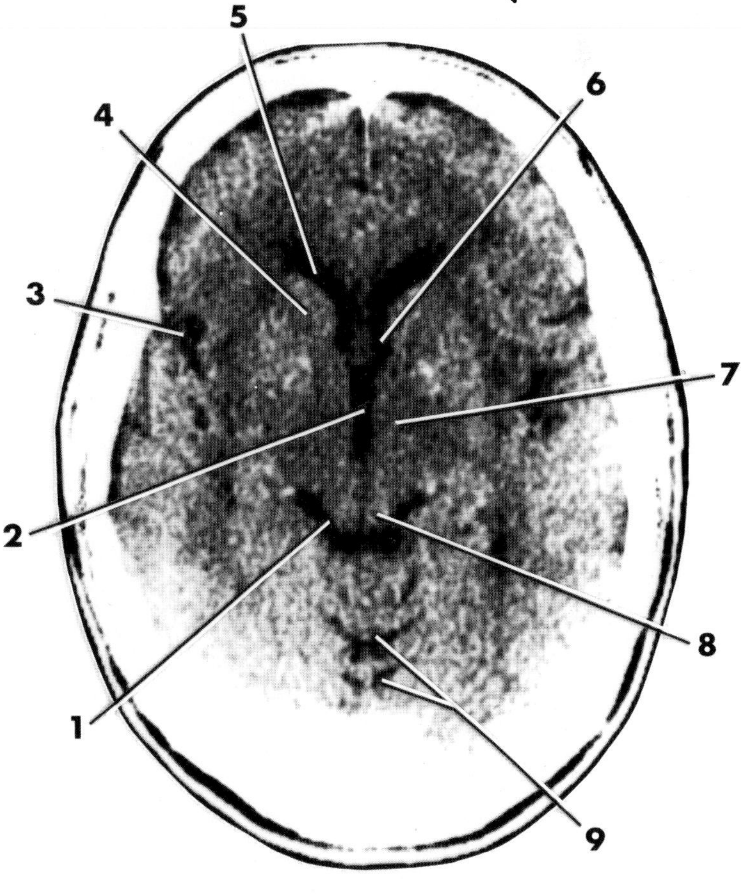

B

Scan A

1. **Posterior and Inferior Part of Falx Cerebri**—It is attached to a variable ridge of bone on the inner surface of the posterior part of the skull.
2. **Cisterna Ambiens** (upper part - L. *ambo*, both sides)—on each side of the midbrain of the ambient cistern (subarachnoid space) there is a connection with the cistern of the quadrigeminal plate posteriorly and interpeduncular cistern anteriorly.
3. **Thalamus (Superior Posterior Part)**—compare with nos. **10** and **11** in Figure 73*B* or no. **1** in Figure 74*B*.
4. **External Capsule**—compare with no. **4**, Figure 73*B* or with no. **5**, Figure 74*B*.
5. **Septum Pellucidum**—compare with no. **8**, Figure 72*A* or with no. **5**, Figure 73*A*.
6. **Anterior Horn of Lateral Ventricle**—compare with no. **8**, Figure 73*A*.
7. **Genu of Corpus Callosum**—compare with no. **7**, Figure 72 or with no. **6**, Figure 73*A*.
8. **Head of Caudate Nucleus**—compare with no. **9**, Figure 72 and with no. **7**, Figure 73*A*.
9. **Anterior Limb of Internal Capsule**—compare with no. **6**, Figure 73*B*.
10. **Lentiform Nucleus**—compare with no. **5**, Figure 72 and with no. **5**, Figure 73*B*.
11. **Posterior Limb of Internal Capsule**—compare with no. **8**, Figure 73*B*.
12. **Calcified Pineal Body** (shaped like a pine cone)—serves as a useful neuroradiological and neurosurgical landmark. It becomes calcified in approximately 75% of North American adults. In Figure 74*B*, it lies between the pulvinar (**1**) of each thalamus.
13. **Glomus of Choroid Plexus (Calcified)**—the calcified globular enlargement of the choroid plexus appears as a white dot in the collateral trigone of the lateral ventricle.
14. **Straight Sinus**—formed by the union of the inferior sagittal sinus with the great cerebral vein (of Galen). It courses along the line of attachment of the falx cerebri to the tentorium cerebelli. It is triangular in cross-section and becomes continuous with the tranverse sinus, usually the left.

Scan B

1. **Internal Occipital Protuberance—**an irregular elevation on the interior of the occipital bone which more or less matches the external occipital protuberance.
2. **Anterior Cerebral/Anterior Communicating Artery Complex (Opacified)—**this cluster of arteries is superior to the diverging optic nerves in the cistern of the lamina terminalis.
3. **Crista Galli** (L. crest)—the elevated ridge of the perpendicular plate of the ethmoid bone that provides an attachment of the falx cerebri.
4. **Lateral Part of Sphenoid Ridge—**the lesser wing of the sphenoid bone presents a sharp posterior margin (ridge) which overhangs the anterior part of the middle cranial fossa.
5. **Cisterna Ambiens—**this subarachnoid space courses inferiorly and rostrally on each side of the midbrain. In Figure 76, it would occupy the space on each side of the midbrain.
6. **Incisura Tentori** (one edge of)—the free left and right concave anteromedial borders of the tentorium cerebelli form and opening into the posterior cranial fossa from the anterior and middle cranial fossa. This oval opening surrounds the midbrain.
7. **The Straight Sinus (Opacified)—**the posterior portion of the falx cerebri is attached to the midline of the tentorium cerebelli. The straight sinus is located at the junction of these two.

Figure 84 Two prints (**A** and **B**) of a CT scan taken at approximately 10° to the horizontal plane.
Scan A was made through the frontal horns and the region of the great cerebral vein (of Galen).
Scan B was made through the tuberculum sellae and the midbrain.

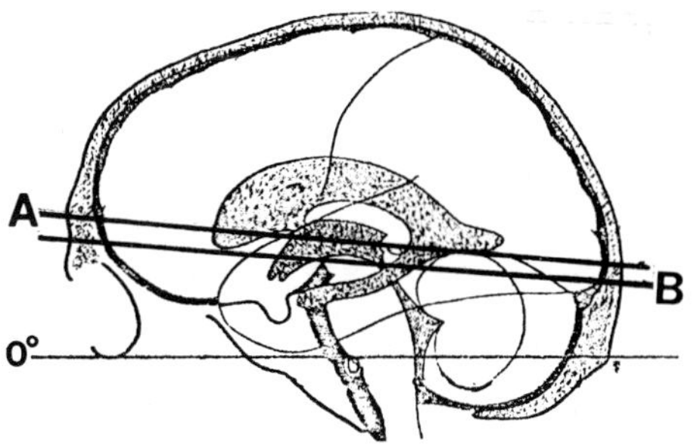

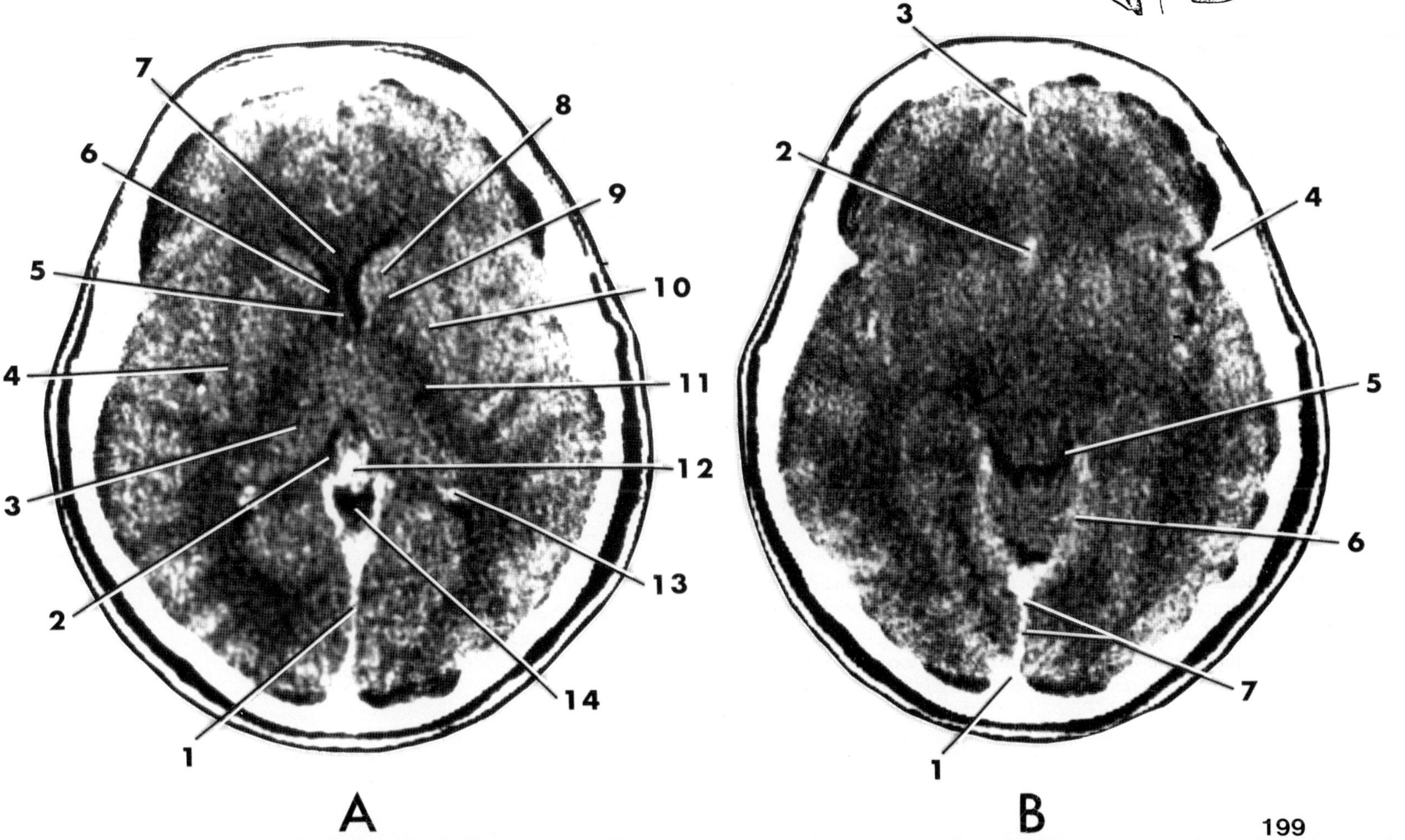

11

Coronal (Frontal) Serial Sections of the Brain

Coronal (frontal) serial sections were cut through a whole brain, approximately 12 mm in thickness. The sections were then surface-stained by the modified Mulligan technique (blue, gray matter; white, white matter), photographed, mounted, and the important structures in each section numbered. In sections where there were more than 15 important structures illustrated, a duplicate photograph was used to identify the additional structures.

Throughout the series, a small drawing of the brain appears in the upper right-hand corner of each figure with a line drawn through the brain to indicate the level through which the section was taken. These sections were cut at the angles indicated to demonstrate the important structures.

1. **Lateral Sulcus** (anterior end) **(Fissure of Sylvius)**—this deep furrow is an important landmark on the lateral surface which separates the frontal and temporal lobes. It extends superiorly and posteriorly into the inferior parietal lobe (see also no. **2**, Fig. 86, and no. **10**, Fig. 87).
2. **Insular Cortex** (L. *insula,* island)—buried area of cerebral cortex concealed from surface view and lying at the bottom of lateral sulcus (**1**).
3. **Inferior Frontal Gyrus**—located below inferior frontal sulcus. Consists of pars opercularis, pars triangularis, and pars orbitalis (not all shown here; see also no. **9**, Fig. 7*A*).
4. **Anterior Horn of Lateral Ventricle** (anterior end)—located in medullary center of frontal lobe. It is bounded in front and above by genu and body of corpus callosum, respectively.
5. **Cingulate Gyrus**—begins beneath the genu and continues above the corpus callosum as far posteriorly as the splenium (see also no. **8**, Fig. 86).
6. **Longitudinal Cerebral Fissure**—separates the cerebral hemispheres. The falx cerebri is contained in it.
7. **Superior Frontal Gyrus**—located between the superior frontal and cingulate sulci. It extends from superior lateral surface on to the superior medial surface.
8. **Medullary Center**—consists of a solid mass of myelinated association, commissural, and projection fibers, neuroglia, and blood vessels.
9. **Callosal Sulcus (Sulcus of the Corpus Callosum)**—separates the cingulate gyrus from the corpus callosum.
10. **Genu of Corpus Callosum** (L. genu, knee)—anterior end of corpus callosum where reciprocal commissural fibers radiate into frontal lobes as forceps minor (see also no. **7**, Fig. 72 and no. **6**, Fig. 73).
11. **Head of Caudate Nucleus**—part of a cerebral basal ganglion. It bulges into anterior horn of lateral ventricle (**4**) (see also no. **10**, Fig. 87).
12. **Gyrus Rectus**—on orbital surface of frontal lobe, medial to the olfactory sulcus.

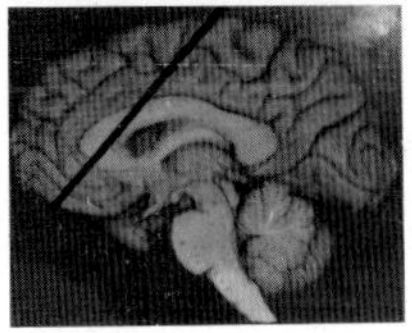
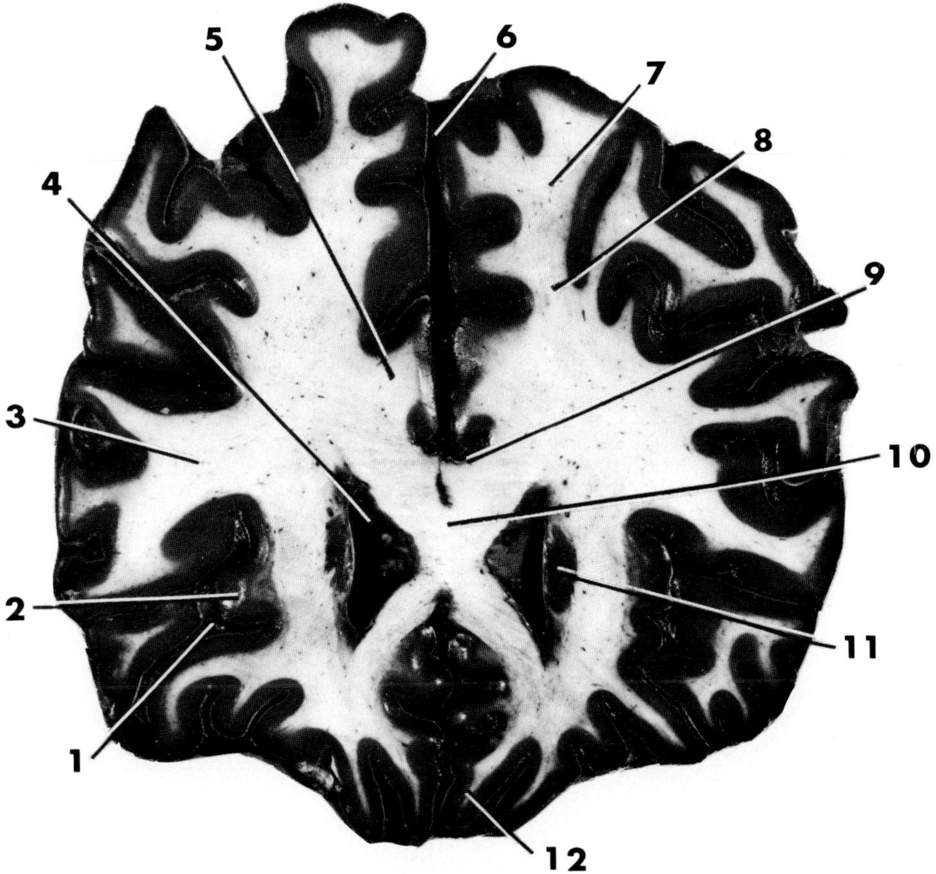

Figure 85

1. **Septum Pellucidum**—a double membrane located between the anterior part of corpus callosum and fornix. Here it is separating the posterior parts of the anterior horns (**9**) of the lateral ventricles (see also no. **3**, Fig. 87).
2. **Lateral Sulcus (Fissure of Sylvius)**—consists of three rami: a main part, the long posterior ramus (shown here) extending into the parietal lobe, and the short anterior and ascending rami (not shown here) projecting into the frontal lobe.
3. **Claustrum**—thin sheet of grey matter located medial to insula between the extreme and external capsules. Claustrum is a Latin word meaning "a barrier."
4. **Anterior Limb of Internal Capsule**—consists of projection fibers and is located between head of caudate nucleus and lentiform nucleus (see also no. **2**, Fig. 87).
5. **Body of Corpus Callosum**—composed of reciprocal commissural fibers that cross in the midline from one cerebral hemisphere to the other.
6. **Superior Frontal Gyrus**—located between the superior frontal and cingulate sulci. It extends from superior lateral surface on to the superior medial surface.
7. **Longitudinal Cerebral Fissure**—separates the cerebral hemispheres. The **falx cerebri** is contained in it.
8. **Cingulate Gyrus**—begins beneath the genu of corpus callosum and continues above the body of the corpus callosum as far posteriorly as the splenium of this commissure (see also no. **5**, Fig. 85).
9. **Anterior Horn of Lateral Ventricle**—located in medullary center of frontal lobe. It is bounded in front and above by genu and body of corpus callosum, respectively.
10. **Head of Caudate Nucleus**—part of a cerebral basal ganglion. It bulges into anterior horn of lateral ventricle (**9**) (see also no. **1**, Fig. 87).
11. **External Capsule**—consists mainly of projection fibers but has commissural and association fibers. It is situated between putamen (**12**) and claustrum (**3**) (see also no. **9**, Fig. 87).
12. **Putamen** (L. shell)—lateral portion of lentiform nucleus separated from globus pallidus (not shown in this section) by lateral medullary lamina.
13. **Rostrum of Corpus Callosum**—thin anterior part of corpus callosum beneath the genu. It is continuous with the lamina terminalis.

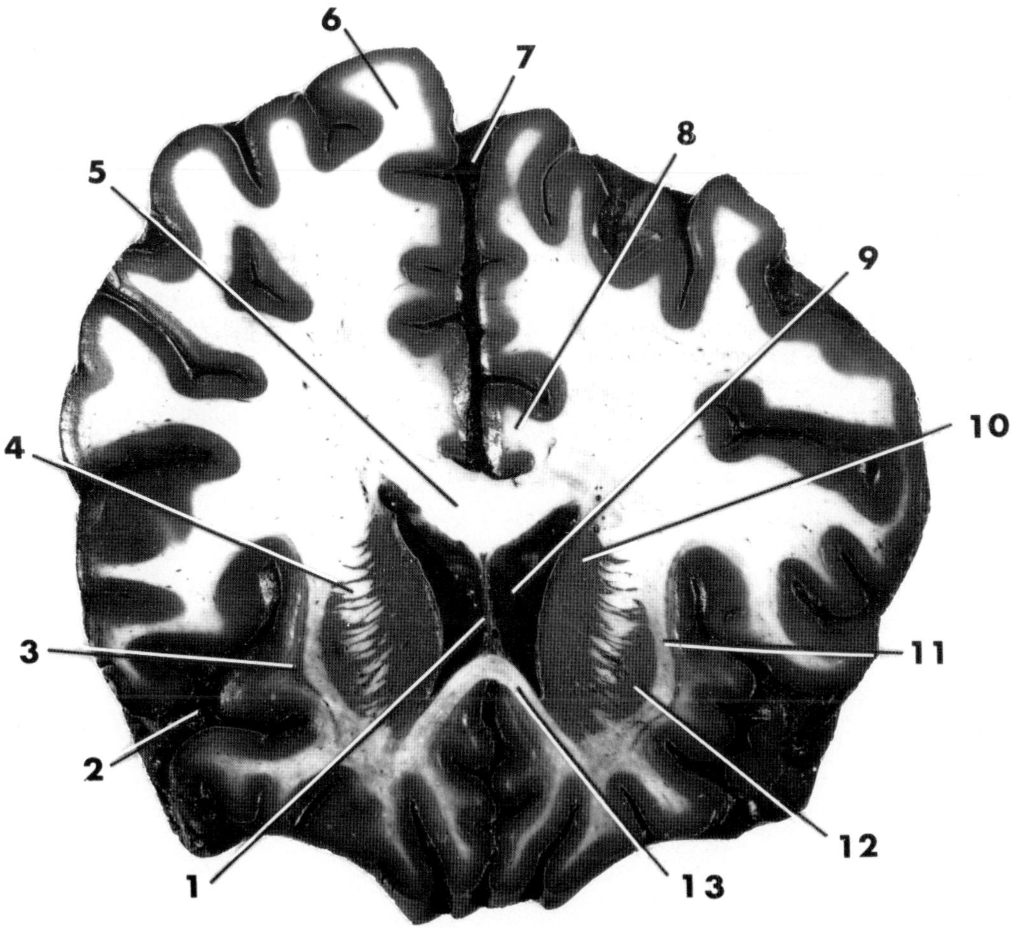

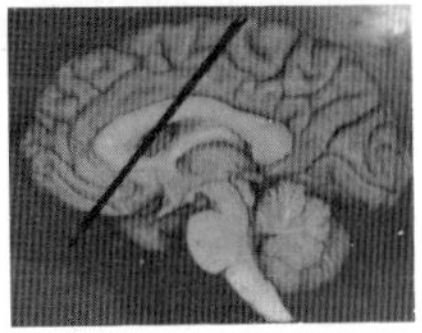

Figure 86

1. **Head of Caudate Nucleus**—part of a cerebral basal ganglion. It bulges into the anterior horn of lateral ventricle (**4**). Note its continuity with the inferior part of the putamen (**12**) (see also no. **10**, Fig. 86).
2. **Anterior Limb of Internal Capsule**—consists of projection fibers and is located between head of caudate nucleus and lentiform nucleus (see also no. **6**, Fig. 73*B*).
3. **Septum Pellucidum**—a double membrane located between the anterior part of corpus callosum and fornix. It separates the anterior horns of lateral ventricles (**4**) (see also no. **1**, Fig. 86).
4. **Anterior Horn of Lateral Ventricle**—located in medullary center of frontal lobe. It is bounded in front and above by genu and body of corpus callosum, respectively.
5. **Superior Frontal Gyrus**—located between the superior frontal and cingulate sulci. It extends from superior lateral surface on to the superior medial surface.
6. **Callosal Sulcus (Sulcus of the Corpus Callosum)**—separates the cingulate gyrus from the corpus callosum (see also no. **9**, Fig. 85).
7. **Cingulate Gyrus**—begins beneath the genu of the corpus callosum and continues above the body of the corpus callosum as far posteriorly as the splenium of this commissure (see also no. **8**, Fig. 86).
8. **Body of Corpus Callosum**—composed of reciprocal commissural fibers that cross in the midline from one cerebral hemisphere to the other.
9. **External Capsule**—consists mainly of projection fibers, but has commissural and association fibers. It is situated between putamen (**12**) and claustrum (**11**) (see also no. **11**, Fig. 86 and no. **2**, Fig. 73*B*).
10. **Lateral Sulcus (Fissure of Sylvius)**—consists of three rami: a main part, the long posterior ramus (shown here) extending into the parietal lobe, and the short anterior and ascending rami (not shown here) projecting into the frontal lobe (see also no. **2**, Fig. 86).
11. **Claustrum** (L. barrier)—a thin sheet of grey matter located medial to insula between the extreme and external capsules.
12. **Putamen** (L. shell)—lateral portion of lentiform nucleus separated from globus pallidus by lateral medullary lamina.

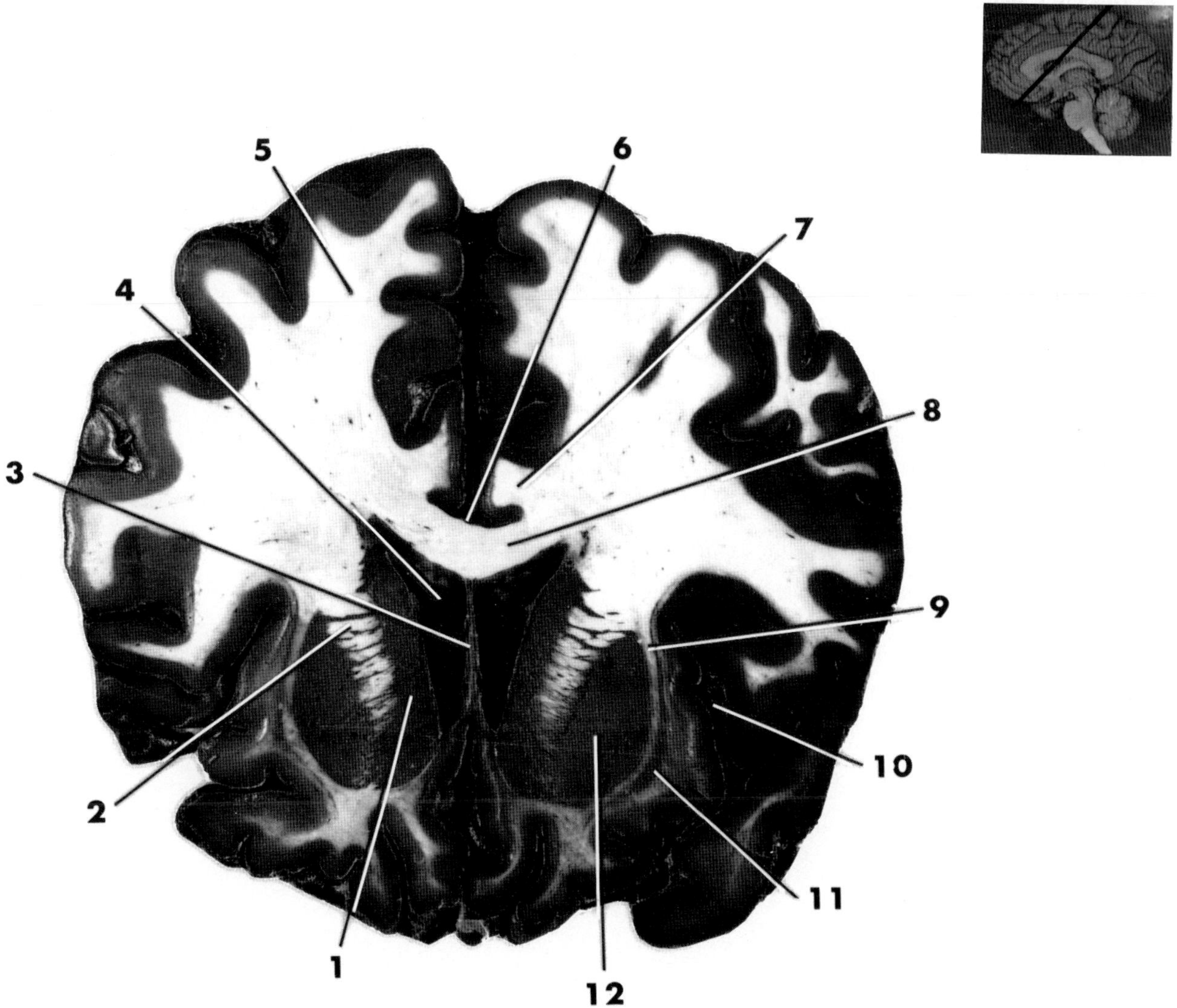

Figure 87

1. **Column of Fornix**—is a continuation of the body of the fornix (L. arch) which curves ventrally from the dorsal surface of thalamus and passes in front of the interventricular foramen and into the hypothalamus to end in the mammillary body.
2. **Putamen** (L. shell)—lateral portion of lentiform nucleus.
3. **Lateral Sulcus (Fissure of Sylvius)**—its long posterior ramus extends into the parietal lobe (see also no. **10**, Fig. 87).
4. **Anterior Thalamic Nucleus (Tubercle)**—responsible for thalamic tubercle with which the fornix bounds the interventricular nucleus. It is part of the limbic system.
5. **Tail of Caudate Nucleus**—extends from the head, backwards as a slender mass of gray matter located on the dorsolateral surface of thalamus, then forwards into the temporal lobe to terminate at the amygdaloid nucleus. The tail (L. *cauda*) is the basis for the name caudate nucleus.
6. **Body of Corpus Callosum**—composed of reciprocal commissural fibers that cross in the midline from one cerebral hemisphere to the other.
7. **Cingulate Sulcus**—intervenes between cingulate gyrus and superior frontal gyrus.
8. **Body of Lateral Ventricle**—located between body of corpus callosum forming its roof and the dorsal surface of thalamus forming its floor. Several other structures are also located in its floor, *e.g.*, tail of caudate (**5**) and body of fornix (**9**).
9. **Body of Fornix**—formed by a continuation of fibers from each crus of the fornix which lies on the medial side of dorsal surface of each thalamus (see also no. **3**, Fig. 89*B*).
10. **Posterior Limb of Internal Capsule**—composed of projection fibers separating lentiform nucleus from thalamus (*i.e.*, corticospinal, corticobulbar, corticopontine, and thalamocortical tracts) (see also no. **8**, Fig. 89*A* and no. **8**, Fig. 73*B*).
11. **External Capsule**—consists mainly of projection fibers, but has commissural and association fibers. It is situated between putamen (**2**) and claustrum (**12**) (see also no. **9**, Fig. 87 and no. **4**, Fig. 73*B*).
12. **Claustrum**—thin sheet of gray matter located medial to insula between the extreme and external capsules. Claustrum is the Latin word for a barrier.
13. **Anterior Commissure** (of left side)—consists of reciprocal commissural fibers that cross the midline and course through corpus striatum (head of caudate nucleus and lentiform nucleus) to end in temporal pole cortex (see also no. **7**, Fig. 74*A*, and no. **11**, Fig. 89*A*).

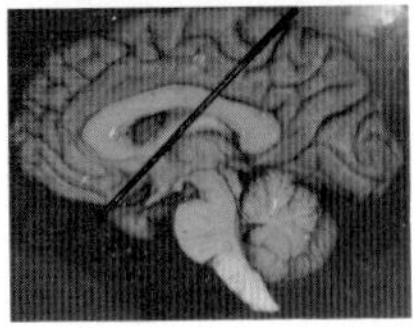

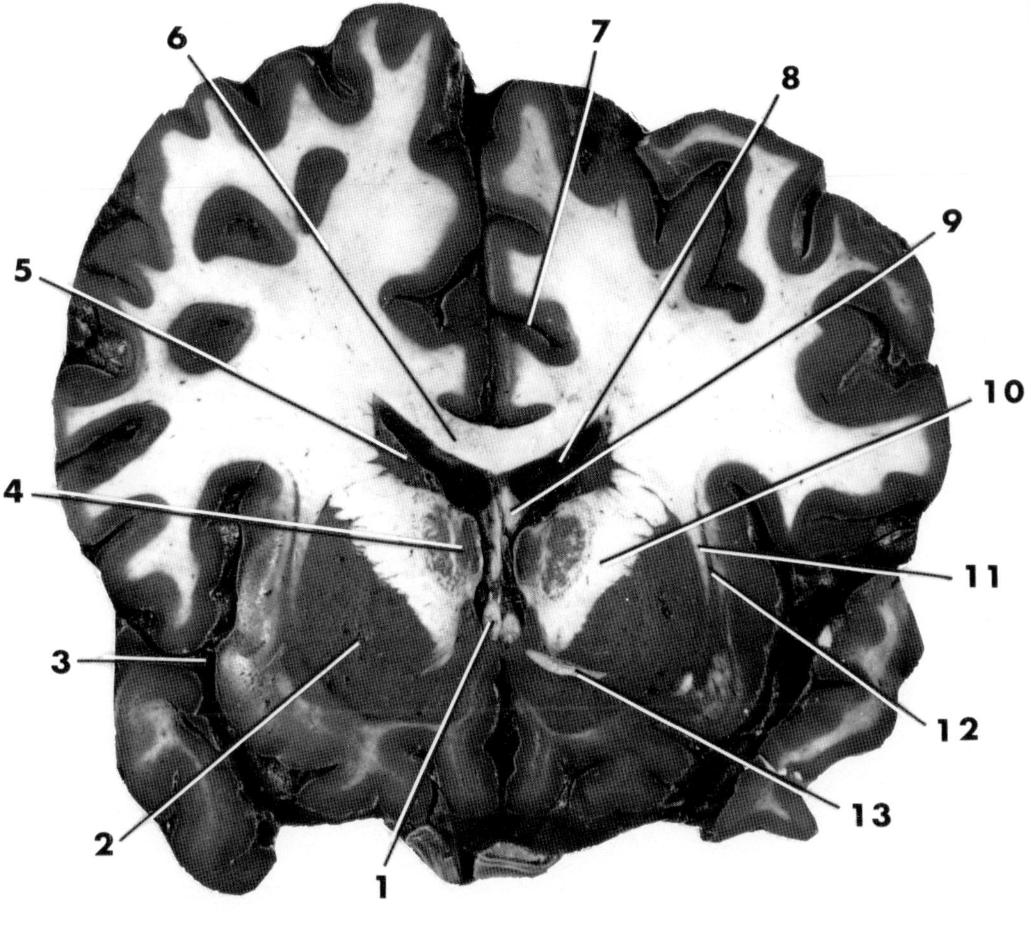

Figure 88

1. **Hypothalamic Area**—surrounds basal area of third ventricle, visible in the midline, and is separated from thalamus by hypothalamic sulcus. Fibers of columns of fornix (right one labelled **12**) demarcate the medial and lateral areas.
2. **Globus Pallidus** (L. a ball + pale)—the medial part of the lentiform nucleus. It is separated from putamen (**10**) by the lateral medullary lamina and from the thalamus by the posterior limb of internal capsule (**8**). It is paler than the putamen (lateral part of lentiform nucleus) in freshly cut brains because it contains large neurons and many myelinated nerve fibers.
3. **Medial Medullary Lamina**—consists of nerve fibers that divide the globus pallidus (**2**) into medial and lateral parts.
4. **Extreme Capsule**—separates the claustrum (**9**) from insular cortex (no. **2**, Fig. 73*B*).
5. **Lateral Medullary Lamina**—consists of nerve fibers in lentiform nucleus that separate putamen (**10**) from globus pallidus (**2**).
6. **External Capsule**—consists mainly of projection fibers, but has commissural and association fibers. It is situated between putamen (**10**) and claustrum (**9**) (see also no. **4**, Fig. 73*B* and no. **9**, Fig. 87).
7. **Tail of Caudate Nucleus**—located on dorsal surface of thalamus in lateral area of floor of body of lateral ventricle (see also no. **5**, Fig. 88, and no. **9**, Fig. 74*A*).
8. **Posterior Limb of Internal Capsule**—composed of projection fibers separating lentiform nucleus from thalamus (*i.e.,* corticospinal, corticobulbar, corticopontine, and thalamocortical tracts) (see also no. **10**, Fig. 88, and no. **8**, Fig. 73*B*).
9. **Claustrum**—thin sheet of gray matter located medial to insula forming a barrier (L. *claustrum*) between the extreme and external capsules.
10. **Putamen** (L. shell)—lateral portion of lentiform nucleus separated from globus pallidus by lateral medullary lamina.
11. **Anterior Commissure** (part of)—consists of reciprocal commissural fibers that cross midline and course through corpus striatum (head of caudate nucleus and lentiform nucleus) to end in temporal pole cortex (see also no. **13**, Fig. 88, and no. **7**, Fig. 74*A*).
12. **Fibers of Fornix**—the column of the fornix extends into hypothalamus (**1**) and terminates on the mammillary body, dividing this area into medial and lateral nuclear areas.

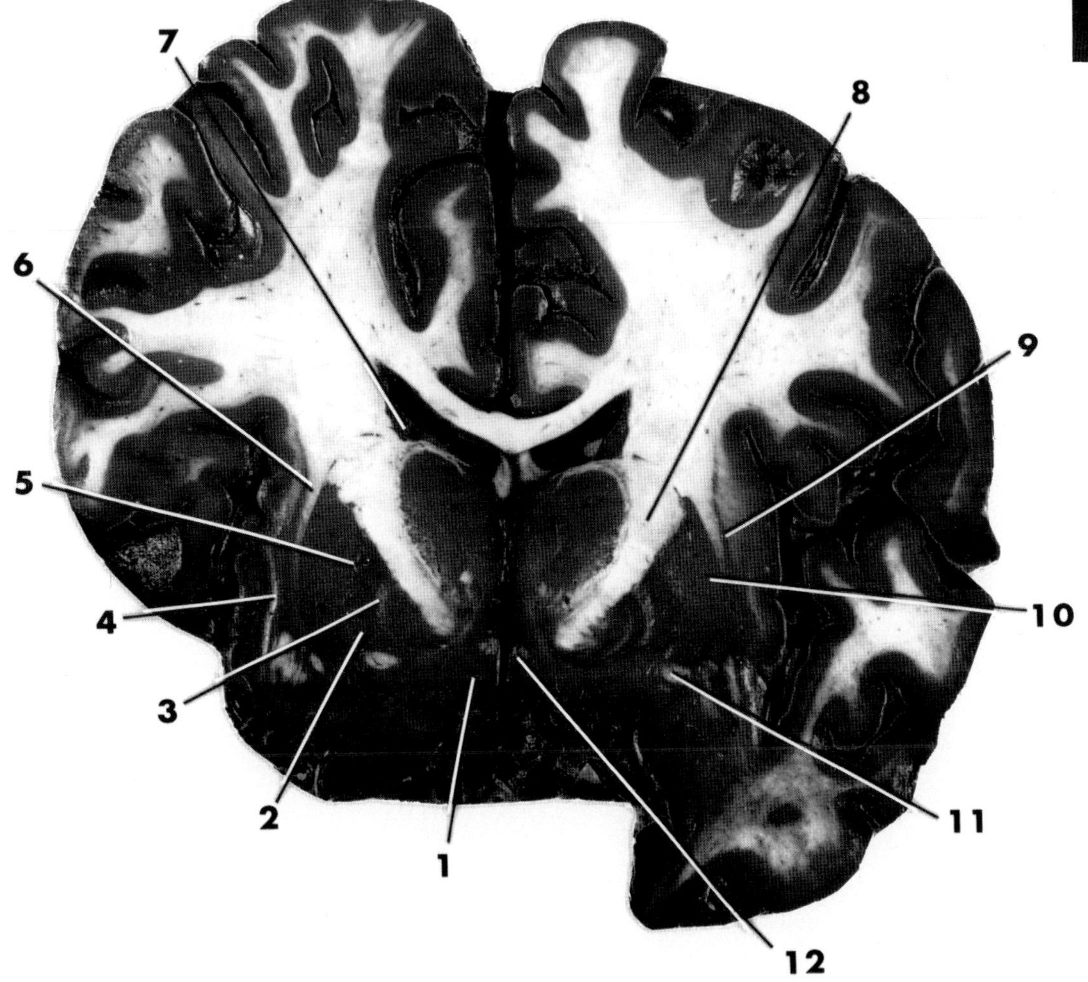

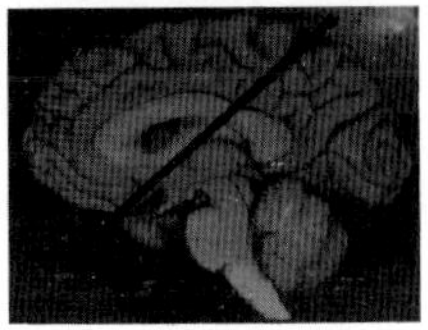

Figure 89*A*

1. **Hypothalamic Sulcus**—separating medial thalamic area (superior) from medial hypothalamic nuclei (inferior).
2. **Third Ventricle**—diencephalic part of the ventricular system located between left and right thalami and hypothalamic areas.
3. **Body of Fornix**—formed by a continuation of fibers from each crus of the fornix which lie on the medial side of dorsal surface of each thalamus (see also no. **9**, Fig. 88, and no. **2**, Fig. 72).
4. **Body of Corpus Callosum**—composed of reciprocal commissural fibers that cross in the midline from one cerebral hemisphere to the other.
5. **Cingulate Gyrus**—begins beneath the genu of the corpus callosum and continues above the body of the corpus callosum as far posteriorly as the splenium of this commissure (only the middle part is shown here) (see also no. **7**, Fig. 87).
6. **Body of Lateral Ventricle**—located between body of corpus callosum forming its roof and the dorsal surface of thalamus forming its floor. Several other structures are also located in its floor, e.g., tail of caudate (no. **8**, Fig. 88) and body of fornix (**3**).
7. **Anterior Thalamic Nucleus**—responsible for thalamic tubercle with which the fornix bounds the interventricular foramen. It is part of the limbic system.
8. **Lateral Thalamic Area**—separated from medial thalamic nucleus by internal medullary lamina. The lateral area consists of ventral and dorsal tiers of nuclei and is bounded laterally by the internal capsule.
9. **Lateral Sulcus (Fissure of Sylvius)**—consists of three rami: a main part, the long posterior ramus, extending into the parietal lobe, and the short anterior and ascending rami projecting into the frontal lobe.
10. **Medial Thalamic Area**—separated from lateral thalamic area (**8**) by internal medullary lamina. Above the hypothalamic sulcus this nuclear area, along with midline nuclei, forms the lateral wall of the third ventricle.

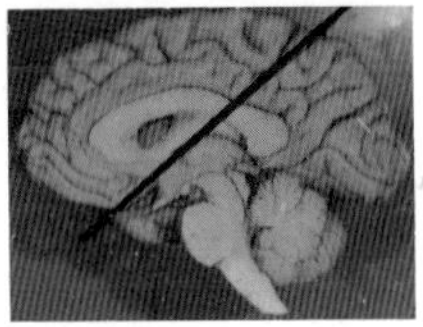

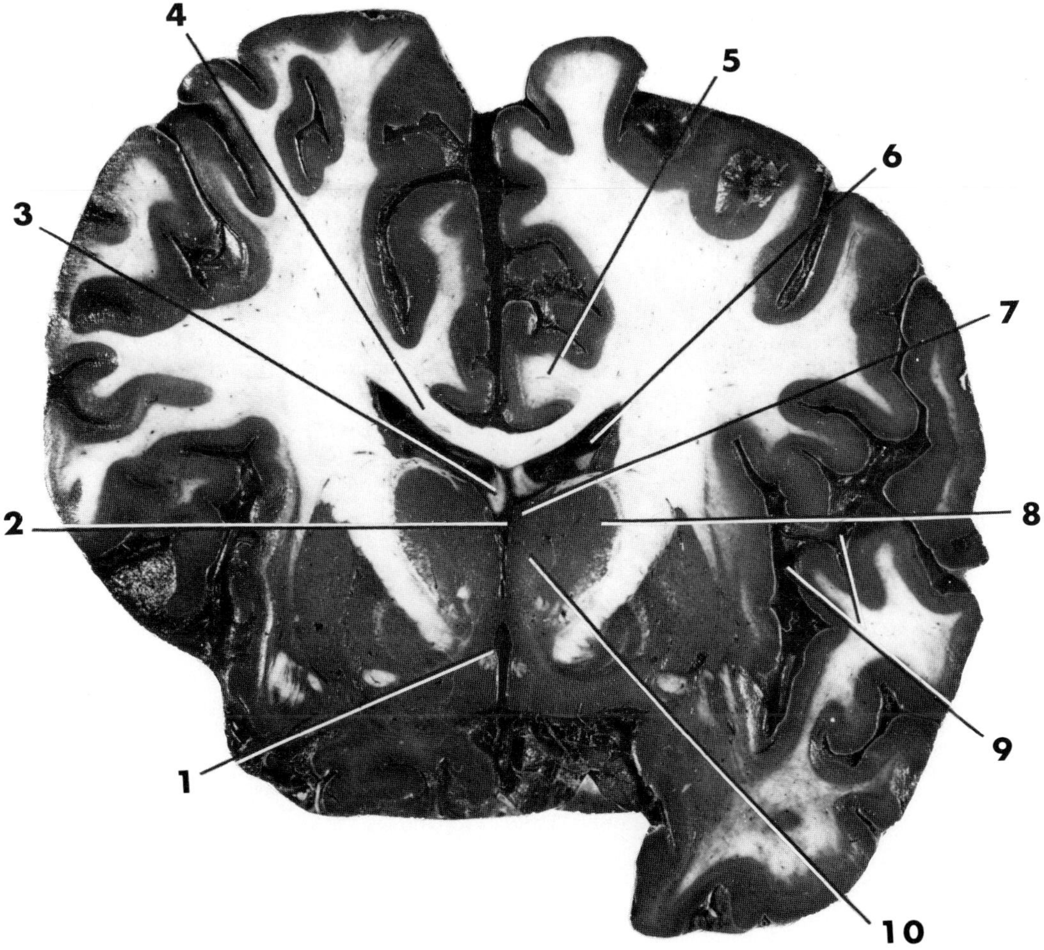

Figure 89*B*

1. **Mammilothalamic Tract (of Vicq d'Azyr)**—part of limbic system, consists of reciprocal tract fibers connecting anterior thalamic and mammillary nuclei (see also no. **4**, Fig. 74*A*).
2. **Fibers of Fornix**—extend from column of the fornix through the hypothalamus, dividing it into medial and lateral nuclear areas before terminating in the mammillary body (see also Fig. 89*B*).
3. **Fibers of Superior Cerebellar Peduncle (Brachium Conjunctivum)**—fibers from cerebellar nuclei of one hemisphere leave the cerebellum as a dense fiber bundle, course into, then decussate (cross) in the midbrain at the level of the inferior colliculus to end on the ventral lateral nucleus of the thalamus and red nucleus. At this level the fibers are passing through the subthalamic area to the ventrolateral nucleus.
4. **Medial Medullary Lamina**—consists of nerve fibers that divide the globus pallidus into medial and lateral parts (see also no. **4**, Fig. 74*B*).
5. **Extreme Capsule**—separates claustrum and insular cortex (see also no. **2**, Fig. 73*B*).
6. **Subthalamic Region**—located ventral to lateral part of the thalamic nuclear area. It separates the hypothalamus from the internal capsule.
7. **Body of Lateral Ventricle**—located between the body of the corpus callosum, forming its roof, and the dorsal surface of the thalamus, forming its floor. The choroid plexus (**9**) is located in it.
8. **Body of Fornix**—formed by a continuation of fibers from the two crura of the fornix which originate in the hippocampus. Each crus fornix curves onto the dorsomedial surface of the thalamus from the inferior horn of the lateral ventricle.
9. **Choroid Plexus**—located in the inferior horns and body of each lateral ventricle and supplied by the choroidal arteries. Its cells produce cerebrospinal fluid.
10. **Lateral Thalamic Area**—separated from medial thalamic area (no. **10**, Fig. 89*B*) by internal medullary lamina. It lies adjacent to the posterior limb of the internal capsule. It is subdivided into dorsal and ventral nuclear regions.
11. **Optic Tract**—composed of optic nerve fibers located between the optic chiasma and the lateral geniculate body. The optic tract winds around the rostral end of the cerebral peduncle enroute to the lateral geniculate body and pretectal nuclear area.
12. **Hypothalamic Region**—surrounds basal area of the third ventricle. Fibers of the columns of the fornix and of the mammillothalamic tract course through this area.

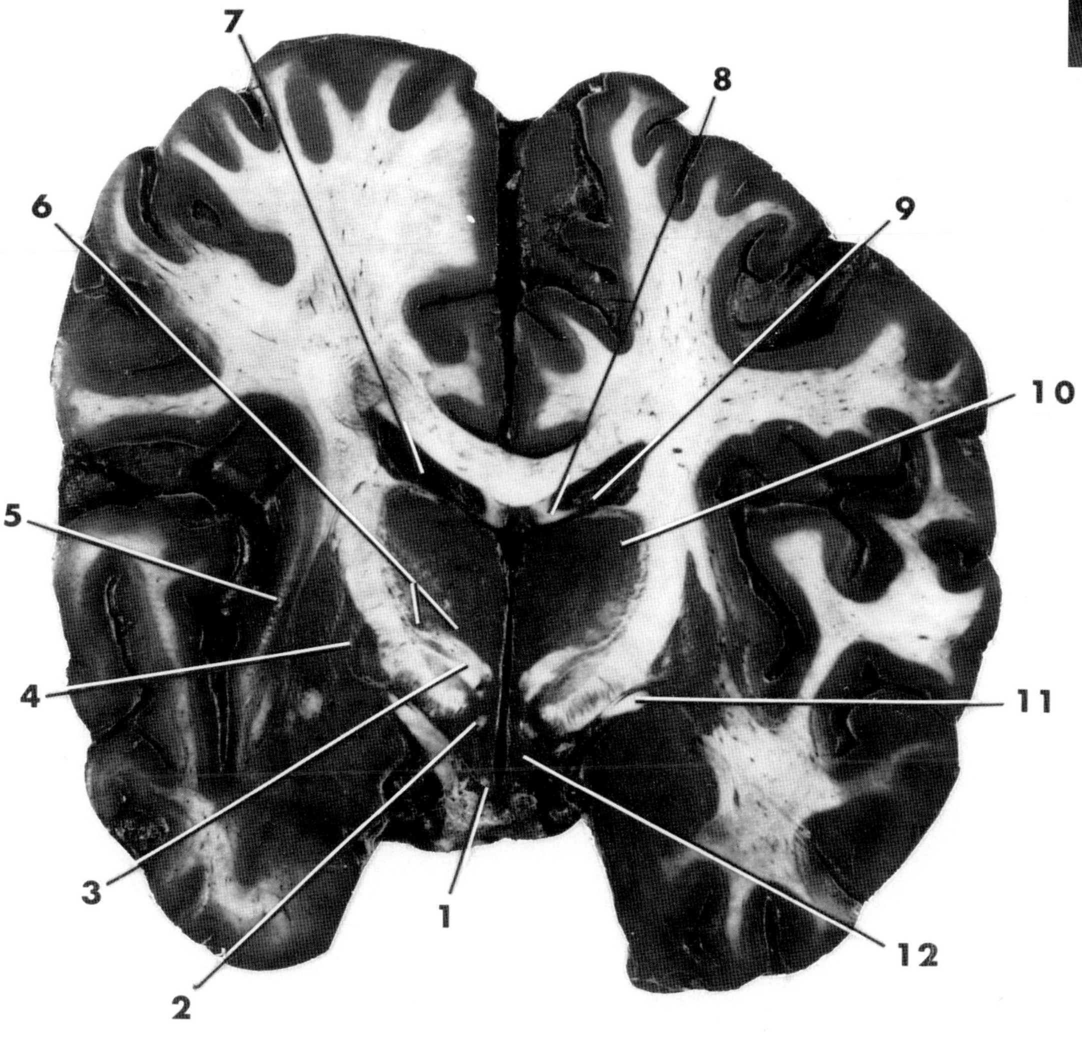

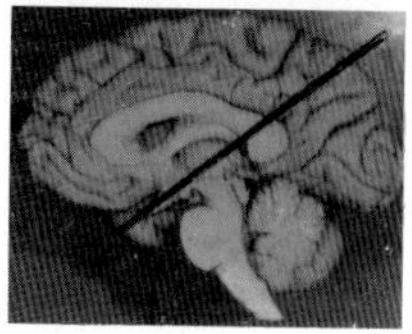

Figure 90*A*

1. **Globus Pallidus** (L. a ball + pale)—the medial part of the lentiform nucleus which appears pale in a freshly cut brain. It is separated from putamen (**3**) by the lateral medullary lamina and from the thalamus by the posterior limb of internal capsule (see also no. **8**, Fig. 73*B* and no. **2**, Fig. 74*B*).
2. **Lateral Medullary Lamina**—consists of nerve fibers in lentiform nucleus that separate putamen (**3**) from globus pallidus (**1**).
3. **Putamen** (L. shell)—lateral portion of lentiform nucleus separated from globus pallidus by lateral medullary lamina.
4. **Claustrum**—thin sheet of gray matter located medial to insula forming a barrier (L. *claustrum*) between the extreme and external capsules.
5. **Lateral Sulcus (Fissure of Sylvius)**—consists of three rami: a main part, the long posterior ramus (shown here), extending into the parietal lobe, and the short anterior and ascending rami (not shown), projecting into the frontal lobe.
6. **Tail of Caudate Nucleus**—located on dorsal surface of thalamus in lateral area of floor of body of lateral ventricle (see also no. **5**, Fig. 88 and no. **6**, Fig. 91*B*).
7. **Body of Corpus Callosum**—composed of reciprocal commissural fibers that cross in the midline from one cerebral hemisphere to the other.
8. **Medial Thalamic Nuclear Area**—separated from lateral thalamic nuclei (no. **10**, Fig. 90*A*) by internal medullary lamina. Above the hypothalamic sulcus this nuclear area, along with midline nuclei, forms the lateral wall of the third ventricle.
9. **External Capsule**—consists mainly of projection fibers, but has commissural and association fibers. It is situated between putamen (**3**) and claustrum (**4**) (see also no. **11**, Fig. 88 and no. **4**, Fig. 73*B*).
10. **Third Ventricle**—Diencephalic part of ventricular system located between left and right thalami and hypothalamic areas. Observe that it is a median, cleft-like space.
11. **Basis Pedunculi (Crus Cerebri)** (beginning of)—projection fibers from internal capsule continue into this ventral part of cerebral peduncle of the midbrain.

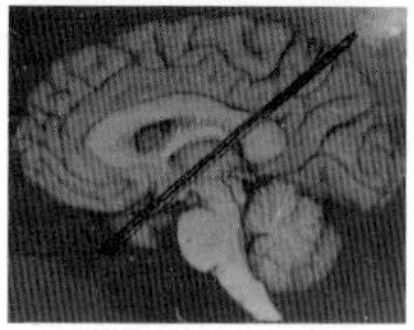

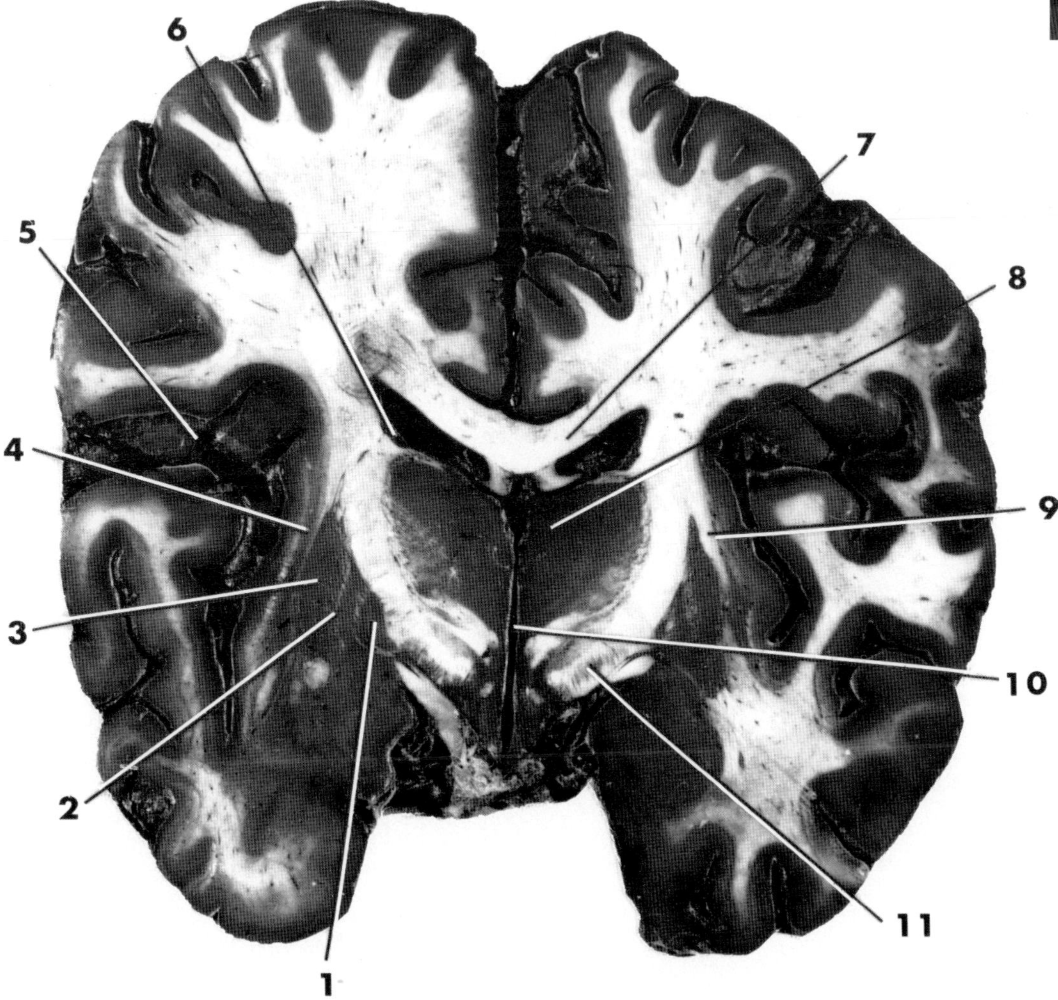

Figure 90*B*

1. **Substantia Nigra**—located in midbrain and extends into subthalamic area. The crus cerebri and midbrain tegmentum are on each side of it. Its black (L. *niger*) appearance results from the melanin granules its cells contain.
2. **Subthalamic Area**—is located ventral to the ventral lateral part of the thalamus. The hypothalamus is medial and the internal capsule is lateral to it.
3. **Pulvinar** (L. cushioned seat)—is the cushion-like posterior part of the thalamus that overhangs the medial and lateral geniculate bodies. Each pulvinar rests on the dorsolateral aspect of the midbrain.
4. **Habenular Trigone** (L. dim. of *habena*—strap, rein)—is a small triangular swelling in the epithalamus, adjacent to the posterior end of the roof of the third ventricle.
5. **Cingulate Gyrus**—begins beneath the genu of the corpus callosum and continues above the body of the corpus callosum as far posteriorly as the splenium of this commissure (only the middle portion is shown here) (see also no. **8**, Fig. 86 and no. **7**, Fig. 87).
6. **Body of Fornix**—formed by a continuation of fibers from each crus of the fornix which lie on the medial side of dorsal surface of each thalamus (see also no. **8**, Fig. 90*A* and no. **3**, Fig. 89*D*).
7. **Third Ventricle** (posterior part)—diencephalic part of ventricular system located between left and right thalami and hypothalamic area.
8. **Superior Cerebellar Peduncle (Brachium Conjunctivum)**—cerebellothalamic fibers (axons) from each dentate, emboliform, and globose nucleus leave the cerebellum as a dense fiber bundle (peduncle) which courses into the tegmentum of the midbrain, where they decussate in the midline at the level of the inferior colliculus.
9. **Mammillary Body** (L. *mamilla,* nipple)—basilar portion of hypothalamic nucleus that has a nipple-like appearance. It has an important function in the limbic system and the autonomic nervous system.

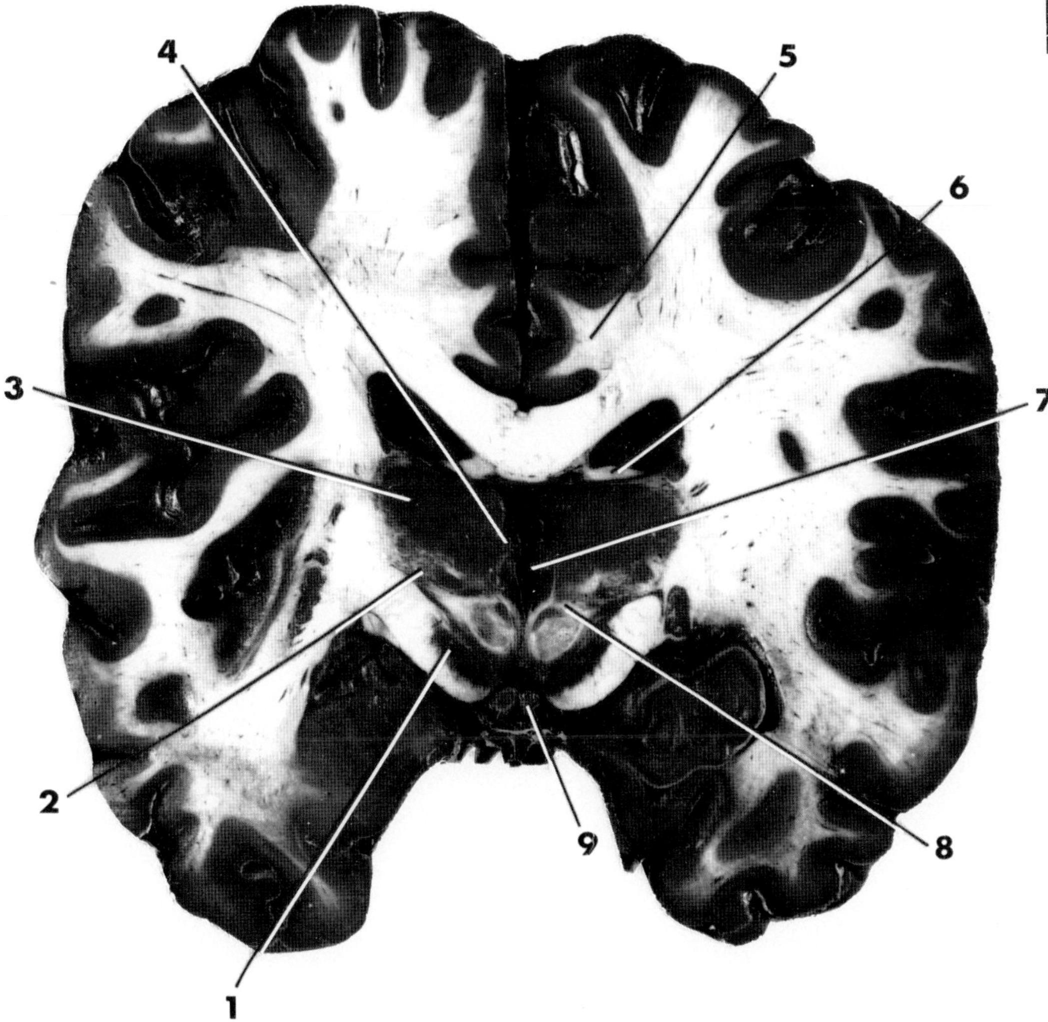

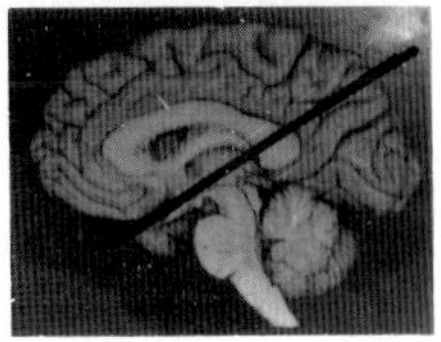

Figure 91*A*

1. **Red Nucleus**—prominent brain stem motor nucleus located in tegmentum of rostral midbrain. Fibers of the superior cerebellar peduncle encapsulate it or terminate in it (see also no. **6**, Fig. 75*A*).
2. **Putamen** (the caudal tip)—of the lentiform nucleus. At this point it is still bounded by the external and internal capsules (see also no. **2**, Fig. 88 and no. **3**, Fig. 90*B*).
3. **Body of Lateral Ventricle**—located between body of corpus callosum forming its roof and the dorsal surface of thalamus forming its floor. Several other structures are located in its floor, *e.g.*, tail of caudate nucleus (**6**) and body of fornix (visible here and in no. **6**, Fig. 89*B*).
4. **Callosal Sulcus (Sulcus of the Corpus Callosum)**—separates the cingulate gyrus from the corpus callosum.
5. **Body of Corpus Callosum**—composed of reciprocal commissural fibers that cross in the midline from one cerebral hemisphere to the other.
6. **Tail of Caudate Nucleus**—located on dorsolateral surface of thalamus in the floor of body of lateral ventricle (see also no. **7**, Fig. 89*A* and no. **6**, Fig. 90*B*).
7. **Inferior Horn of Lateral Ventricle**—extends downwards and then forwards into the temporal lobe. The tail of the caudate nucleus and the stria terminalis are located in its roof and the hippocampus (**8**) in its floor.
8. **Hippocampus** (G. seahorse)—gyrus located in floor of inferior horn. It is part of the limbic system, and its fibers form the alveus, fimbria, and fornix which end in the mammillary body.
9. **Basis Pedunculi (Crus Cerebri)**—located on ventral surface of cerebral peduncle. Projection fibers from internal capsule continue into midbrain to form this rope-like bundle of corticopontine and corticospinal fibers.

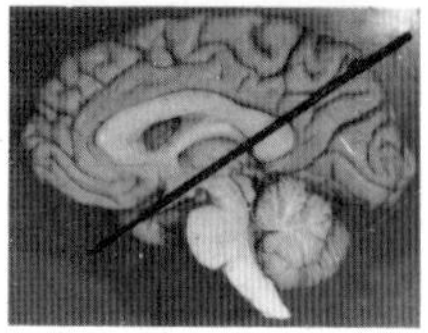

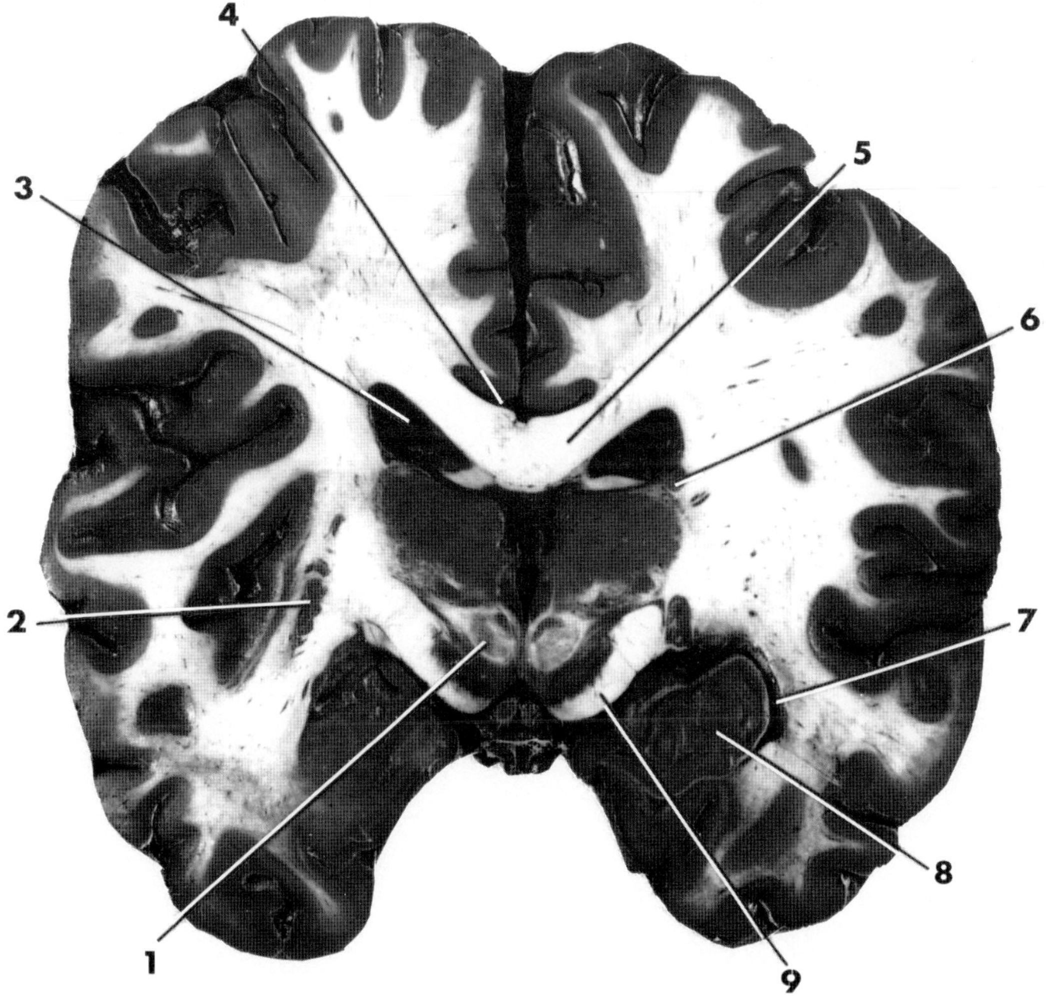

Figure 91*B*

1. **Basis Pedunculi (Crus Cerebri)**—located on ventral surface of cerebral peduncle. Projection fibers from internal capsule pass into midbrain to form this massive fiber bundle.
2. **Hippocampus** (G. seahorse)—located in floor of inferior horn. It is part of limbic system, and its fibers form the alveus, fimbria, and fornix which end in the mammillary body.
3. **Medial Lemniscus** (G. ribbon, band)—ascending sensory tract that originates in contralateral nucleus gracilis and cuneatus and terminates in ventral posterior nucleus of thalamus. It transmits discriminative touch, proprioception, and vibration sense (see also no. **3**, Fig. 77 and no. **3**, Fig. 93).
4. **Medial Geniculate Body**—nuclear swelling beneath the pulvinar of posterior surface of thalamus. It is part of auditory pathway.
5. **Central Gray Matter**—poorly organized region of gray matter that surrounds the cerebral aqueduct (**11**).
6. **Crus of Fornix** (L. *crus,* leg)—consists of hippocampal fibers (axons) that are a continuation of the fimbria.
7. **Pineal Body** (gland)—part of epithalamus resting on tectum of midbrain. Shaped like a pine (L. *pinus*) cone.
8. **Superior Colliculus** (L. small elevation)—nerve cell mass in the rostral half of dorsal surface of midbrain. It is a relay station in visual system for eye and head turning movements (see also no. **9**, Fig. 75*A*).
9. **Trigone of Lateral Ventricle** (beginning portion)—the posterior and inferior horns emerge from the caudal part of the body of the lateral ventricle. The posterior horns extend into the medullary center of the occipital lobes (see also no. **5**, Fig. 34).
10. **Pulvinar** (L. cushioned seat)—the posterior cushion-like part of the thalamus that overhangs the medial and lateral geniculate bodies. Each pulvinar rests on the dorsolateral aspect of the midbrain.
11. **Cerebral Aqueduct (of Sylvius)**—canal located beneath the tectum of midbrain. It connects the third and fourth ventricles.
12. **Superior Cerebellar Puduncle (Brachium Conjunctivum)**—fibers (axons) from each dentate, emboliform, and globose nuclei leave the cerebellum as a dense fiber bundle which courses into the tegmentum of the midbrain, where they decussate in the midline at the level of the inferior colliculus.
13. **Substantia Nigra**—located in midbrain and extends into subthalamic area. The crus cerebri and midbrain tegmentum are on each side of it.

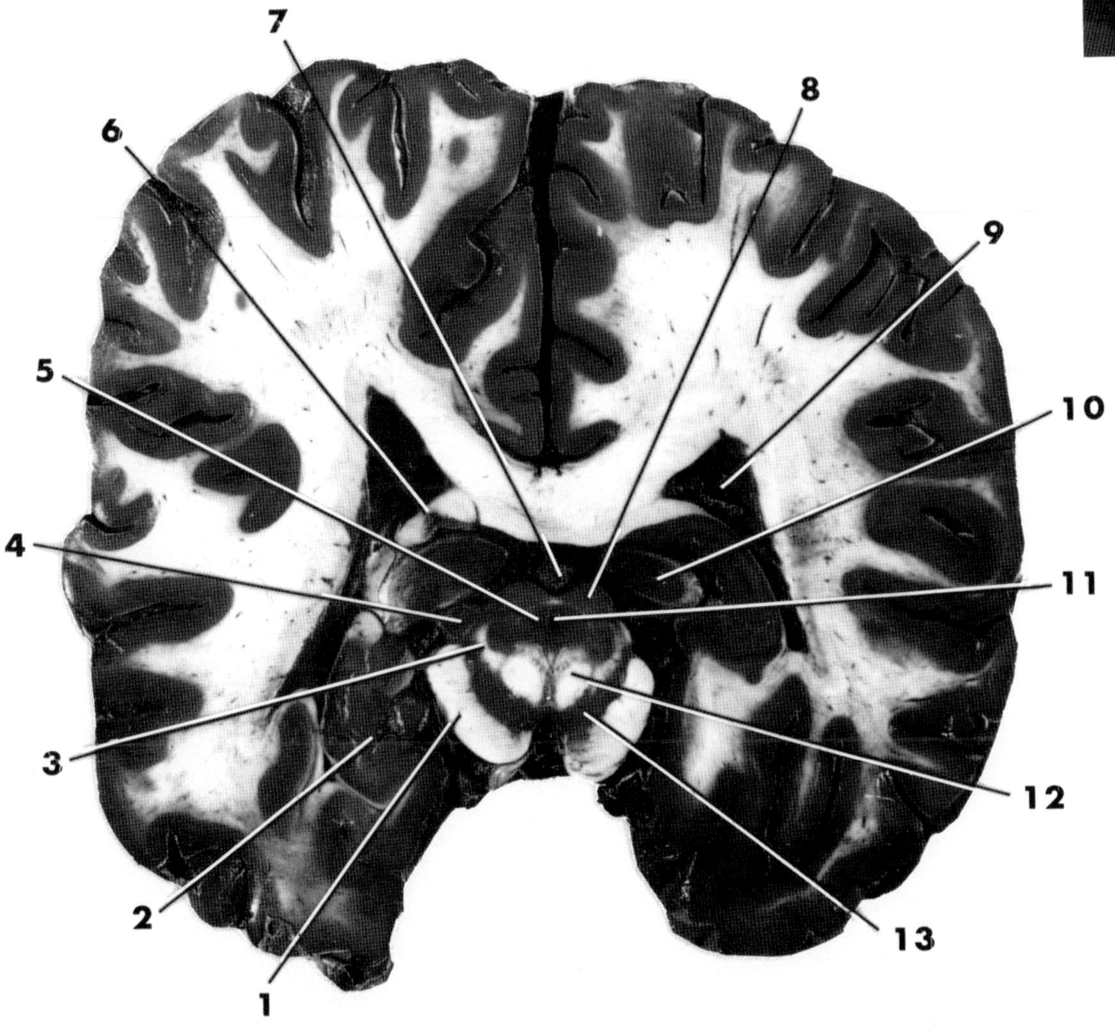

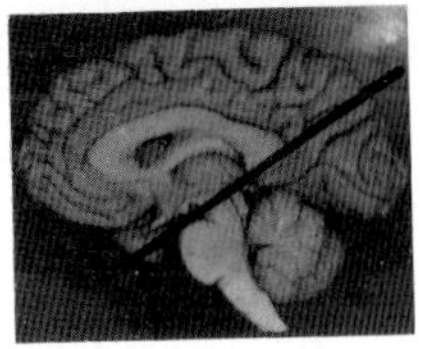

Figure 92

1. **Corticospinal Fibers**—course uninterrupted through basal pons in bundles (fasciculi) to form the pyramids in the medulla (see also no. **1**, Fig. 94 and no. **1**, Fig. 95).
2. **Pontocerebellar Fibers**—axons of pontine neurons in contralateral basal pons course transversely through pons and form the middle cerebellar peduncle (brachium pontis).
3. **Medial Lemniscus**—this ascending sensory tract is horizontally positioned in the tegmental pons and emerges laterally in the midbrain tegmentum (see also no. **3**, Fig. 94).
4. **Medial Longitudinal Fasciculus**—axons from vestibular nuclei form a discrete bundle of fibers that are located close to midline, directly beneath cranial nerve nuclei. This fasciculus functions in extraocular movements in response to vestibular stimuli.
5. **Inferior Colliculus** (L. small elevation)—nerve cell mass in the caudal half of the tectum of midbrain. It is a relay station in the auditory pathway and also functions in head turning movements in response to sound.
6. **Cerebral Aqueduct (of Sylvius)**—duct located beneath the tectum of midbrain. It connects the third and fourth ventricles.
7. **Posterior Horn of Lateral Ventricle**—posterior extension of lateral ventricle into medullary center of the occipital lobe.
8. **Central Gray Matter**—poorly organized region of gray matter that surrounds the cerebral aqueduct.
9. **Decussation of Superior Cerebellar Peduncles (Decussation of Brachia Conjunctiva)**—fibers of these peduncles cross in the midline of the midbrain tegmentum to course to the contralateral lateral ventral nucleus of thalamus and red nucleus. The decussation is located in the midbrain at the level of the inferior colliculus.
10. **Pontine Nuclei**—aggregations of pontine neurons are scattered among longitudinal and transverse fibers in basal pons. Axons of these neurons, known as pontocerebellar fibers (**2**), course transversely in basal pons and form the middle cerebellar peduncle (brachium pontis).

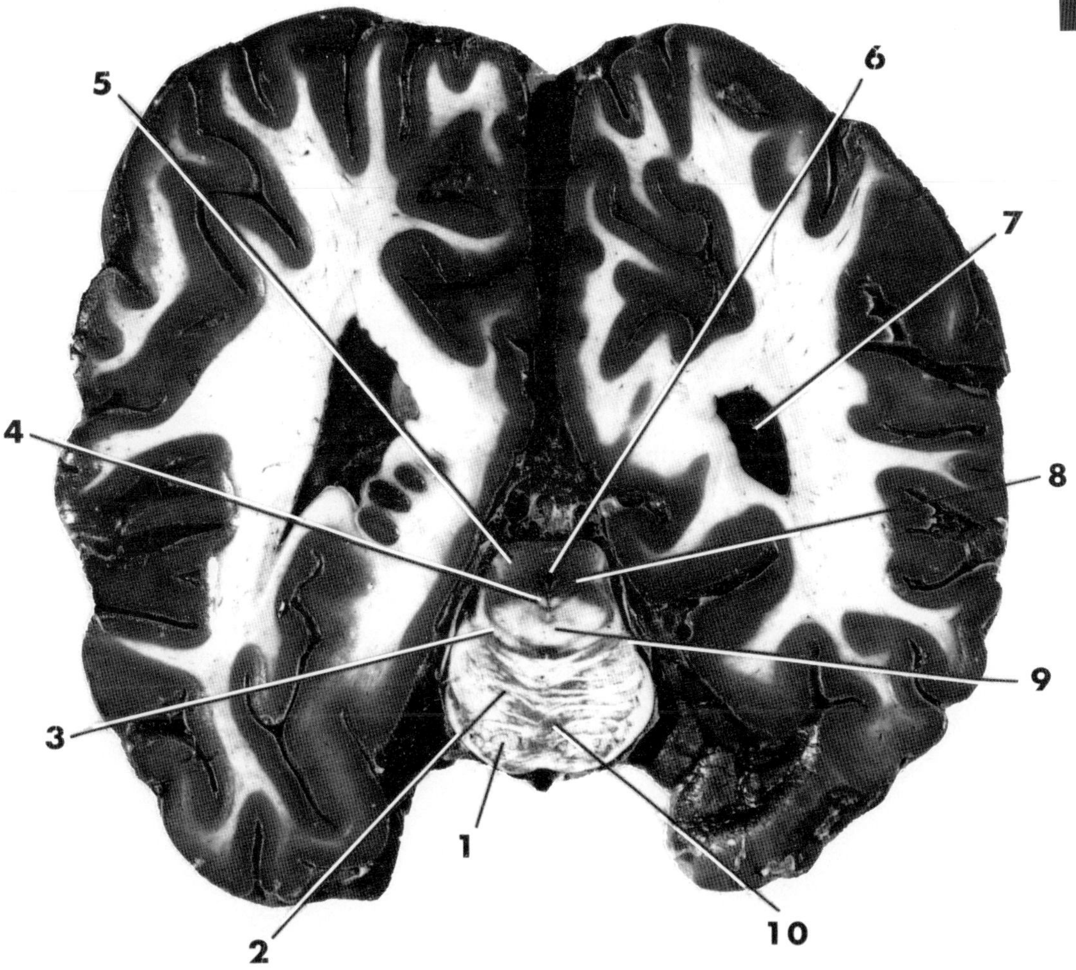

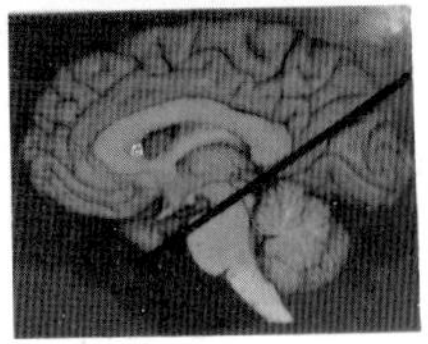

Figure 93

1. **Corticospinal and Corticobulbar Fibers**—course uninterrupted through basal pons in bundles (fasciculi) to form the pyramids in the medulla (see also no. **1**, Fig. 93, and no. **1**, Fig. 95).
2. **Pontocerebellar Fibers**—axons of pontine neurons in contralateral basal pons course transversely through pons and form the middle cerebral peduncle (brachium pontis).
3. **Medial Lemniscus**—this ascending sensory tract is horizontally positioned in the tegmental pons and emerges laterally in the midbrain tegmentum.
4. **Lateral Lemniscus** (G. band, ribbon)—part of auditory pathway between cochlear nuclei and inferior colliculus. It is located in dorsolateral wall of rostral pons and midbrain.
5. **Fourth Ventricle** (rostral portion)—the superior medullary velum (**8**) and superior cerebellar peduncle (**9**) form its roof and lateral wall, and the pons tegmentum its floor.
6. **Posterior Horn of Lateral Ventricle**—posterior extension of lateral ventricle into the medullary center of the occipital lobe.
7. **Calcarine Sulcus** (L. *calcar,* spur)—prominent sulcus on medial surface of cerebral hemisphere. It courses beneath the splenium of the corpus callosum to the occipital pole and is an important landmark for visual cortex (see also no. **6**, Fig. 95).
8. **Superior Medullary Velum** (L. veil)—consists of a thin sheet of ependyma and pia mater that bridges the space between the superior cerebellar peduncles (**9**). It forms the roof of the rostral part of fourth ventricle.
9. **Superior Cerebellar Peduncle (Brachium Conjunctivum)**—axons from dentate, emboliform, and globose nuclei form this compact bundle that courses to midbrain tegmentum. At the midline, the fibers decussate to the contralateral side.
10. **Medial Longitudinal Fasciculus**—axons from vestibular nuclei form a discrete bundle of fibers that are located close to midline directly beneath cranial nerve nuclei. This fasciculus functions in extraocular movements in response to vestibular stimuli (see also no. **4**, Fig. 93).
11. **Middle Cerebellar Peduncle (Brachium Pontis)**—beginning portion. Pontocerebellar fibers (axons of pontine neurons) cross transversely to the contralateral basal pons and course posteriorly and laterally into medullary center of cerebellar hemisphere which forms this prominent compact fiber bundle—the middle cerebellar peduncle.
12. **Pontine Nuclei**—aggregations of pontine neurons are scattered among longitudinal and transverse fibers in basal pons. Axons of these neurons, known as pontocerebellar fibers (**2**), course transversely in basal pons and form middle cerebellar peduncle (**11**).

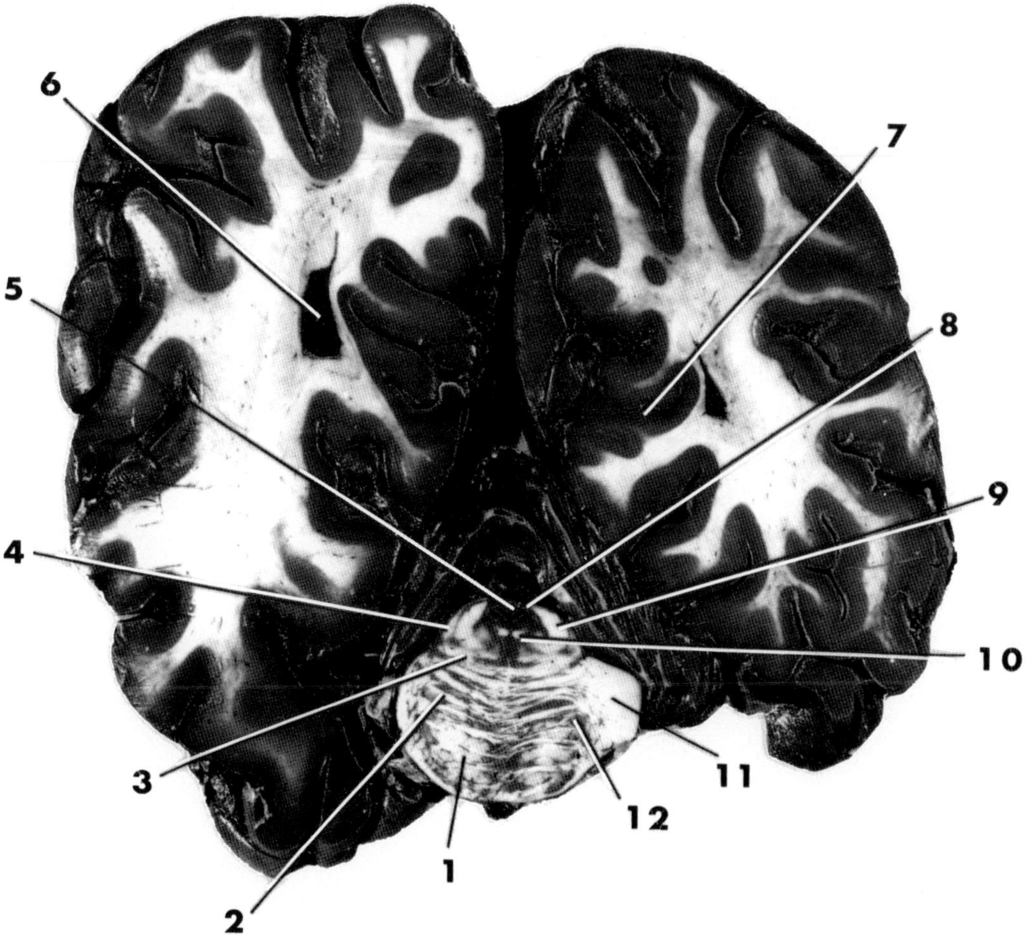

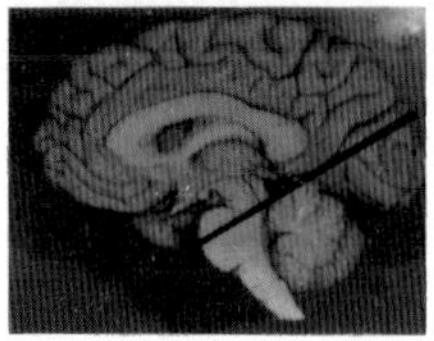

Figure 94

1. **Corticospinal Fibers**—converge and course uninterrupted through basal pons in bundles (fasciculi) to form the pyramids in the medulla (see also no. **1**, Fig. 93 and no. **1**, Fig. 94).
2. **Medial Lemniscus**—this ascending sensory tract is horizontally positioned in the tegmental pons and emerges laterally in the midbrain tegmentum.
3. **Tegmentum of Pons** (L. *tegmentum,* cover)—dorsal portion of the pons lying between basal pons and fourth ventricle.
4. **Visual Cortex**—surrounds the calcarine sulcus (**6**); also known as area 17 of Brodmann classification of cortical areas.
5. **Posterior Horn of Lateral Ventricle**—posterior extension of lateral ventricle towards occipital pole.
6. **Calcarine Sulcus** (L. *calcar,* spur)—prominent sulcus on medial surface of cerebral hemisphere. It courses beneath the splenium of the corpus callosum to the occipital pole and is an important landmark for visual cortex (see also no. **7**, Fig. 94 and no. **6**, Fig. 96).
7. **Superior Medullary Velum** (L. veil)—consists of a thin sheet of ependyma and pia mater that bridges the space between the superior cerebellar peduncles (**9**). It forms the roof of rostral part of fourth ventricle (see also no. **8**, Fig. 94).
8. **Fourth Ventricle** (rostral portion)—the superior medullary velum (**7**) and superior cerebellar peduncles (**9**) form its roof and lateral wall, and the pons tegmentum its floor.
9. **Superior Cerebellar Peduncle (Brachium Conjunctivum)**—axons from dentate, emboliform, and globose nuclei form this compact bundle that courses to midbrain tegmentum. At the midline, the fibers decussate to the contralateral side (see also no. **9**, Fig. 94).
10. **Middle Cerebellar Peduncle (Brachium Pontis)**—beginning portion. Pontocerebellar fibers (axons of pontine neurons) cross transversely to the contralateral basal pons and course posteriorly and laterally into medullary center of cerebellar hemisphere to form this prominent compact fiber bundle, the middle cerebellar peduncle (see also no. **11**, Fig. 94).
11. **Pontocerebellar Fibers**—axons of pontine neurons in contralateral basal pons course transversely through pons and form the middle cerebellar peduncle (see also no. **3**, Fig. 94 and no. **2**, Fig. 93).

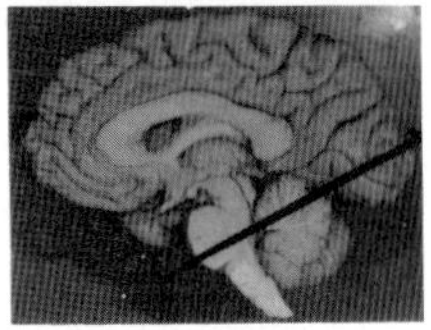

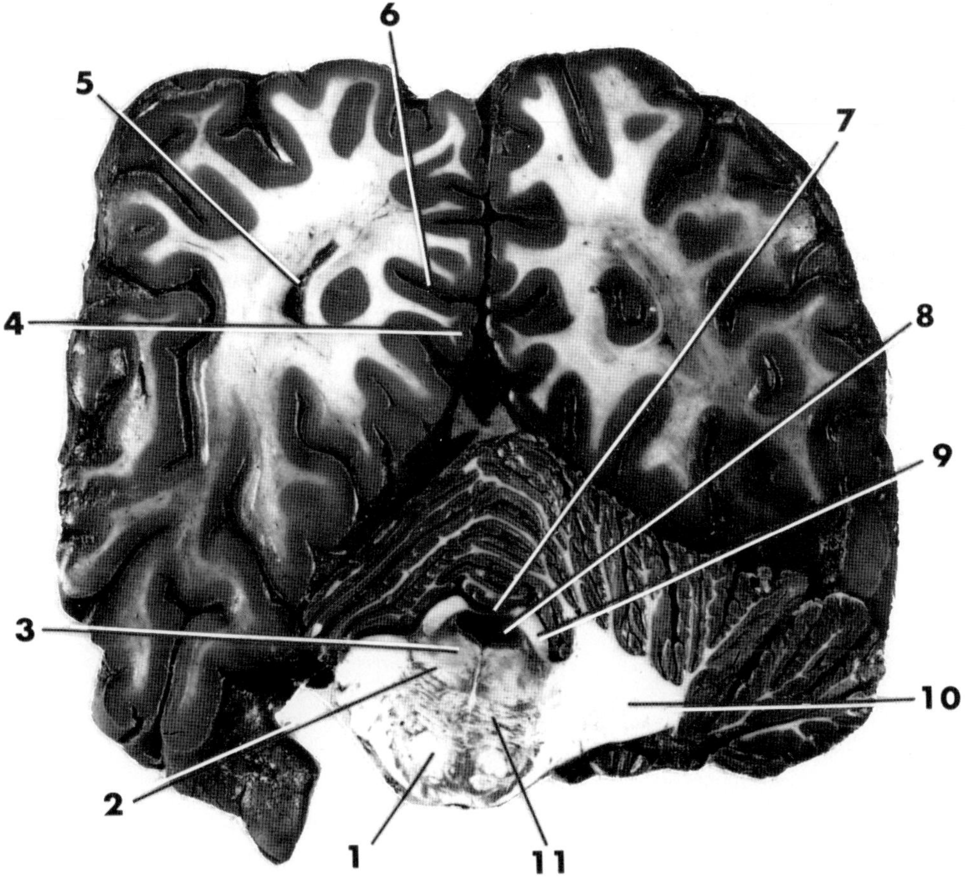

Figure 95

1. **Pyramid**—located on ventral surface of medulla between ventral median fissure and ventrolateral sulcus. It consists of corticospinal tract fibers which continue from internal capsule through crus cerebri (basis pedunculi) and basal pons.
2. **Olive**—oval bulging on lateral wall of medulla. It contains the inferior, accessory, and superior olivary nuclei which function with motor system.
3. **Floor of Fourth Ventricle (Rhomboid Fossa)**—formed by the dorsal surface of the tegmentum of pons and open portion of medulla.
4. **Fourth Ventricle**—is located between the cerebellum and the tegmental pons and the medulla. Its floor (**3**) is broad in its midportion, but narrows toward cerebral aqueduct and obex (L. barrier)—between caudal end of this ventricle and central canal of spinal cord).
5. **Occipital Lobe**—on the lateral surface is limited in front by a line which joins the parietooccipital sulcus with the preoccipital notch. On the medial surface it is limited in front by the parietooccipital sulcus.
6. **Calcarine Sulcus** (L. *calcar,* spur)—prominent sulcus on medial surface of cerebral hemisphere. It courses beneath the splenium of corpus callosum to the occipital lobe and is an important landmark for visual cortex (see also no. **7**, Fig. 94 and no. **6**, Fig. 95).
7. **Visual Cortex**—surrounds the calcarine sulcus (**6**); also known as area 17 of Brodmann classification of cortical areas.
8. **Dentate Nucleus** (L. *dentatus,* toothed)—shaped like a wrinkled sac that has toothed appearance. Largest of the cerebellar nuclei, located deep in medullary center of each cerebellar hemisphere. Axons of neurons in this nucleus converge to form the superior cerebellar peduncle.
9. **Vestibular Area (Area Acoustica)**—located in lateral area of floor of fourth ventricle, lateral to sulcus limitans. It contains the vestibular nuclear complex (superior, medial, lateral, and inferior nuclei).
10. **Medial Longitudinal Fasciculus**—axons from vestibular nuclei form a discrete bundle of fibers that are located close to midline, directly beneath cranial nerve nuclei. This fasciculus functions in extraocular movements in response to vestibular stimuli (see also no. **3**, Fig. 97).

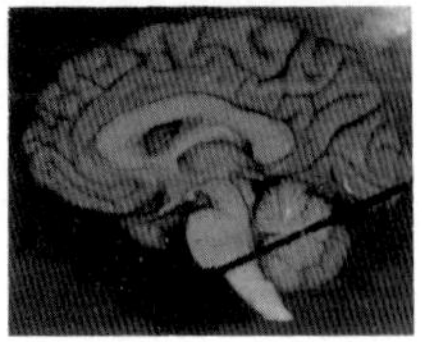

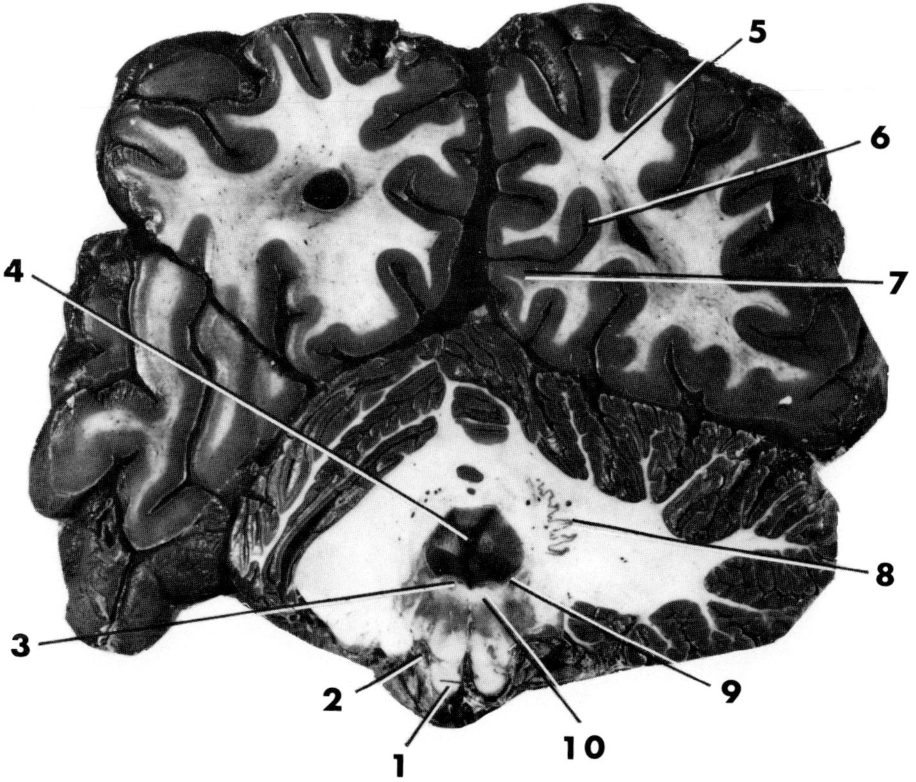

Figure 96

1. **Inferior Olivary Nucleus**—located in the olive which lies between the pyramid (**8**) and the tuberculum cinereum. It functions with the motor system and has extensive cerebellar connections.
2. **Inferior Cerebellar Peduncle (Restiform Body)**—main mass of this rope-like (L. *restiform*) structure consists of cerebellar afferents from brain stem and spinal cord.
3. **Medial Longitudinal Fasciculus**—axons from vestibular nuclei form a discrete bundle of fibers that are located close to midline, directly beneath cranial nerve nuclei. This fasciculus functions in extraocular movements in response to vestibular stimuli.
4. **Dentate Nucleus** (L. *dentatus,* toothed)—the largest of the cerebellar nuclei that has the shape of a wrinkled sac with a toothed edge. Located deep in the medullary center of each cerebellar hemisphere. Axons of neurons in this nucleus converge to form the superior cerebellar peduncle (see also no. **8**, Fig. 96, and no. **1**, Fig. 79).
5. **Vestibular Nuclei (Area Acoustica)**—located in lateral area of floor of fourth ventricle, lateral to sulcus limitans. It contains the vestibular nuclear complex (superior, medial, lateral, and inferior nuclei).
6. **Spinal Tract and Nucleus of Fifth Cranial Nerve**—these two structures comprise the tuberculum cinereum in the dorsolateral sulcus of the medulla. Fibers from the trigeminal nerve enter the lateral pons and descend into the medulla and cephalic end of the spinal cord, where they turn into and synapse on neurons of the spinal nucleus of C.N. V which lies immediately adjacent to it.
7. **Medial Lemniscus**—consists of vertical column of fibers on each side of the midline in tegmentum of medulla superior to the pyramid. These fibers originate in nucleus gracilis and nucleus cuneatus and terminate in the contralateral ventral posterior nucleus of thalamus (see also no. **7**, Fig. 79, and no. **3**, Fig. 80).
8. **Pyramid**—located on ventral surface of medulla between ventral medial fissure and ventrolateral sulcus. It consists of corticospinal tract fibers which continue from internal capsule through basis pedunculi and basal pons into the medulla.

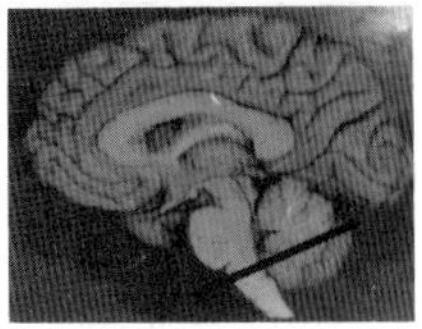

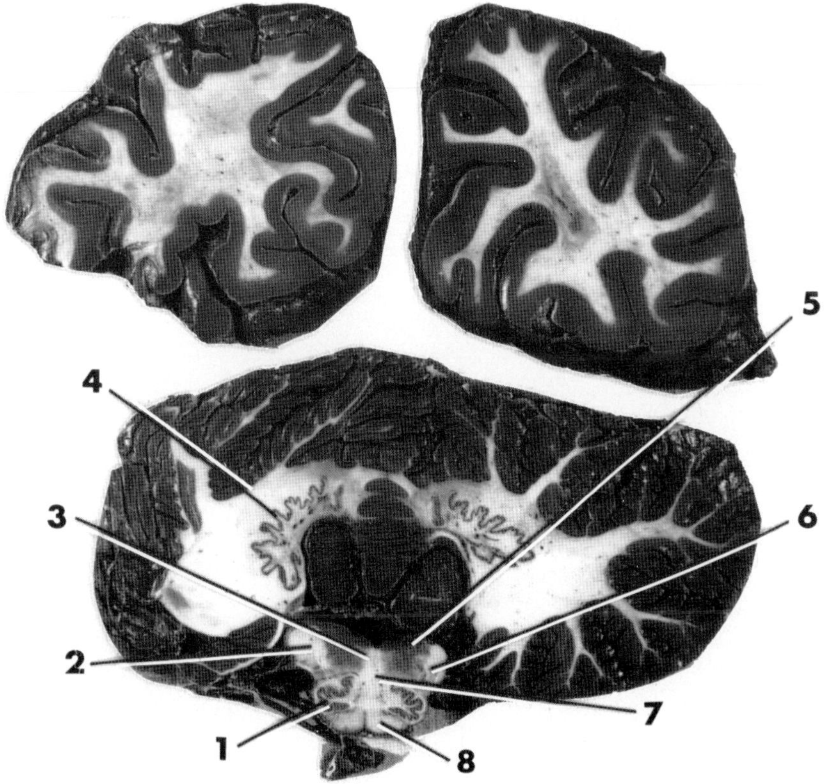

Figure 97

1. **Pyramid**—located on ventral surface of medulla between ventral median fissure and ventrolateral sulcus. It consists of corticospinal tract fibers which continue from internal capsule through basis pedunculi and basal pons into the medulla.
2. **Inferior Olivary Nucleus**—located in the olive which lies between the pyramid (**1**) and the tuberculum cinereum. It functions with the motor system and has extensive cerebellar connections.
3. **Spinal Tract and Nucleus of Trigeminal Nerve**—these two structures comprise the tuberculum cinereum in the dorsolateral sulcus of the medulla. Fibers from the trigeminal nerve enter the lateral pons and descend into the medulla and cephalic end of the spinal cord, where they turn into and synapse on neurons of the spinal nucleus of C.N. V which lies immediately adjacent.
4. **Dentate Nucleus** (L. *dentatus,* toothed)—largest of the cerebellar nuclei. Has the shape of wrinkled sac with a toothed edge. Located deep in medullary center of each cerebellar hemisphere. Axons of neurons in this nucleus converge to form the superior cerebellar peduncle (see also no. **1**, Fig. 79, and no. **4**, Fig. 97).
5. **Fourth Ventricle**—located between cerebellum and the tegmental pons and medulla. Its floor (rhomboid fossa) is broad in its midportion, but narrows toward obex and cerebral aqueduct.
6. **Inferior Cerebellar Peduncle (Restiform Body)**—rope-like (L. *restiform*) mass of fibers consists of cerebellar afferents from brain stem and spinal cord.
7. **Medial Longitudinal Fasciculus**—axons from vestibular nuclei form a discrete bundle of fibers that are located close to midline directly beneath cranial nerve nuclei. This fasciculus functions in extraocular movements in response to vestibular stimuli.
8. **Decussation of Pyramids**—located in ventral caudal medulla where approximately 85% of the corticospinal fibers of the pyramid cross (decussate) in the ventral median fissure to the opposite side and descend in the lateral column of white matter of the spinal cord (see also no. **6**, Fig. 87).

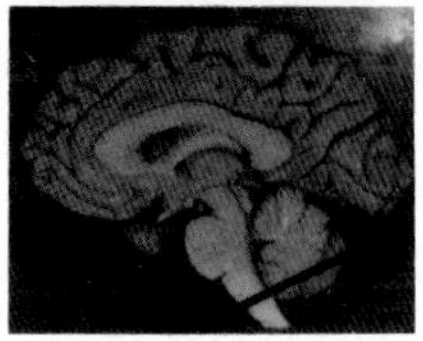

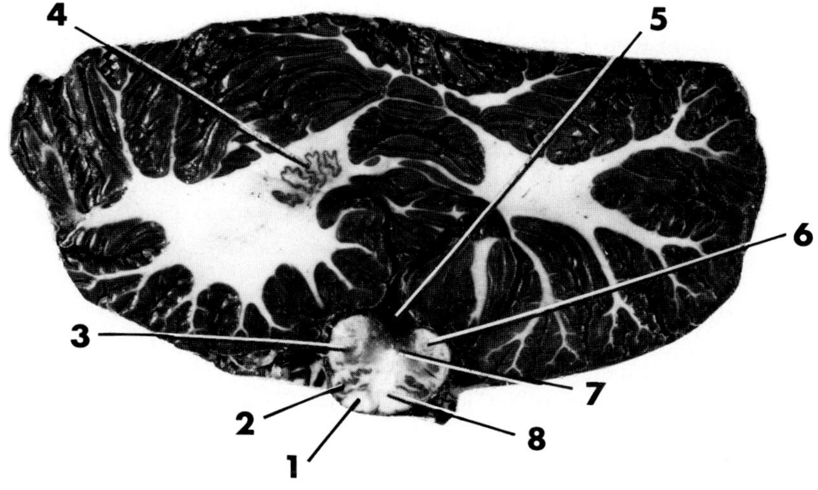

Figure 98

12

Sagittal Serial Sections of the Brain

Sagittal serial sections were cut through half a brain, approximately 12 mm in thickness. The sections were then surface-stained by the modified Mulligan technique (blue, gray matter; white, white matter), photographed, mounted, and the important structures in each section numbered. In sections where there were more than 15 important structures illustrated, a duplicate photograph was used to identify the additional structures.

Throughout the series, a small drawing of the brain appears in the upper right-hand corner of each figure with a line drawn through the brain to indicate the level through which the section was taken.

1. **Superior Temporal Gyrus**—has a large cortical surface forming the floor of lateral sulcus (**2**). The *transverse temporal gyrus* (**2**) extends medially from this surface to the insula in the lateral fissure and marks the location of the auditory area of cortex.
2. **Lateral Sulcus (Fissure of Sylvius)**—deep fissure which begins on the inferior surface and extends laterally between the frontal and temporal lobes.
3. **Central Sulcus (Fissure of Rolando)**—an important landmark in the sensorimotor cortex. It begins approximately 1 cm behind the midpoint between frontal and occipital poles and extends downward and forward on the lateral surface, almost as far as the lateral sulcus.
4. **Precentral Gyrus**—located between central sulcus and precentral sulcus. It is the landmark for the motor area of cerebral cortex.
5. **Postcentral Gyrus**—located between central sulcus and postcentral sulcus. It is the landmark for the general sensory area of cortex.
6. **Superior Temporal Sulcus**—courses parallel to lateral sulcus and extends into inferior parietal lobule.
7. **Middle Temporal Gyrus**—located between superior and middle temporal sulci.

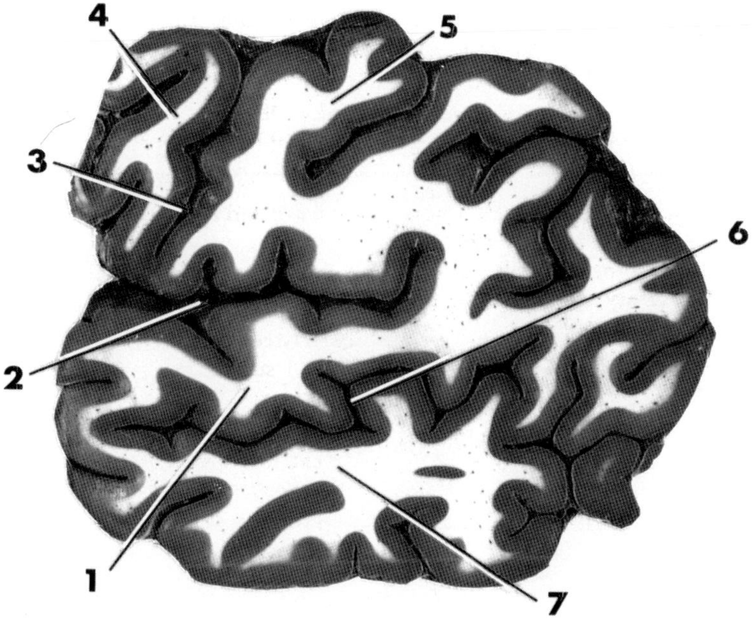

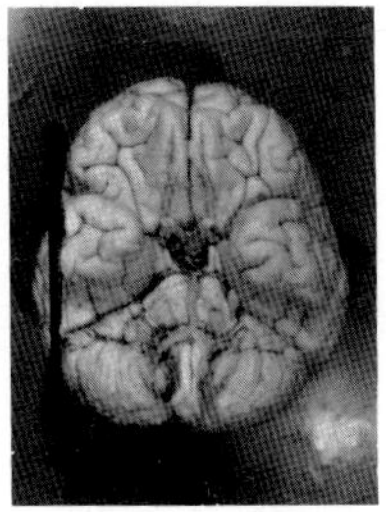

Figure 99

1. **Lateral Sulcus (Fissure of Sylvius)**—this deep fissure is an important landmark on the lateral surface which divides the temporal and frontal lobes. It extends superiorly and posteriorly into the inferior parietal lobule.
2. **Pars Orbitalis**—is the anterior division of the inferior frontal gyrus that is separated into three portions by the ascending and anterior rami of the lateral sulcus.
3. **Pars Triangularis**—is the middle triangular area of the inferior frontal gyrus that is separated into three portions by the ascending and anterior rami of the lateral sulcus.
4. **Pars Opercularis**—is the posterior area of the inferior frontal gyrus that is separated into three portions by the ascending and anterior rami of the lateral sulcus. The motor speech (Broca's) area, usually in the left cerebral hemisphere, occupies the opercular and triangular (**3**) portions of the inferior frontal gyrus.
5. **Medullary Center**—of the cerebral hemisphere is made up of myelinated axons of cortical association, commissural, and projection neurons and axons of thalamic neurons projecting to cortex.
6. **Occipital Pole**—convex posterior end of occipital lobe lying superior to the tentorium cerebelli and cerebellum.
7. **Superior Temporal Gyrus**—located between the lateral sulcus and superior temporal sulcus. Some of its large surface forms the floor of the lateral sulcus.

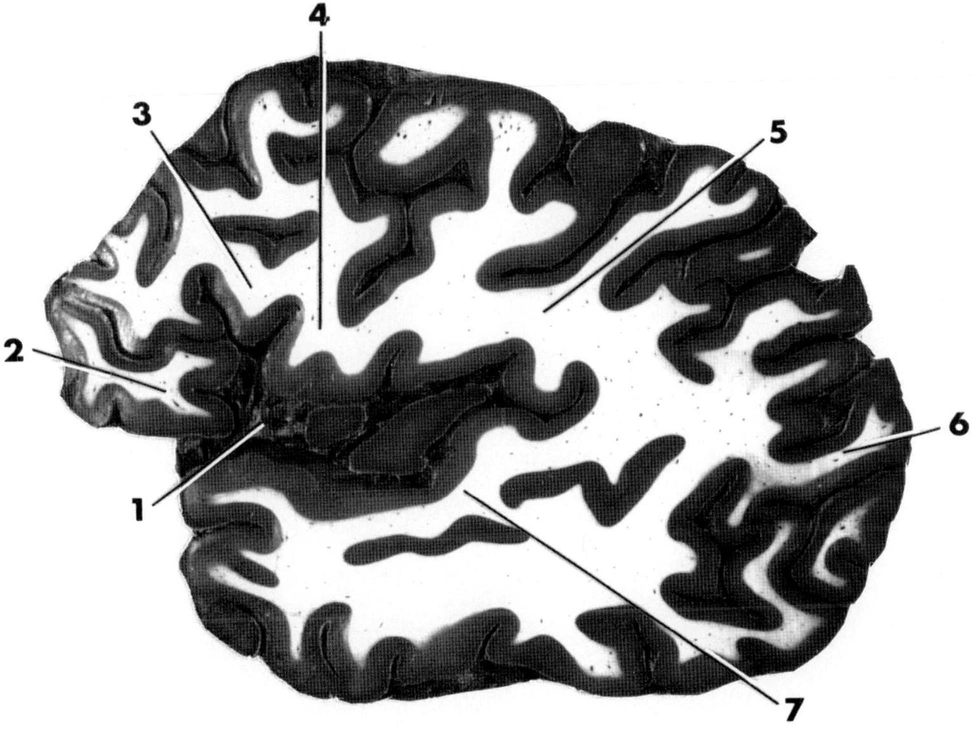

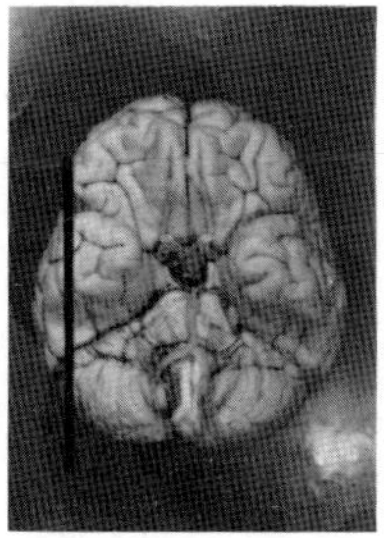

Figure 100

1. **Temporal Lobe** (medullary center indicated)—outlined on lateral surface by the lateral sulcus and an imaginary line extending from the end of it to meet a vertical imaginary line extending from the parietooccipital sulcus (fissure) to the preoccipital notch.
2. **Insula (Island of Reil)**—lies at the bottom of the lateral sulcus and is hidden from view by the frontal, parietal, and temporal opercula (lips of lateral sulcus) (see no. **9**, Fig. 8).
3. **Frontal Lobe** (medullary center indicated)—occupies the entire area in front of the central sulcus and above the lateral sulcus on the lateral surface. On the medial surface it occupies the entire area in front of and above the corpus callosum, as far as an imaginary line drawn inferiorly from the central sulcus to the corpus callosum.
4. **Precentral Gyrus**—located between the central sulcus and the precentral sulcus. It is the landmark for the motor area of cerebral cortex.
5. **Central Sulcus (Fissure of Rolando)**—is an important landmark which divides motor and sensory areas of the sensiomotor cortex. This sulcus extends inferiorly on the lateral surface from the approximate midpoint of the superior border at a 70° angle to almost meet the lateral sulcus.
6. **Parietal Lobe** (medullary center indicated)—is bounded by the lateral sulcus and central sulcus and by two imaginary boundaries; the first of these is by a line extending from the parietooccipital sulcus inferiorly in the preoccipital notch and the second, an imaginary line which is an extension of the lateral sulcus to meet the above established line.
7. **Medullary Center**—of the cerebral hemisphere is made up of myelinated axons of cortical association, commissural, and projection neurons, and axons of thalamic neurons projecting to the cortex.
8. **Occipital Pole**—convex posterior end of occipital lobe lying superior to the tentorium cerebelli and cerebellum. It is related to the upper fossa in the squamous part of the temporal bone.

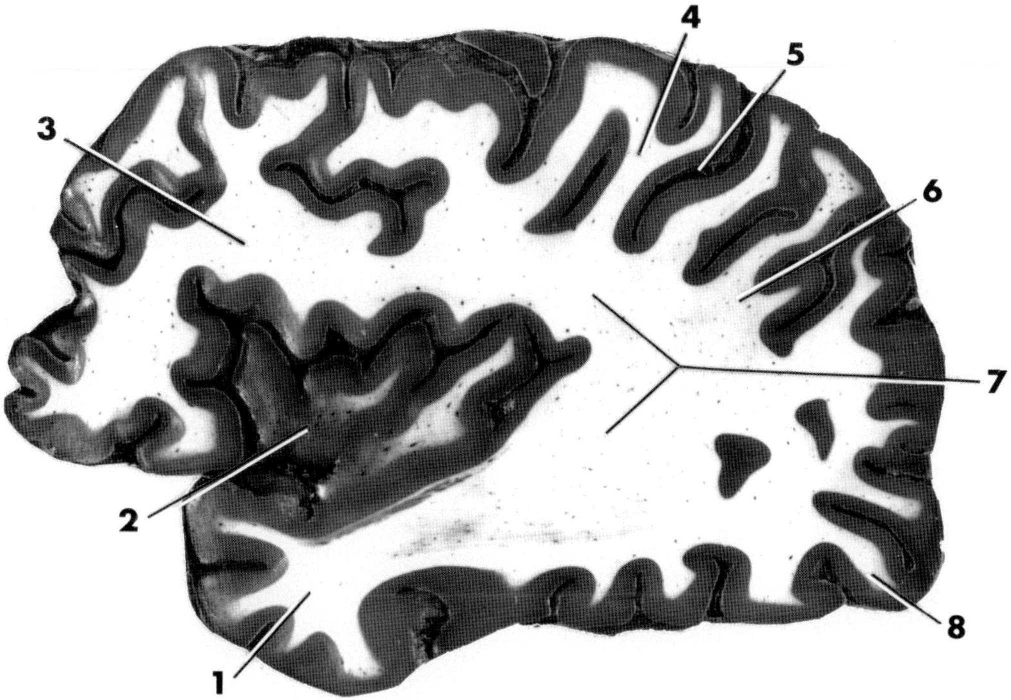

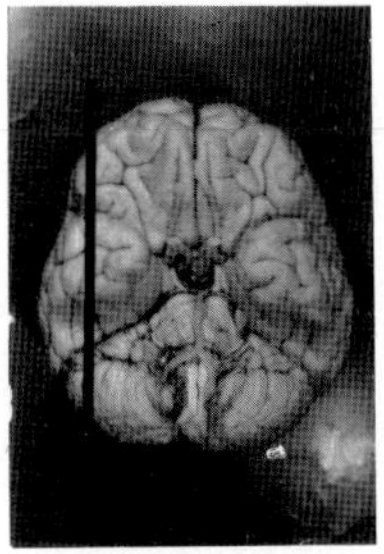

Figure 101

1. **Inferior Horn of Lateral Ventricle**—this part of the roughly C-shaped ventricle extends from the body of the lateral ventricle into the temporal lobe. The tail of the caudate nucleus (**10**) is located in its roof and the hippocampus (**11**) is located in its floor.
2. **Putamen** (L. shell)—the larger and lateral part of lentiform nucleus of the corpus striatum.
3. **Precentral Sulcus**—located in frontal lobe, courses parallel with the central sulcus, and separates motor cortex (in precentral gyrus) from premotor cortex (in superior and middle frontal gyri).
4. **Precentral Gyrus**—located between central sulcus and precental sulcus **(3).** It is the landmark for the motor area of the cerebral cortex.
5. **Central Sulcus**—located on lateral surface of the cerebral hemisphere. It extends inferiorly and anteriorly (approximately 70° angle) from about 1 cm behind the midpoint of the superior border to end near the lateral sulcus. It separates frontal and parietal lobes.
6. **Postcentral Gyrus**—located between central sulcus and postcentral sulcus. It is the landmark for general sensory area of cortex.
7. **Postcentral Sulcus**—located in parietal lobe, courses parallel with the central sulcus. The sensory area of cortex is anterior to it and the somesthetic association cortex is posterior to it in superior parietal lobule.
8. **Medullary Center**—of the cerebral hemisphere is made up of myelinated axons of cortical association, commissural, and projection neurons and axons of thalamic neurons projecting to the cortex.
9. **Body of Lateral Ventricle (Collateral Trigone)**—this posterior part of the body of lateral ventricle will branch into its inferior and posterior horns.
10. **Tail of Caudate Nucleus**—located in roof of inferior horn of lateral ventricle (**1**). The tail (L. *cauda*) curves around the lateral area in floor of body of lateral ventricle. At that point the tail is resting on the dorsal surface of the thalamus and then curves around the posterior part of thalamus to extend into inferior horn of the lateral ventricle.
11. **Hippocampus** (G. seahorse)—located in floor of inferior horn of lateral ventricle. It is part of the limbic system, and its fibers terminate mainly in mammillary bodies (also other hypothalamic areas) via the alveus, fimbria, and fornix (see also no. **8**, Fig. 91*B* and no. **9**, Fig 103).

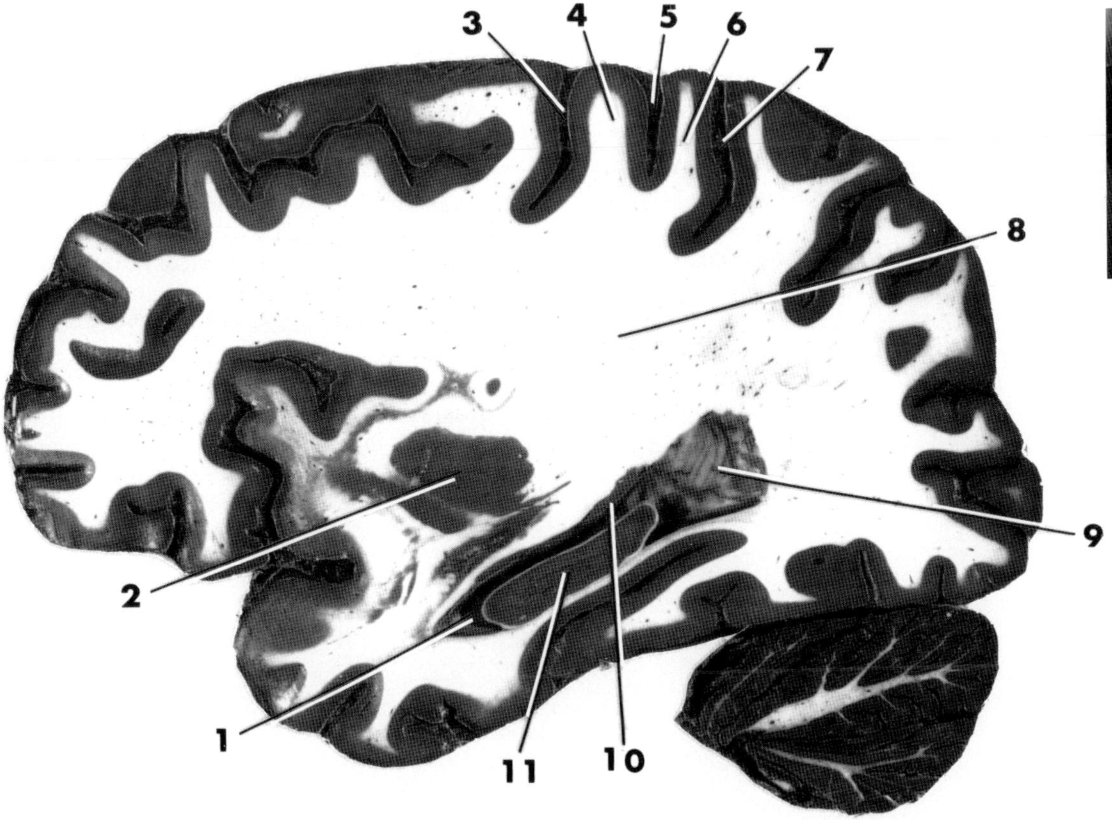

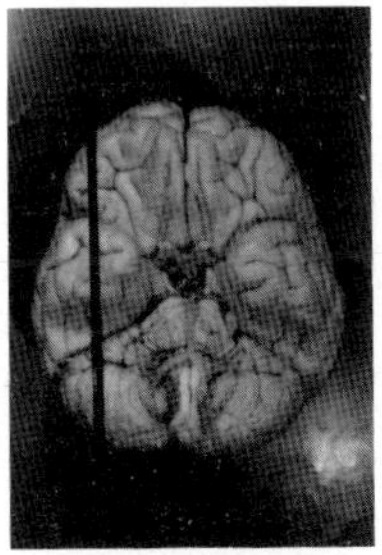

Figure 102

1. **Inferior Horn of Lateral Ventricle**—this part of the lateral ventricle extends from the body of lateral ventricle into the temporal lobe. The tail of the caudate nucleus (no. **10**, Fig. 102) is located in its roof and the hippocampus (**9**) forms an elevation in its floor.
2. **Temporal Lobe**—outlined on lateral surface by the lateral sulcus and an imaginary line extending from the end of it to meet as a vertical imaginary line extending from parietooccipital sulcus to the preoccipital notch. On the inferior surface the temporal lobe is outlined by a line drawn between the anterior end of calcarine sulcus and preoccipital notch.
3. **Anterior Commissure**—composed of reciprocal commissural fibers that cross the midline in the lamina terminalis and column of the fornix, then course laterally through the corpus striatum to end in temporal lobe cortex (see also no. **3**, Fig. 105*A*).
4. **Putamen** (L. shell)—the larger and lateral part of the lentiform nucleus (see also no. **2**, Fig. 102 and no. **3**, Fig. 104).
5. **Internal Capsule** (posterior limb)—composed of projection fibers separating lentiform nucleus from thalamus. Corticospinal, corticobulbar, and corticopontine tract fibers are examples of projection fibers in this area (see also no. **13**, Fig. 104 and no. **1**, Fig. 105*B*).
6. **Parietooccipital Sulcus**—deep sulcus or fissure on medial surface that extends from calcarine sulcus upwards to intersect the superior border approximately 4 cm from occipital pole. It continues for a short distance on the lateral surface (see also no. **2**, Fig. 5).
7. **Choroid Plexus** (G. *chorioeidēs*, like a membrane)—located in the body of lateral ventricle. It is seen here at the collateral trigone (area of lateral ventricle where posterior and inferior horns diverge from the body; see **c**, Fig. 26).
8. **Posterior Horn of Lateral Ventricle**—extends posteriorly from body of lateral ventricle at level of collateral trigone into the medullary center of the occipital lobe.
9. **Hippocampus** (G. seahorse)—located in floor of inferior horn of lateral ventricle. It is part of limbic system, and its fibers terminate mainly in mammillary bodies (also other hypothalamic areas) via the alveus, fimbria, and fornix (see also no. **11**, Fig. 102 and no. **8**, Fig. 91*B*).

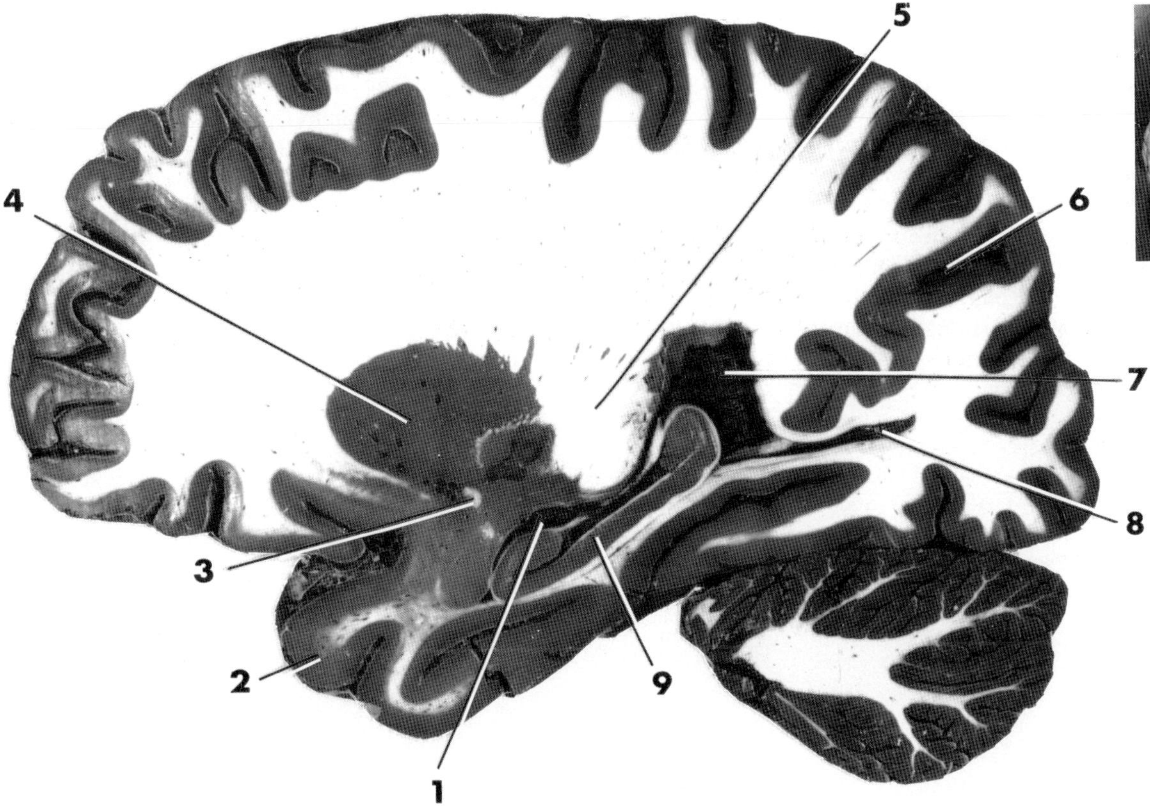

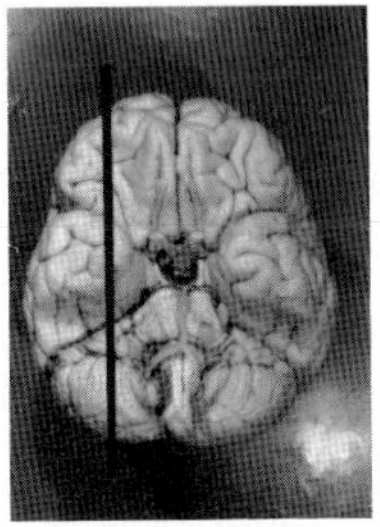

Figure 103

1. **Optic Tract**—optic nerve fibers coursing between the optic chiasma and lateral geniculate body. The optic tract fibers curve around the cerebral peduncle and most of them synapse on neurons in the lateral geniculate body (see also no. **2**, Fig. 105*A*).
2. **Globus Pallidus**—medial part of lentiform nucleus. The lateral medullary lamina separates it from the putamen, the lateral part of the lentiform nucleus. **Note**—because the lentiform nucleus is lens-shaped and the putamen forms its outer shell, the anterior part of the putamen can lie rostral to the globus pallidus in a sagittal section through the lentiform nucleus.
3. **Putamen** (L. shell)—the larger and lateral part of the lentiform nucleus, see no. **2** for explanation of why putamen appears rostral to globus pallidus (**2**) in this figure.
4. **Lateral Medullary Lamina**—consists of nerve fibers that separate globus pallidus (**2**) from putamen (**3**). See also no. **5**, Fig. 89*A* and no. **2**, Fig. 90*B* for divisions of lentiform nucleus.
5. **Corona Radiata** (small segment)—composed of converging projection fibers from cerebral cortex coursing inferiorly and medially, above thalamus and lentiform and caudate nuclei. These fibers continue between lentiform nucleus, caudate nucleus (**6**), and thalamus as the internal capsule.
6. **Caudate Nucleus**—consists of an anterior portion or head which tapers into a slender tail extending backward and then forward into the temporal lobe. The caudate nucleus has an extensive relationship with the lateral ventricle and extends from its anterior horn into its body and into the roof of its inferior horn. (see also no. **2**, Fig. 105 and no **10**, Fig. 86).
7. **Posterior Horn of Lateral Ventricle (Collateral Trigone)**—the inferior and posterior horns branch from this area of the lateral ventricle.
8. **Parietooccipital Sulcus**—deep sulcus or fissure on medial surface that extends from calcarine sulcus upwards to intersect the superior border approximately 4 cm from occipital pole. It continues for a short distance on the lateral surface.
9. **Crus of Fornix**—a continuation of the fimbria which is composed of fibers that emerge from hippocampus. These fibers merge with those of the opposite side to form the body of the fornix.
10. **Pulvinar of Thalamus** (L. cushioned seat)—this dorsal and posterior cushion-like portion of the thalamus overhangs the medial and lateral geniculate bodies. The pulvinar bulges onto the dorsal surface of the midbrain.
11. **Lateral Geniculate Body**—located beneath lateral area of pulvinar (**10**). Many fibers of optic tract synapse on neurons in lateral geniculate nucleus.
12. **Hippocampus** (G. seahorse)—located in the floor of inferior horn of lateral ventricle. It is part of limbic system and its fibers terminate mainly in mammillary bodies (also other hypothalamic areas) via the alveus, fimbria, and fornix (see also no. **11**, Fig. 102 and no. **9**, Fig. 103).
13. **Internal Capsule** (posterior limb)—composed of cortical projection fibers which are a continuation of corona radiata (**5**). The posterior limb separates thalamus from lentiform nucleus.

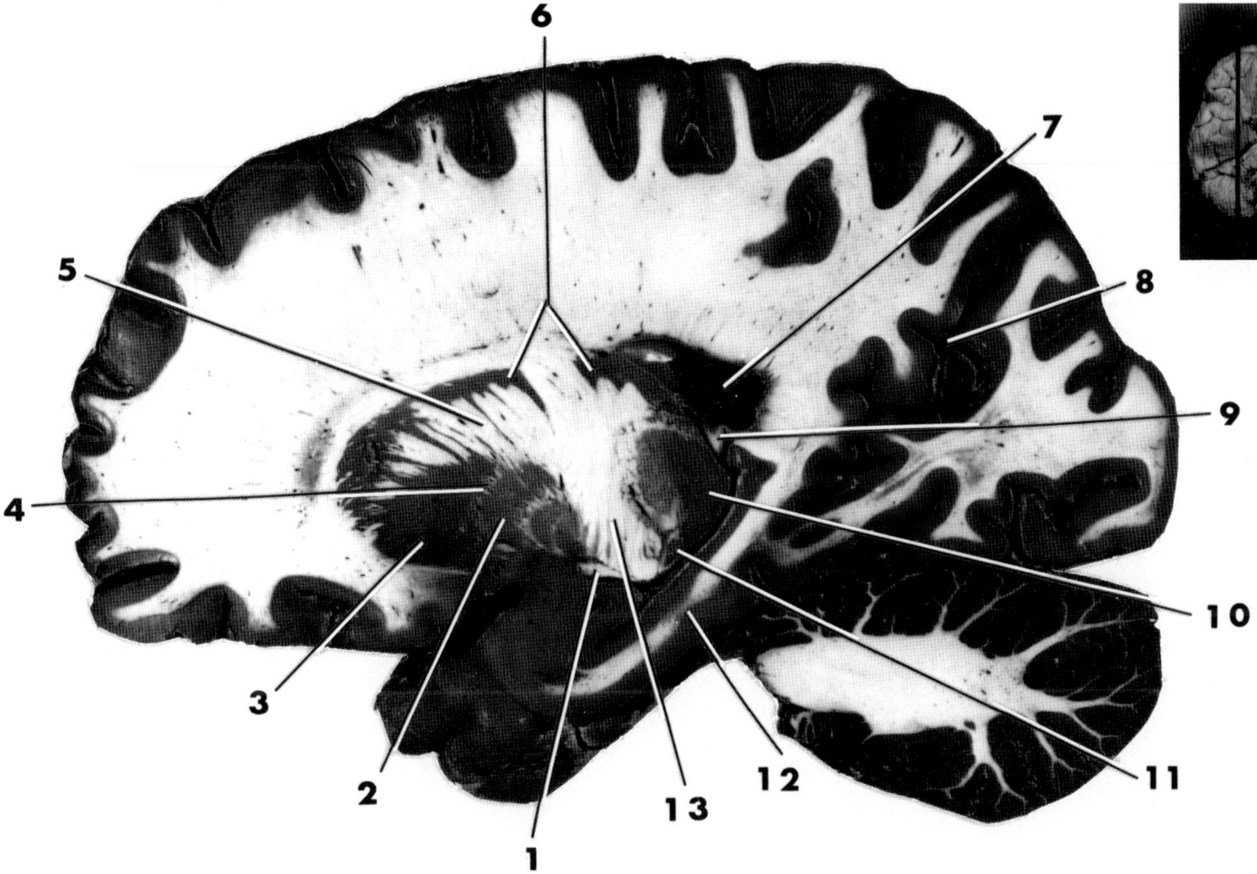

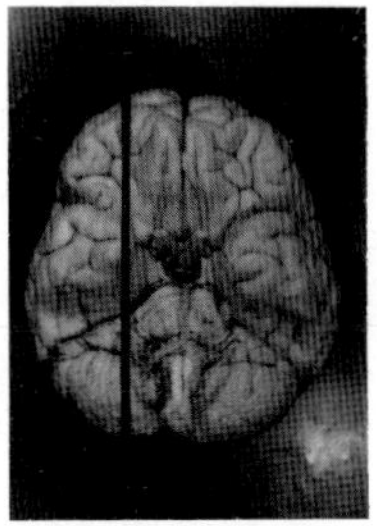

Figure 104

1. **Uncus** (L. hook)—the hooked-back portion of the rostral end of the parahippocampal gyrus in the temporal lobe, constituting a landmark for the lateral olfactory area.
2. **Optic Tract**—composed of optic nerve fibers from optic chiasma that course around cerebral peduncle to end predominately in the lateral geniculate body. Some fibers continue into the tectal and pretectal areas of midbrain.
3. **Anterior Commissure**—composed of reciprocal commissural fibers that cross the midline between column of fornix and lamina terminalis and then course through the corpus striatum on their way to the temporal lobes.
4. **Red Nucleus**—prominent brain stem motor nucleus located in the rostral midbrain between substantia nigra (**5**) and tegmentum. It has an extrapyramidal function in motor movements.
5. **Substantia Nigra**—a large brain stem motor nucleus located in basal tegmental area of midbrain. It has extensive connections with the globus pallidus of the corpus striatum and ventral lateral thalamic nucleus. This nucleus gets its name from its black (L. *niger*) color in a freshly cut brain.
6. **Basis Pedunculi (Crus Cerebri)**—ventral part of the cerebral peduncle which is a continuation of the internal capsule (see no. **13**, Fig. 104) which consists of cortical projection fibers (*i.e.*, corticospinal, corticobulbar, corticopontine tracts, etc.).
7. **Dentate Nucleus** (L. *dentatus*, toothed)—the largest of the four pairs of cerebellar nuclei. It is embedded deep in the medullary center of each cerebellar hemisphere (see also no. **7**, Fig. 106*A*).
8. **Middle Cerebellar Peduncle (Brachium Pontis)**—the arm (L. *brachium*)-like bridge (L. pons) composed of axons (**9**) of contralateral basal pontine neurons which leave the basal pons and course posteriorly and laterally into the medullary center of the cerebellar hemisphere.
9. **Pontocerebellar Fibers**—consist of axons of pontine neurons that course transversely in the midline of the basal pons to form the contralateral middle cerebellar peduncle.
10. **Basal Pons** (L. bridge)—lower part of the pons ventral to the tegmentum which appears to form a bridge between the right and left halves of the cerebellum.

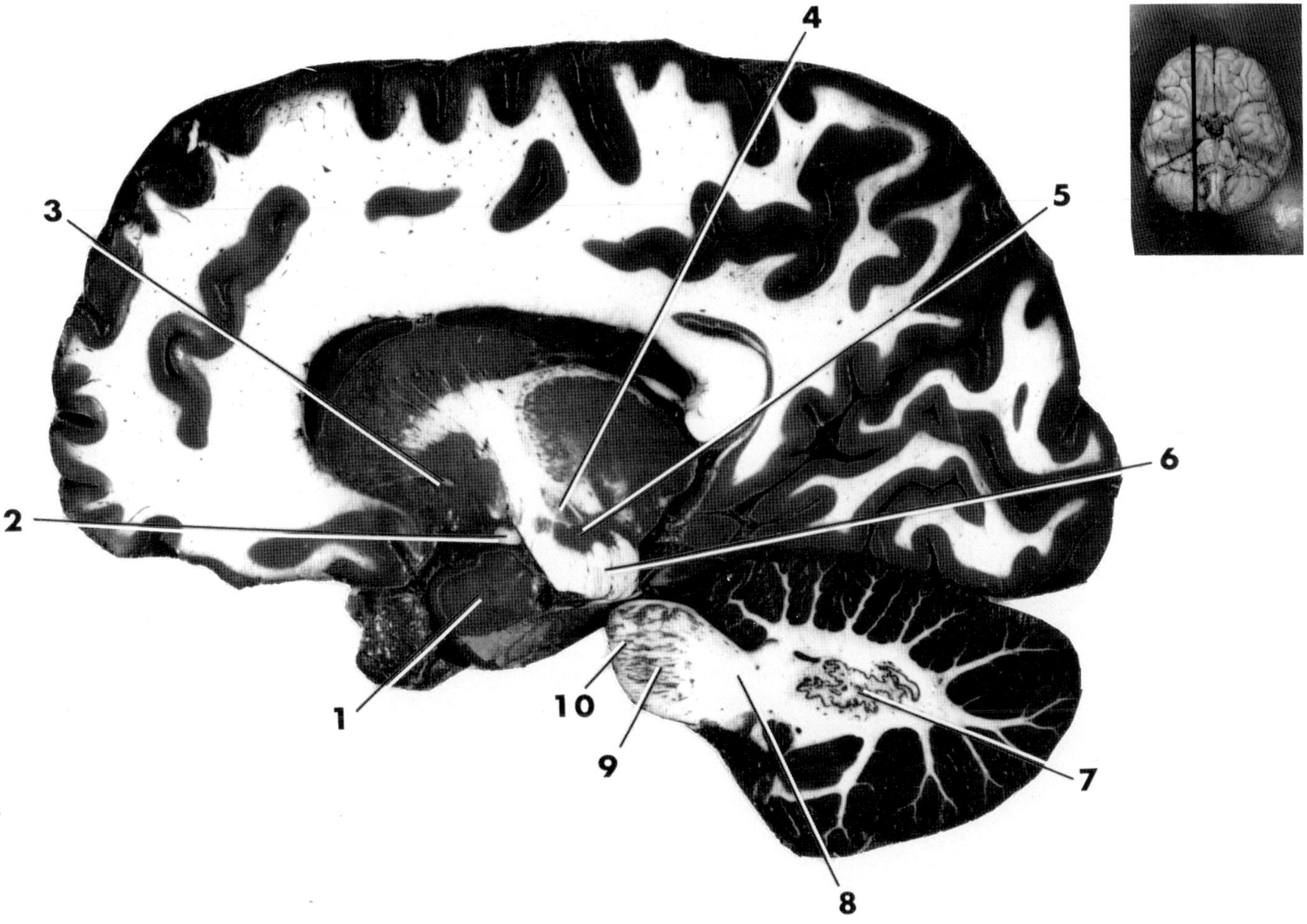

Figure 105*A*

1. **Genu of Internal Capsule**—The internal capsule consists of an anterior limb, a genu (L. knee), and a posterior limb. The *genu* is medial to the apex of the lentiform nucleus and is composed of cortical and thalamic projection fibers.
2. **Head of Caudate Nucleus**—bulges into the anterior horn of the lateral ventricle. It tapers posteriorly into the tail of the caudate nucleus. Inferiorly and laterally it is continuous with the putamen to form the corpus striatum.
3. **Anterior Horn of Lateral Ventricle**—extends forward from the body of the lateral ventricle (**4**) as far as the genu of the corpus callosum (**1**).
4. **Body of Lateral Ventricle**—each lateral ventricle consists of a body in the region of the parietal and frontal lobes from which anterior, posterior, and inferior horns extend. It is located beneath the body of the corpus callosum.
5. **Dorsolateral Thalamic Area**—consists of the pulvinar, lateral posterior nucleus, and lateral dorsal nucleus. This area is adjacent to the internal capsule and has reciprocal connections with association cortex.
6. **Crus of Fornix**—consists of hippocampal fibers (axons of hippocampal neurons) that first form the fimbria of the fornix and continue as the crus. The left and right crura join to form the body of the fornix.
7. **Splenium of Corpus Callosum** (G. *splēnion,* bandage)—thickened posterior portion of corpus callosum. Consists of commissural fibers radiating into occipital lobes as the forceps major.
8. **Calcarine Sulcus**—on medial surface of cerebral hemisphere. It courses from beneath the splenium (**7**) to the occipital pole and forms an important landmark for the visual cortex.
9. **Pulvinar** (L. cushioned seat)—this cushion-like dorsal and posterior portion of the thalamus overhangs the medial and lateral geniculate bodies and bulges onto the dorsal surface of the midbrain (see also no. **10**, Fig. 104).

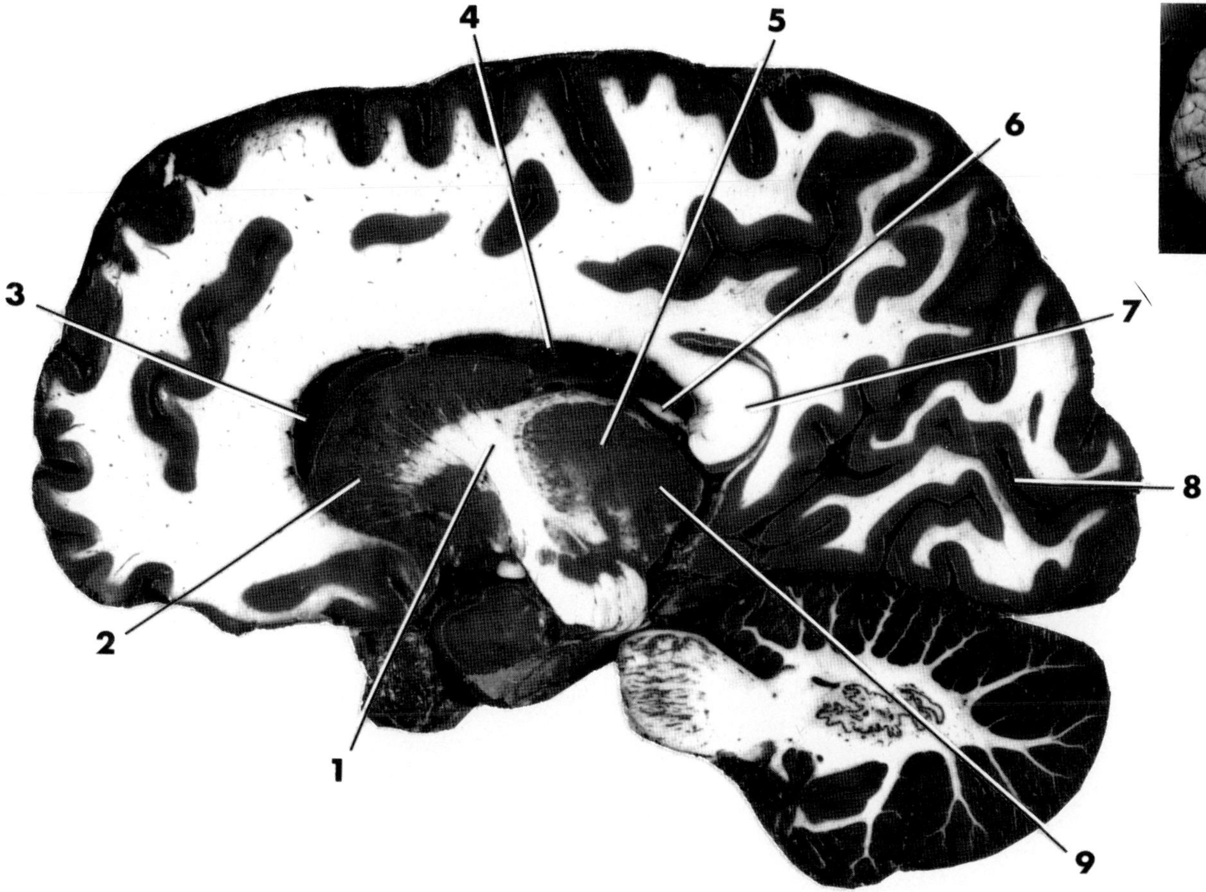

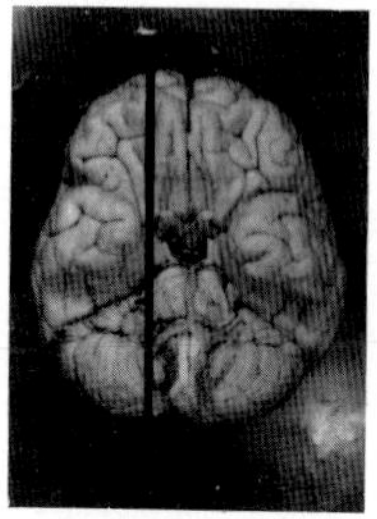

Figure 105*B*

1. **Genu of Corpus Callosum**—anterior end of corpus callosum with the angular shape of a flexed knee (L. *genu*). It tapers inferiorly into the rostrum (L. beak) of the corpus callosum. It consists of commissural fibers that radiate into the frontal lobes forming the forceps minor.
2. **Cingulate Gyrus**—located on medial surface of cerebral hemisphere, immediately adjacent to the corpus callosum. Having the form of a girdle or band (L. *cingulum*), it begins beneath the genu and continues above the corpus callosum as far back as its splenium.
3. **Body of Corpus Callosum**—composed of compact reciprocal commissural fibers that cross at the midline into the medullary center of each cerebral hemisphere.
4. **Body of Fornix**—formed by a continuation of fibers from each crus of fornix. The fornix is part of the limbic system connecting hippocampus with mammillary bodies and other hypothalamic areas.
5. **Splenium of Corpus Callosum**—bandage (G. *splēnion*)-like, posterior portion of corpus callosum. Consists of commissural fibers radiating into occipital lobes as forceps major.
6. **Superior and Inferior Colliculi (Corpora Quadrigemina)**—these four rounded small elevations (L. *colliculi*) make up the tectum (L. roof) of the midbrain.
7. **Dentate Nucleus** (L. *dentatus,* toothed)—the largest of the four pairs of cerebellar nuclei. It is deeply embedded in the medullary center of each cerebellar hemisphere (see also no. **7**, Fig. 105*A*).
8. **Superior Cerebellar Peduncle (Brachium Conjunctivum)**—axons of neurons from each dentate, emboliform, and globose nucleus leave the cerebellum, forming a dense fiber bundle which courses into the tegmentum of the midbrain. These fibers decussate in the midline at the level of the inferior colliculus.
9. **Inferior Olivary Nucleus**—found in the olive of the medulla oblongata. It lies between the pyramid and the tuberculum cinereum.
10. **Corticospinal and Corticopontine Tracts**—cortical projection fibers pass into the basal pons from internal capsule and basis pedunculi. Some of these longitudinal fibers terminate on pontine neurons (corticopontine fibers) and others pass through basal pons uninterrupted into the medulla and spinal cord (corticospinal fibers).

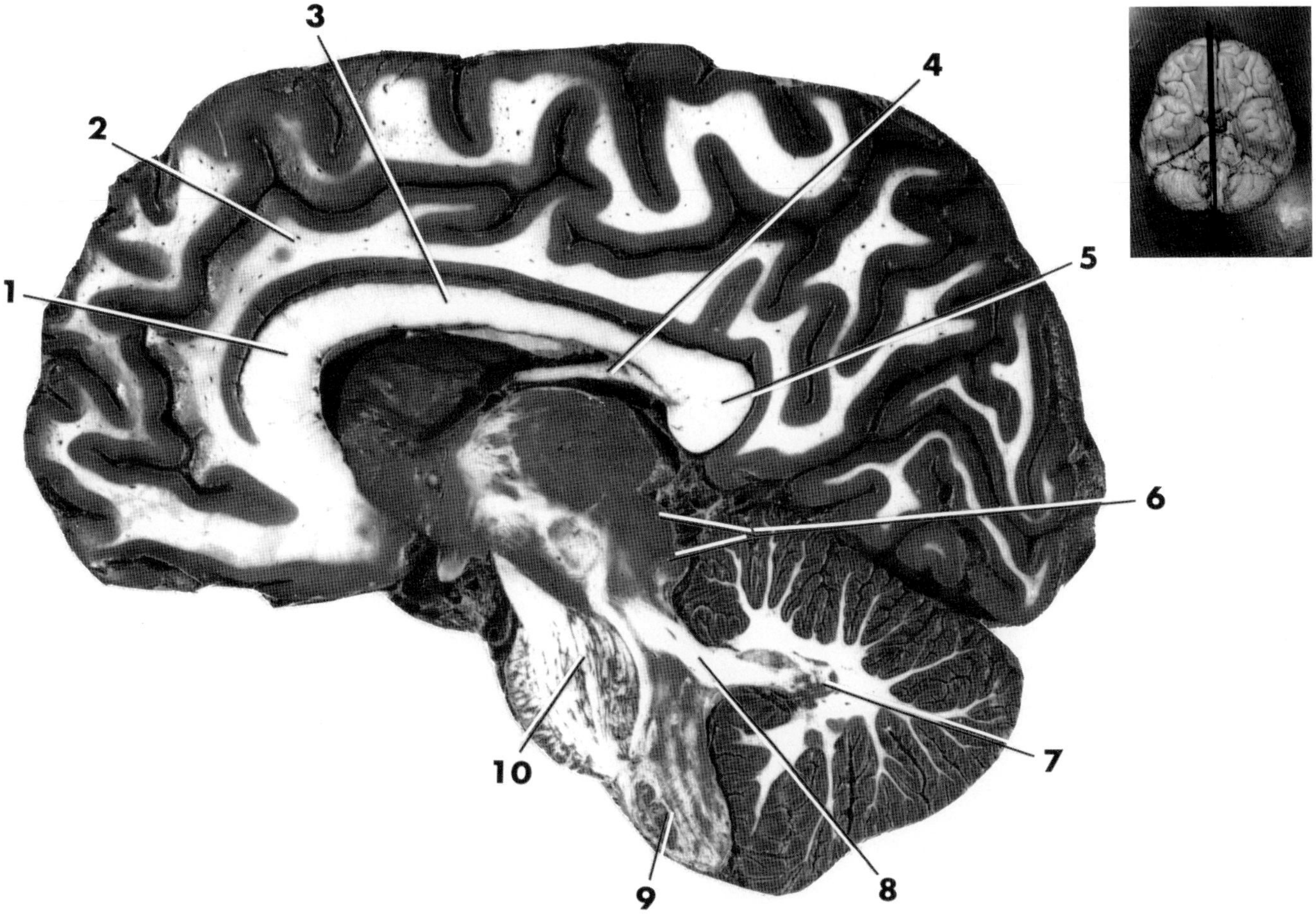

Figure 106*A*

1. **Basis Pedunculi (Crus Cerebri)**—ventral aspect of cerebral peduncle. It consists of cerebral projection bundles (*i.e.*, corticospinal, corticobulbar, corticopontine tracts, etc.) that continue from internal capsule into that part of the midbrain (see also no. **11**, Fig. 90*B* and no. **2**, Fig. 75*A*).
2. **Optic Tract**—composed of optic nerve fibers from optic chiasma that course around cerebral peduncle to end predominately in the lateral geniculate body. Some fibers continue into tectal and pretectal areas of midbrain.
3. **Hypothalamic Area**—surrounds the third ventricle ventral to the hypothalamic sulcus on each side. The hypothalamic area is subdivided in several nuclear areas which have an important influence on the autonomic nervous system.
4. **Anterior Commissure**—consists of reciprocal commissural fibers that cross the midline between the column of fornix and lamina terminalis and course through the corpus striatum into the temporal lobes (see also no. **13**, Fig. 88 and no. **11**, Fig. 89*A*).
5. **Head of Caudate Nucleus**—bulges into anterior horn of lateral ventricle; inferiorly it is continuous with the putamen to form the corpus striatum (see also no. **2**, Fig. 105*B*).
6. **Medial Thalamic Nucleus**—is separated from the lateral thalamic nuclear area by the internal medullary lamina. The medial thalamic nucleus and midline nuclei form the lateral walls of the third ventricle above the hypothalamic sulcus.
7. **Pulvinar** (L. cushioned seat)—this dorsal and posterior portion of the thalamus overhangs the medial and lateral geniculate bodies. The pulvinar bulges onto the dorsal surface of the midbrain.
8. **Red Nucleus**—prominent brain stem motor nucleus located in the tegmentum of the rostral midbrain. Fibers of the superior cerebellar peduncle end in or encapsule it (see no. **6**, Fig. 75*A*). The nucleus gets its name from its pink color in a freshly cut midbrain.
9. **Rubrospinal and Rubroreticular Tracts**—axons of neurons from the red nucleus descend into contralateral brain stem and spinal cord as part of the extrapyramidal motor pathways.
10. **Pontine Nuclei**—consist of patches of pontine neurons scattered between fibers in basal pons. Axons of these neurons cross to contralateral side and into cerebellum as pontocerebellar fibers.
11. **Substantia Nigra**—located in midbrain between basis pedunculi and tegmentum. This nucleus has connections with globus pallidus and ventral lateral thalamic nucleus and functions in motor movements. The black (L. *niger*) appearance of this nucleus results from the melanin granules it contains (see also no. **5**, Fig. 105*A*).

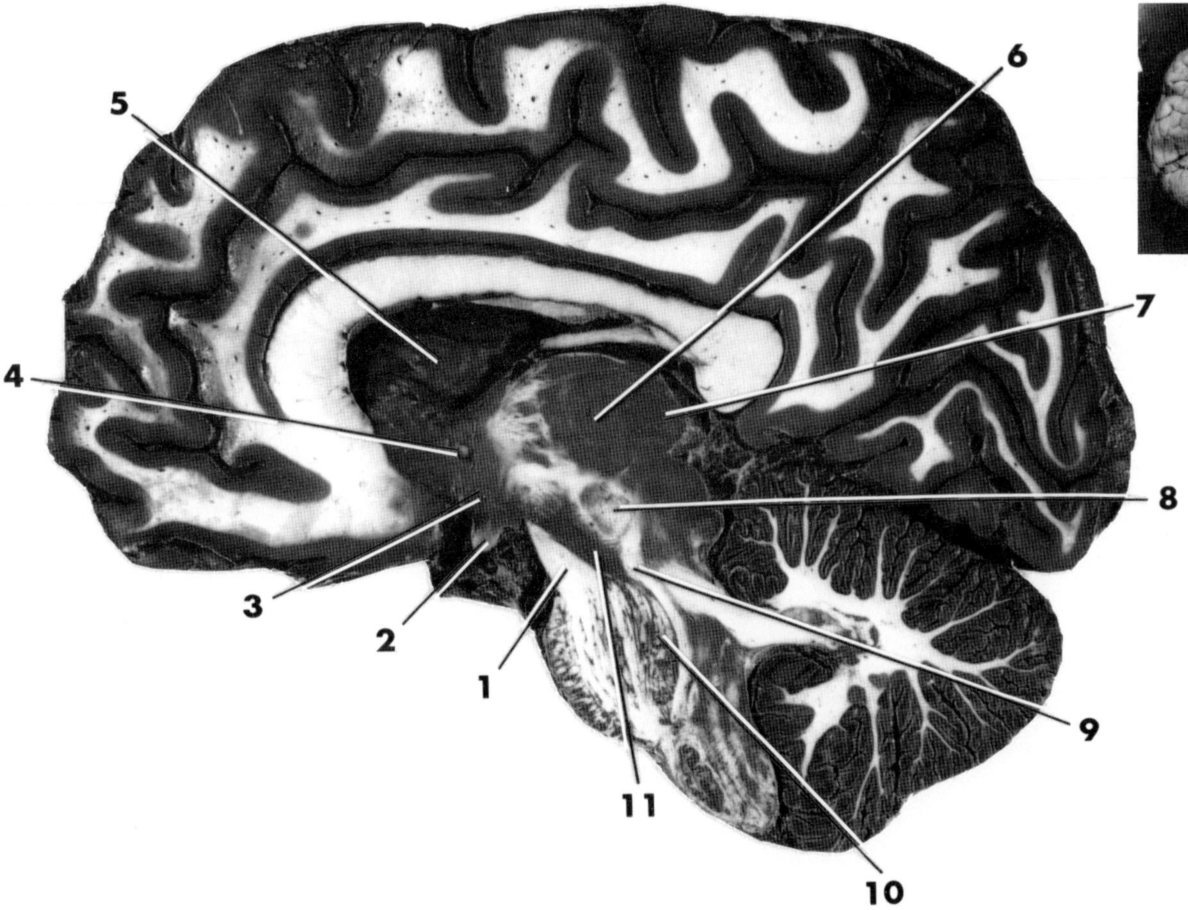

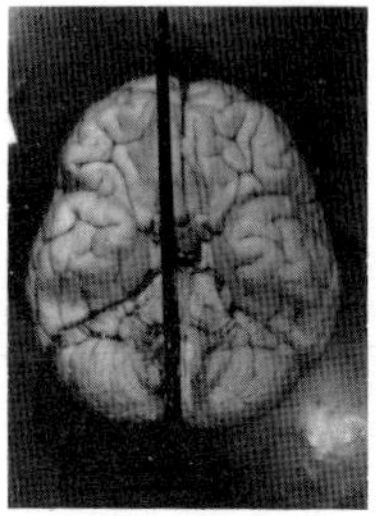

Figure 106*B*

1. **Mammillary Body** (L. *mammilla,* dim. of *mamma,* breast)—one of two small swellings on the ventral surface of the hypothalamus. Has an important function with the limbic system.
2. **Lamina Terminalis**—this thin terminal plate passes upward from the optic chiasma and forms the anterior wall of the third ventricle.
3. **Anterior Commissure**—is composed of reciprocal commissural fibers that cross the midline between lamina terminalis (**2**) and column of fornix enroute to each temporal lobe cortex.
4. **Septum Pellucidum** (L. partition + transparent)—separating much of the body and part of anterior horn of lateral ventricle.
5. **Genu of Corpus Callosum** (L. *genu,* knee)—anterior knee-like end of corpus callosum where commissural fibers radiate into frontal lobes forming forceps minor.
6. **Interventricular Foramen (of Monro)**—connects the lateral ventricles with the third ventricle. It is bounded by the fornix and anterior tubercle of thalamus.
7. **Body of Corpus Callosum**—composed of compact reciprocal commissural fibers that cross in the midline to each cerebral hemisphere.
8. **Body of Fornix**—located on floor of body of lateral ventricle. It rests on dorsomedial surface of thalamus.
9. **Splenium of Corpus Callosum** (G. *splēnion,* bandage)—posterior thickened portion of corpus callosum.
10. **Pineal Body** (L. *pineus,* relating to pine)—this part of the epithalamus, shaped like a pine cone, is separated from midbrain by a cistern.
11. **Posterior Commissure**—located at entrance to cerebral aqueduct. Reciprocal fibers cross midline of midbrain and connect pretectal and tectal nuclear areas.
12. **Superior and Inferior Colliculi (Corpora Quadrigemina)**—these four rounded elevations (L. *colliculi*), make up the tectum (L. roof) of the midbrain.
13. **Cerebral Aqueduct (of Sylvius)**—in midbrain connecting IIIrd and IVth ventricles (see also no. **2**, Fig. 76 and no. **11**, Fig. 92).
14. **IVth Ventricle**—space between cerebellum and pons and medulla. A median and two lateral apertures lead from this ventricle to subarachnoid space.
15. **Decussation of Superior Cerebellar Peduncle (Brachium Conjunctivum)**—dentothalamic fibers from each side cross the midline of midbrain tegmentum at the level of the inferior colliculus to course to red nucleus and ventral lateral thalamus (see also no. **12**, Fig. 92).

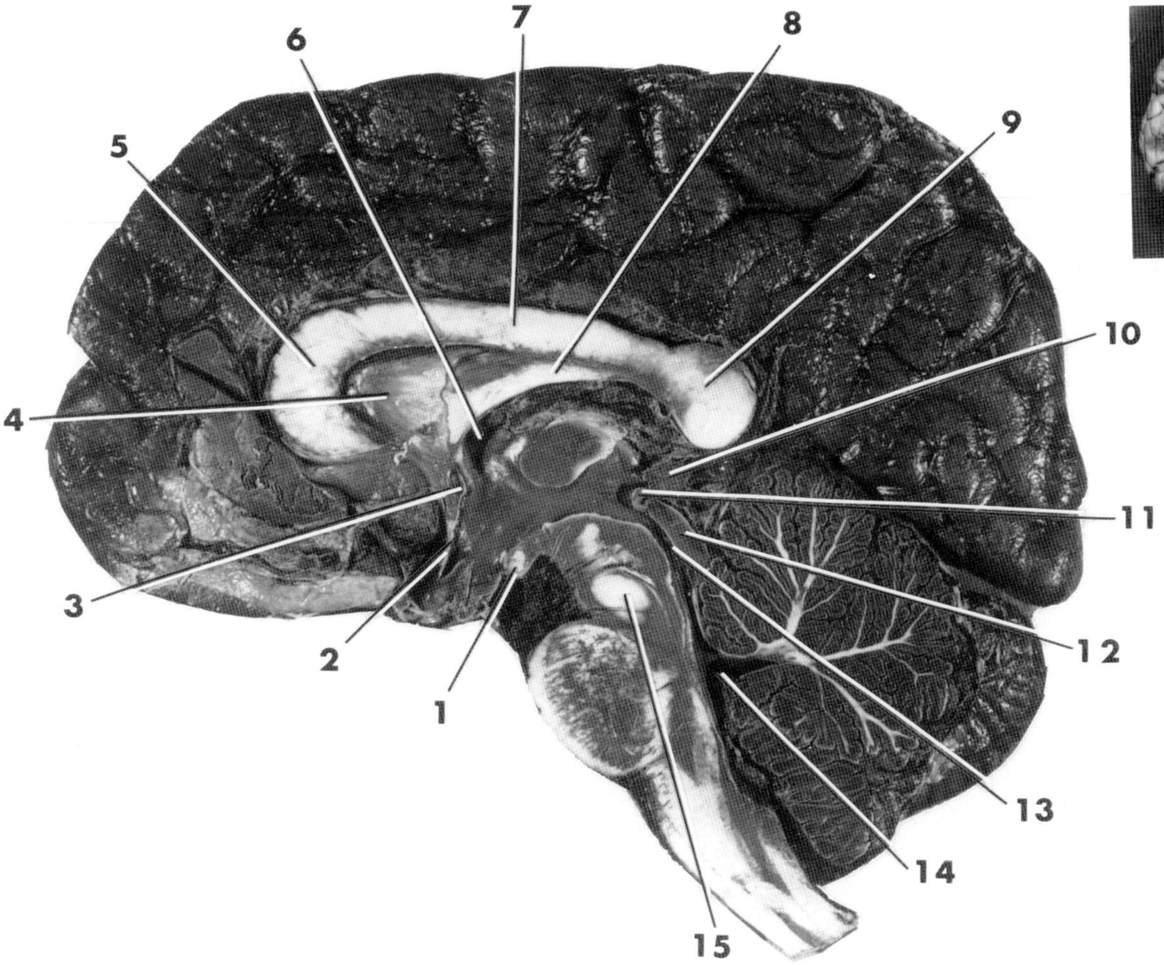

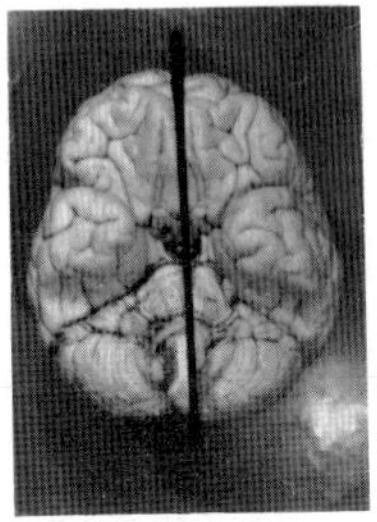

Figure 107

Bibliography

Barr, M. L.: *The Human Nervous System. An Anatomical Viewpoint,* Ed. 3. Harper and Row, Hagerstown, Md., 1979.

Brodal, A.: *The Cranial Nerves: Anatomy and Anatomico-Clinical Correlations.* Blackwell Scientific Publications, Oxford, 1965.

Carpenter, M. B.: *Human Neuroanatomy,* Ed. 7. Williams & Wilkins, Baltimore, 1976.

Carpenter, M. B.: *Core Text of Neuroanatomy,* Ed. 2. Williams & Wilkins, Baltimore, 1978.

DeArmond, S. J., Fusco, M. M., and Dwewy, M. M.: *Structure of the Human Brain: A Photographic Atlas,* Ed. 2. Oxford University Press, New York, 1976.

Ford, D. H., and Schade, J. P.: *Atlas of the Human Brain,* Ed. 2. Elsevier, New York, 1970.

Gluhbegovic, N., and Williams, T. H.: *The Human Brain: A Photographic Guide.* Harper and Row, Hagerstown, Md., 1980.

Montemurro, D. G., and Bruni, J. E.: *The Human Brain in Dissection.* W. B. Saunders, Philadelphia, 1981.

Moore, K. L.: *Clinically Oriented Anatomy.* Williams & Wilkins, Baltimore, 1980.

Nieuwenhuys, R., Voogd, J., and van Huijzen, C.: *The Human Central Nervous System: A Synopsis and Atlas.* Springer, New York, 1978.

Roberts, M., and Hanaway, J.: *Atlas of the Human Brain in Section,* Lea & Febiger, Philadelphia, 1970.

Smith, C. G.: *Serial Dissections of the Human Brain,* Urban & Schwarzenberg, Baltimore, 1981.

Watson, C.: *Basic Human Neuroanatomy: An Introductory Atlas,* Ed. 2. Little, Brown and Co., Boston, 1977.

Zuleger, S., and Straubesand, J.: *Atlas of the Central Nervous System in Sectional Planes.* Urban & Schwarzenberg, Baltimore, 1977.

Index

Main page references are printed in **bold type**. In most cases items are listed under nouns rather than under descriptive adjectives, *e.g.*, the trochlear nerve will not be found under trochlear but under the general heading NERVES. Similarly, all arteries, nuclei, and veins are listed under ARTERIES, NUCLEI, and VEINS, respectively. Common alternate terms are also given, *e.g.*, the superior cerebellar peduncle is also called the brachium conjunctivum.